Get a Life, America!

Get a Life, America!

Your Companion in Achieving Life-long Health

Leonard R. Mees, M.D.

Foreword: Harvey S. Hecht, M.D., F.A.C.C.
Director of Atherosclerotic Detection and Preventive Treatment Center
Chairman, Department of Medicine, Arizona Heart Hospital
Phoenix, Arizona

Cover Photo: Rebecca Mees

Sabec Publishing
P.O. Box 82545
Portland, OR 97282-0545

Publisher's Cataloging-in-Publication
(Provided by Quality Books, Inc.)

Mees, Leonard R.
    Get a life, America! : your companion in
    achieving life-long health / Leonard R. Mees ;
    foreword: Harvey S. Hecht. -- 1st ed.
    p. cm.
    Includes bibliographical references and index.
    LCCN: 99-73857
    ISBN: 0-9675500-0-9

    1. Health. 2. Health behavior.   I. Title.

RA776.M5 2000   613
                          QBI99-1968

Attention Organizations, Corporations, Medical facilities, Nursing homes, etc.:
Quantity discounts are available on bulk purchases of this book for educational purposes or fund raising. Special books or book excerpts can also be created to fit specific needs. For information, please contact Sabec Publishing Company, P.O. Box 82545, Portland, OR 97282-0545 or visit us at www.Getalifeamerica.com.

Acknowledgments

The most rewarding section of the book to write, acknowledgment of those persons, without whose help this book would never have seen the light of day, gives me great satisfaction. It also means the book is done. Whoopee!

My younger daughter, Becky Mees, provided encouragement and emotional support during some of the difficult, doubting times, and deserves great credit for her technical expertise. She conceived and designed the cover, took the cover photograph(s), wrote the subtitle (steadfastly insisting against commercial hype), edited the book, generally consulted on issues of philosophy and ethic, and ran endless errands for the final production of *Get a Life, America!* Thanks Beck.

My older daughter, Sarah Mees, provided long-term emotional support and encouragement from the beginning of the project. Often we don't understand that we effect the lives of others by how we support them. Sarah deserves special credit for reinforcing my belief in the principles and philosophy of *Get a Life, America!* Thanks Sarah.

My parents, Joe and Irene Mees, agreed that my concept of pursuing health rather than running from disease makes good sense. They generously financed this project. Thanks Mom and Dad.

Harvey Hecht, M.D., was kind enough to carefully and critically read *Get a Life, America!,* and then to write a very complimentary Foreword. I'm particularly pleased that Harvey wrote the Foreword because I respect him as a cardiologist and respect the Arizona Heart Institute, where Harvey is director of Preventive Treatment Center. Thanks Harvey.

Fred Katz, my life-long friend, advisor, confessor, and reviewer of the book surprised me with his enthusiasm for *Get a Life, America.!* He likened its motivational value to the movie, *Hurricane.* Thanks, Fred.

Anne Bell, M.S., R.D., reviewed the final writing of *Get a Life, America!* and offered the very kind words found on the back cover. Annie also provided emotional support and friendship during the doubtful times. Thanks Annie.

My friend, David Delgado, coined the title, saying, "You think it's easy to eat right, exercise, and manage your stress? Come on, get a life!" We turned the frustration of the exclamation, "Get a life," into an ultimately positive message in *Get a Life, America!* Thanks Dave.

Without question, I've forgotten someone, and I apologize. I sincerely appreciate every comment, criticism, and kind ear that I have met along my journey of writing *Get a Life, America!* Thanks all.

Finally, I wish to thank the University of Rochester School of Medicine and Dentistry, an institution who selflessly shared its ethic of public service with each of us students. For me, it made all the difference in the world.

Table of Contents

Preface   **1**

Jacks or Better   **5**

It's a poker axiom, "You must have jacks or better to open." The author certainly does as he draws upon twenty years of intense medical experience, five years of research, and a professional lifetime of writing and speaking, to chronicle his reasoning that illness is sick. He states that we can achieve life-long health, and that our nation can, too, as we learn to *Get a Life, America!*

Chapter I
A Change of Heart   **17**

Few of us would argue that we Americans lead unhealthy lives. Few would debate the benefits of adopting healthy lifestyles. Unfortunately, a rare few know how to make the necessary changes to achieve health. To counter the lack of information, "A Change of Heart" lays the foundation for achieving life-long health by teaching you the process of change – behavior modification.

As the car designer who doesn't understand the workings of the gas combustion engine can't build a fine car, if you don't understand how you work and change, you won't build a healthy you. "A Change of Heart" launches you on your journey to life-long health. *Bon voyage.*

Chapter II
What's Eating You?   **45**

"What's Eating You?" serves as Your Survival Guide to the Russian Roulette of American Cuisine. Nutrition, long taught and thought boring, is a key member among the Major League Players of Health. Without good nutrition, sooner or later, we'll be in serious health jeopardy.

Statistics document that over 90% of us eat poorly. "What's Eating You?" provides education to reverse those dismal statistics. This chapter teaches food fundamentals, how to accomplish healthful supermarket shopping, how to eat well at home, and how to survive the Russian Roulette of Restaurant Dining. And, do you know what? It's fun! Tasty, too!

Chapter III
Use it or Lose it!   **91**

Muscles, memory, or sex – use it or lose it! Here we focus on muscles, on the benefits of using them for a life-time, on how they work, and on how you can take control and write your own exercise prescription. We discover the two muscle fiber types and that each type responds to a different training stimulus. That's why no single exercise or machine trains the entire body. The whats, whys, and hows of exercise reveal themselves not as mysteries, but as friends for life.

Chapter IV
Through the Eye of the Tiger   **137**

Stress! Yipes! Everyone has it, yet most of us deny its existence. Somehow, we have accepted it as a norm in our society. Normal or not, stress kills. This chapter looks at stress through the eye of the tiger. It examines the origins of stress, listens to the masters of stress teaching, and closes with a presentation of how we may live in harmony with the stressors of our worlds.

Chapter V
Denial is Not Just a River in Egypt   **187**

Even more steadfastly than we deny the presence of our stressors, we abdicate any knowledge of depression in our lives. We distance ourselves from it emotionally by treating it metaphorically, as Winston Churchill dubbed his depression, "the black dog." Still viewed as a social stigma, fully one in five of us Americans suffers from this malady. Using George Washington's principle of, "Once aware, half solved," we address the gargantuan nature of this problem. We acknowledge its presence, learn about its insidious nature, discover coping behaviors, and better yet, illuminate preventive strategies.

Chapter VI
A Matter of Fat   209

Fat in our diets and fat on our bodies, both kill. That's a matter of fact! Here we learn to become astute managers of the fat in our lives. We look at the simple chemistry of fat, learn how exercise counters build-ups of body and dietary fats, understand the critical relationship between cholesterol and saturated fats, and find fat management to be a simple matter of education and choice.

Chapter VII
Eating to Live, Not Living to Eat   231

Body weight and composition is an expression of the balance of food intake and energy output. It's that simple. Really! This chapter offers the concept of eating to match our energy needs.

We examine the components of energy usage – resting energy needs, the energy needed to process food, and the energy we need for physical activity. We learn to take advantage of each of these components as we choose to live more active lives, and to change our body composition to favor muscle over fat.

Chapter VIII
Vitamins Been Beriberi Good to Me   265

Without adequate vitamins and minerals in our diets, we become sick and we may die. With sufficient vitamins and minerals, we find our lives beriberi good. Quietly, amidst the din of the hype of supplementation, we learn that the wisest consumption of vitamins and minerals is through the food we eat. Yes, as a nation, we eat poorly and are probably at risk for relative vitamin deficiency. Until we learn to eat well, and that's after we've had a chance to digest *Get a Life, America!*, the author recommends supplementation for those of us who think we may not eat healthfully.

Chapter IX
Bringing All the Chickens Together to Take Their Picture 283

Referencing his mother's oft-offered simile about accomplishing a multi-task endeavor, the author and *Get a Life, America!* present a real "how" chapter. This is where we learn how to integrate all of the information we have garnered about the Major League Players of Health. This is where synergy flourishes. The whole of our efforts becomes greater than the sum of the parts. Some would call this magic!

Chapter X
Get a Life, America! 299

Why stop with individual health? *Get a Life, America!* poses innovative methods to improve the health of our nation. Not pipe dreams, readily available techniques at our finger-tips, these functional ideas may be implemented now for our common benefit. As our current Surgeon General, David Satcher, MD, says, "I'm worried about the doing now." Let's do. Let's **Get a Life, America!**

Appendix   333

Glossary   344

References   347

Index   367

About the Author – inside back cover

Foreword

"An ounce of prevention is worth a pound of cure." Who hasn't heard that without inwardly groaning? "Get real," is our response. How about "A stitch in time saves nine?" The boos are equally loud. And yet, is there any question that the average American, after a heart attack, wishes that he had heeded the wisdom of these trite aphorisms? Why is it that we do not appreciate the truth of the medical equivalent of the real estate prescription for success of, "Location, location, and location," i.e., "Prevention, prevention, and prevention?" Is it fatalism, fear, denial, ignorance, laziness, self-indulgence, a death-wish, or indifference? Clearly, the answer is different for each person, but the result is the same: catastrophic illness, death, family disruption, financial ruin. And, more often than not, it could have been prevented. How sad, how foolish, how wasteful!

This is not entirely the patient's fault. Most physicians, sadly, would rather treat disease than prevent it. Most cardiologists would prefer to perform angioplasty than to control the disease process by practicing prevention. The government places a ceiling on what it considers economical to save a year of life, and if an effective prevention program costs more than $35,000 per year of life saved, well, you just aren't worth it. The junk food and tobacco industry would rather have you consume their products even if doing so means you will depart this planet years too soon. Is it any wonder, then, that the average American follows the path of least resistance and does nothing to help himself?

Well, Americans, it need not be this way. As Dr. Leonard Mees has pointed out in his excellent new book, *Get a Life, America!*, we can take control of our own destiny and, rather than living (or not living) to regret our passivity, can actively take steps to prolong our lives! In chapter after chapter of clear, entertaining, accurate, and helpful advice, Dr. Mees provides Americans with an opportunity to change their destinies.

There is no lack of "How to ..." books, promoting the entire spectrum of medical cures from the sublime to the ridiculous, from the most conventional to the lunatic fringe. However, there is a great need for a comprehensive, yet eminently readable resource that does not talk down to the reader, but rather provides encouragement along with sound medical advice. How many times have we picked up books and put them down in 5 minutes (or have them slip through our fingers as they put us to sleep)? How often do we read about the "only way to do things is my way?" when the recommendations are so severe that they can only be adhered to by people who did not heed the advice to begin with? Dr. Mees personalized his message and provides the answers to a wealth of questions regarding diet, exercise, and stress in an easily implemented fashion, utilizing sound, medically accepted principles.

As a cardiologist of many years of dealing with the sequelae of disease, I, quite frankly, would much rather never see another patient with a heart attack. This is not because I choose no to care for sick people, but, rather, because I would like to render my acute care services obsolete by preventing the heart attack from occurring. My best intentions and efforts notwithstanding, however, the most essential component is a motivated person who has some understanding of the threats to health imposed by modern day living and the possibility of averting disease by practicing sound prevention. It is precisely this information that is imparted by Dr. Leonard Mees in *Get a Life, America!*

Harvey S. Hecht, MD, FACC
Director of Atherosclerotic Detection and Preventive Treatment Center
Director of Cardiac Imaging
Chairman, Department of Medicine, Arizona Heart Hospital
Phoenix, Arizona

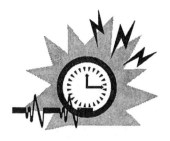

Preface

Fortunate, in my opinion, to have attended the University of Rochester School of Medicine and Dentistry in Rochester, New York, I was steeped early in my medical career in an ethic of service and in the mind-body-spirit model for treating patients. Dr. George Engel, nationally renowned psychiatrist, had established the Med-Psych liaison department in the mid-1960s. That department recognized and championed the inexorable connection between mind, body and spirit. We medical students were taught to view patients as whole people; not as charts, not as numbers, not as diseases, and certainly not as meal tickets.

This patient-service ethic seared itself into my practice of medicine as I made house calls in an era of medical isolationism; as I worked hand-in-hand with the police and fire departments at accident scenes; as I traveled on the Coast Guard "forty-four footer" seven miles off-shore at two in the morning to rescue a sick deck hand from a fishing trawler in ten foot seas; and as I learned first hand what it meant to be sea-sick. Willfully, I accommodated most any request.

Still, only two years into my twenty-year medical practice I began to sense dissatisfaction with my chosen career and how I delivered care. Something wasn't right, but I was unable to discover my *ennui* and to articulate it then. I observed that people brought me illnesses, accidents and deaths that, in my judgment, did not have to occur. Stress related diseases were alarmingly common, overweight persons were the rule, and of course, exercise was a rarity. If only my patients had managed their lives better.

Well-educated and economically stable, they, like most every patient in the country, were medically ignorant and unsophisticated. Many of their illnesses could have been treated by someone with far less professional training than I. In fact, many of the individuals who sought my services could have taken care of themselves if only they had some basic medical acumen and a modicum of self-confidence. To compound their plight, they lived terribly unhealthy lifestyles; lifestyles which led to more than eighty percent of their diseases.

Could these individuals change their unhealthy lifestyles? Could they learn how to care for themselves? I always thought, "Yes," although no one ever told them that they could. Quite to the contrary, they thought change impossible.

Change, of necessity, had to begin with me. Precariously perched to drone mindlessly through twenty years of practice, I began to *Get a Life!*, in medicine. Certainly I continued to provide the best treatment that I could. I treated illnesses, but it was like attempting to put out a grass fire with my jacket. I would knock down one flame and, oops, there's another, and another. I adopted a preventive philosophy and began to educate myself about preventive philosophies and techniques (something never taught in medical school). I maintained files of articles about diseases and their causes, alternative methods of treatment, health promotion efforts like nutrition, exercise and stress management; thinking that someday I would write a book to integrate all of this information in a logical manner. I listened to patients, especially to their ideas about prevention. I sought out positive thinking people with prospective philosophies, asked healthy people how they stayed healthy, and congratulated people for making any healthy change in their lives. I opened my mind, thought, learned, and tried to create a forum for better health. Change began with me.

My favorite challenge in medical practice was the classic overweight, stressed thirty year-old man with high blood pressure. I would examine him, attain all of the necessary data and numbers, then kick back in my chair, smile and say, "Harry, we are going to save your life. No one including you will ever know it, though. We are going to make changes in your lifestyle that will eliminate the heart attack that is staring you in the face. No heroics, no cardiac resuscitation and no surgeons swapping blood vessels on your heart, we are just going to quietly save your life so that you can grow to be a grandfather and enjoy your grandchildren."

Thirty year-old men with high blood pressure frequently don't live to become fifty year-old men. Required to provide, to succeed, to be a father, to be a husband, and to defend their country, young men are commonly ignorant of societal pressures. Society teaches them not to express emotion, but just to "be a man." Blindly, Harry gropes through his life, coping with his stressors in a juvenile manner, internalizing, over-eating and over-working; trying to catch that elusive carrot called success.

That carrot is closer than he realizes, but it's a bit different and tastier carrot. With compassionate teaching, an introduction to awareness and a gradual modification of lifestyle, this thirty year-old man may take control of his life and of his health. He may attain loftier goals and live a healthier, happier, more loving life.

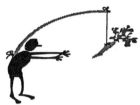

My carrot is teaching Harry, teaching him how not to be stressed, how to manage his body weight and how not to develop high blood pressure, all in a prospective fashion. I want to teach Harry how to avoid the first trip to my office. I want to teach Harry how to *Get a Life!*

My greatest frustration and unhappiness in medical practice was caring for friends and acquaintances whom, out of lifelong ignorance, became the victims of major medical illnesses. The illness might have been a heart attack, a stroke or cancer. Possibly my friend would survive his first heart attack, only to have a second one in a year, and then die. Strokes, fearsome catastrophes, seize a robust person and destroy half of his functioning in a heartbeat. Cancers, many a result of long term, mindless abuse of a healthy body, depress even the most stalwart observer. An inexorable wasting of the miraculous physiology granted us, most major maladies kill unnecessarily.

John, a friendly and personable man, worked all of his life as a painter. I always enjoyed his visits because of his optimistic and happy manner. Unfortunately, he smoked. He combined two major pulmonary risk factors in his life, cigarette-smoke and paint fumes. I assume that you can anticipate the rest of the story. John developed a cough, and his chest film revealed a lemon-sized lung cancer. How do I tell such a delightful man that he has cancer and that he will most likely not see next year?

I have seen too many accidents, unnecessary by my definition. Whether careless, minor ones or catastrophic, life-altering tragedies, accidents result from poor short-term choices, and as such are avoidable.

I recall vividly the night a seventeen year-old boy was brought to our emergency room with a broken neck. He dove from a bridge into shallow water one dark Cape Cod night, "just having fun with the guys." Never to walk again, he might move his arms if he's lucky. His life and that of his family is forever altered. Fighting tears as she undressed this unfortunate lad in the ER, nurse Mary tried to lighten the somber mood of the exam room. She looked at me and said, "Now this is why your mother told you to always wear clean underwear."

The night my fourteen year-old neighbor and her boyfriend lost their lives in an auto accident etched itself indelibly in my memory. Susie and Jack, rushing to reach home before Susie's overbearing father's curfew clanged, careened around a tight corner on a drizzle-slicked road to meet a tree, head on. I attended the accident scene on that cold, foggy Cape night to witness the medical examiner and a state police trooper arguing over whom had jurisdiction. I thought these two "officers" were going to do "odds and evens" to settle their dispute, while two young members of our community lay dead at their feet. Are we so accustomed to, accepting of, deaths among our cherished youth, that we massage our own egos before tending to their needs?

I contend that many, if not most, of the illnesses and accidents that we suffer as individuals and collectively as a nation are unnecessary. I challenge us to change our perspective from one of being passive victims to that of choosing empowerment through knowledge and ability. Given the proper information and a reasonable blueprint of how to apply that information, we can change the face of our nation's health. We can *Get a Life, America!*

Although I attempted to integrate preventive techniques and philosophies into my practice, I found it impossible to practice and preach prospective, preventive management in an atmosphere of illness, reactivity and retroactive thinking. I concluded after much frustration that prevention is best practiced as a specialty.

For twenty years I toiled in the muddy trenches of illness. Now I opt to enjoy the second half of my professional life working with wellness, teaching people how to *Get a Life!* I trust that I can convince you to make an effort to achieve better health, for a world of health, happiness and love beckons you to journey with me through *Get a Life, America!*

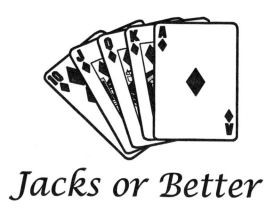

Jacks or Better

*"Education
is the best provision
for old age."*
❖
Aristotle

A Buddhist reclined in the dental operatory adjacent to me one day. I overheard that he didn't want the dentist to use novocaine. He said, "I want to transcend dental medication." Later, I happened upon the same Buddhist at a hot dog stand where he requested of the vendor, "Make me one with everything."

So welcome, folks, as I attempt to make you "one with everything." I invite you to join me and *Get a Life!,* our answer to health, happiness, and love.

That's "Jacks or Better," openers for poker, openers for a radio show, and openers for *Get a Life, America!,* the book. Once you open it, I trust that you will find this book one of the most useful you've ever read. Don't simply allow it to sit on your library shelf, rather place it conspicuously on your coffee table for frequent and easy reference. As with my radio show, I intend *Get a Life, America!* to be your companion in achieving life-long health.

I opened one of my radio programs with that transcendental meditation bit. My guest, a prominent Phoenix cardiologist, had joined me to discuss a very serious topic – early diagnosis and prevention of heart attacks. He didn't have any idea that I would launch the show in that fashion (neither did I until about five minutes before air-time), and I think the levity of the "hook" allowed for a much more relaxed and personal tone to the show.

Before we "went hot," I shared with him that I had chosen classic blues for the theme music of *Get a Life!* the radio show, and I think he was lost in appreciation of the opening piece by Blind Lemon Johnson when I blind-sided him with my adolescent introduction. After the show, I confessed that I suffer from perpetual adolescence, but defended my malady by adding that it serves to keep me young, bright-eyed, and innovative. It helps me to *Get a Life!*

I created the radio show, *Get a Life!,* to serve as a platform for public education about healthy lifestyles. To my knowledge, dedicating a one-hour radio show to public education about healthy lifestyles has never been done, in Phoenix or elsewhere. Yes, some "health shows" address health education, but that attention unveils itself merely to be lip service to wellness, a thinly disguised shill for some worthless product, or an advertisement for some facility's sick care services. At *Get a Life!* we're all about health education.

I'm So Full of It

Sure, I'm dead serious about teaching, and I talk about it a lot. My friends often roll their eyes and say, "Lennie, you're so full of it." I agree. Blessed with my perpetual adolescence, I'm full of ideas, some simple and logical, some downright wacky, about how to teach a sick nation to be healthier. Don't make your judgment about my state of mind yet. Come on down to the airport with me, and I'll share a vision with you.

Flight 1601 crept to a halt at Gate 14. Shortly, as deplaning began my mind's eye whisked me from Sky Harbor International to the Chicago stockyards, where "cattle" plod mindlessly from one holding pen, through narrow restrictive corridors to their next way station. No smiles, no joy, they dutifully accept their lot in life.

An astute observer of human behavior, I sat with double latte in hand, mental camera on auto-wind, photographing this sad procession. I wondered if these "cattle" had any idea of the meaning or quality of their lives. Did they recognize their obesity, stress, depression, poor nutrition, and impending illnesses? So obvious to me, have they ever looked in the mirror to see themselves clearly? Had they any idea that they run on autopilot, mindlessly droning through a murkiness that defines their lives?

I think not. Few of us realize that our lifestyles place us at health risk. Even fewer of us take action to change. Most think that change is impossible.

Many of us seem ignorant of the fact that we lead dangerously unhealthy lives. Epidemiologists have documented that most of the illnesses we experience today result from dysfunctional lifestyles. Our mindless practicing of unhealthy behaviors has earned our position on the precipice of disaster, shoulder to shoulder with the "cattle," heading to the slaughterhouse.

Am I full of it to want to warn these "cattle" of their impending health disaster by posting health warnings and information in airports, on billboards, and on milk cartons? Am I full of it to try to teach them to change their risky lives?

Unfortunately, we don't yet understand how to change our "destiny," but I promise you that we can and will change. I wish to jam a wrench into the gears of the status quo thinking that accepts illnesses as the norm. I focus not on criticism, but on solution. Given that we are a population at risk, I ask for your attention to my message that we as individuals and as a nation must accept and assume responsibility for improving our health. It is we who must *Get a Life!*

Is anything in our lives more precious than health? I can't envision an answer other than, "No." Without good health everything in our lives suffers. With good health our horizons have no limits. We must change! We can change! We will *Get a Life!*

Hey, we're a bright nation, aren't we? We know that we're at risk, don't we? Why, then, have we not effected improved disease statistics? Why do we lose one million American citizens per year to heart disease?

Our health management in the United States as individuals, as a society and through the medical community trumpets a fanfare of failure. The cost of caring for our sick society voraciously consumes one-seventh of our Gross National Product, just about one trillion dollars, with less than 2% of that total directed to preventive services. Of the 2%, only a small fraction apportions specifically to teaching about health and wellness, about getting a life!

While we have risen above the risk of many childhood infectious diseases with the advent of immunizations, the development of antibiotics has allowed us to successfully treat many formerly deadly infections. Sophisticated surgical techniques let many of us live longer than we might have without those operations. Yet in the past forty years our survival rate has plateaued, most of the present diseases being those related to unhealthy lifestyles.

Our lifestyles earn our diseases when 92% of us don't exercise enough to achieve an aerobic training response, 90% of us eat poorly on a day to day basis, 80% of primary care office visits are stress related, 20% of us are depressed, 30-40% of us are obese, the majority of us have cholesterol levels above 200, while many of us futilely attempt to stem the rising tide of risk by simply consuming vitamin and mineral supplements.

Our costs skyrocket, but we don't seem to care. We dutifully accept these human and economic losses as necessary. Is the abject fear accompanying the chest pain of a heart attack necessary? Is the feeling of helplessness and hopelessness associated with a diagnosis of cancer equally requisite?

I say none of this is necessary; not the fear, not the financial losses, not the human losses. *Get a Life, America!* recognizes the crisis, tolls the alarm, and enthusiastically provides the solution for improving individual and national health.

Get a Life, America! articulates a new paradigm for health and wellness. That new paradigm assumes, expects and nurtures our health to the state of grace called wellness. The soon-to-be-old paradigm expects illnesses. While the perceptive difference may seem minor, it looms large in effecting a positive change in individual and societal health.

Get a Life! saves lives. *Get a Life!* saves money. *Get a Life!* reduces taxes. Healthy individuals don't die. Health doesn't cost money. A healthy society doesn't squander unfathomable amounts of tax money on unnecessary illnesses. *Get a Life, America!* works. It works hard for you and for the nation.

Secrets That We Keep

It's no secret that we under-achieve our productive potential in the work place, while we dutifully accept physical and emotional ills as the norm. With illness running rampant, exercise ebbing, gluttony growing, we have become fatter, not fitter, as a nation. Why?

I thought we had some sort of national health initiative, *Healthy People 2000*. Yet, few people have ever heard of it. Unintentionally, I assume, through neglect of vigorous broadcast of its presence and message, it's been kept a secret. A most unfortunate neglect, this "secret" aspired to have 60% of our population exercising by the year 2000. Such an admirable concept, why have we actually ebbed from its goal?

Individually, we're not privy to the "secret" knowledge about wise and judicious, prospective management techniques for our lives. Unaware that individual health management is within our purview, unaware that it is our individual responsibility, we remain ignorant, not stupid. We stagnate, ignorant of our responsibility and of the whats, whys and hows of health management. Searching for the information and drawing up our personal health management plan, our own map to *Get a Life!*, overwhelms most of us. But, once provided with the information for health and wellness, we certainly have the ability to comprehend and apply the knowledge. So that you may plan and live your healthy lifestyle, I give to you *Get a Life, America!*

As a society we're not committed to becoming and remaining healthy. The knowledge for healthier lifestyles is available, but we have been steeped in the tradition of diseases. We have chosen not to disseminate the preventive message as freely as we have chosen to share the repair philosophy. We kept it secret. Even if we do understand that a societal health change will benefit us, the anticipation of change provokes adequate anxiety and apprehension to guarantee the status quo. Society suffers the inertia of the masses, a grudging unwillingness to change, an aversion to creativity and to new ideas. Societal changes only occur when the current norm no longer serves the public need. Evidently, our nation doesn't yet perceive a need to *Get a Life, America!*

Moreover, we teachers keep secrets and thereby fail you. Read the copy of this letter that I send to health promotion colleagues:

Dear Colleague in Health Promotion:

Did Arnold, Jack or Tiger learn to hit a golf ball in one lesson? No, it took a lifetime of learning and practice. Why do we "mortals" expect to learn a new skill, like living healthy lives, quickly? We can't and won't. Learning takes time and practice.

I teach individuals and groups how to achieve health. In developing my philosophy, I wrestled with difficult questions and hammered out positive answers. First, I confronted our national failure of health education. In spite of our attempts to educate the public about health, we have no measurable improvement in disease statistics. Second, I asked how we could provide functional teaching that endures. Third, I queried why our recidivism rate for healthy behavior change approaches 99%. Finally, I addressed why our society seems hell-bent for solutions in "two weeks, five steps, simply by using a magic device, and all with a money back guarantee."

We have failed to educate because we "teachers" have kept much of our knowledge proprietary. Tight-fisted and condescending, we under-estimate public intelligence. We have not freely given health information away. Successful education elevates the student to her point of articulate expertise, to her perception of control. That should be our goal – teaching students well enough that they, too, may teach.

While the perception of control empowers individual success, teaching that endures must be useful and functional, with perceived value and relevance. As Tiger didn't learn to hit a golf ball in one try, and as he practices to maintain his skills, we understand that enduring information must demonstrate a persistent presence. Education must be repetitive throughout our lives, or we risk failure of our intent.

Recidivism, failure of intended behavior change, results from two other errors – ignorance of the process of change and perception that we lack control of our lives. What an easy fix! Let's teach the process of behavior modification while we teach individuals not only how to take control of their lives, but that they must take control.

Let's be forthright about how long the process of behavior modification takes. It's a two-year stewardship, minimum. Why should we think otherwise? We do because we've been brainwashed by product hawkers who spend millions to make billions. They saturate radio, TV and the print media with quick-fix BFL's (big fat lies). Yet, while BFL advertising may make money, I believe honesty always wins. Through honest education, we empower. That's success. That's winning. That's how to *Get a Life, America!*

Sincerely,

Leonard R. Mees, MD

On the heels of this letter, more self-criticism of us preventive medicine types comes to the fore. With all the disease warnings and health information cast upon our waters of awareness, why have we failed to make a dent in disease statistics? As well intentioned as our efforts have been, our silence about certain individually and societally empowering topics keeps secrets, too. We haven't:

➢ focused on how to change to healthy lifestyles
➢ relinquished a sense of personal empowerment to the public
➢ established a persistent educational presence
➢ recognized the necessity of repetition – practice, practice, practice
➢ assumed an assertive position in marketing our message of health

Duke University's wellness program, which incidentally got its roots as a cardiac rehabilitation program, is the only program in the nation to greet their clients with the "Jacks or Better" salutation, "We're here to teach you how to take control of your life and make it a healthy one." At *Get a Life!,* we applaud Duke University's work. It stands as a sentinel for success.

With Duke's wellness program cited as the sole beacon of honesty in health education, we do have a rather scalding indictment of our national health initiative, wouldn't you say?

OK, do we agree that we have a problem? If so, then what's the solution?

Begin With Principles and Philosophy

"Education is the best prescription," quoted C. Everett Koop, MD, former Surgeon General of the United States. "Beyond that wonderful, glorious five second rage, everything is choice," wrote noted thanatologist, Dr. Elizabeth Kubler-Ross. "A problem once recognized is half solved," reasoned our first president, George Washington. "The atherosclerotic process is reversible," proved Dean Ornish, MD, forward thinking, pioneering cardiologist from California. "Don't sweat the small stuff. It's all small stuff," offered Robert S. Eliot, MD, prominent researcher and author about stress and cardiovascular diseases.

These quotes represent some of the principles and philosophy that I present in *Get a Life, America!* In my view, they are part of good health and good living. Education grants power. Without education, we are quite likely doomed to live unenlightened, uninteresting and unhealthy lives. Chaos, anger and frustration often seem to rule our worlds, but in spite of feeling overwhelmed by events and emotions, we always have choices. Cultivating awareness motivates the first steps in solving our problems. Once aware, we can change actions, behaviors and processes that we once thought to be cast in stone. In the end, nothing is as ominous or onerous as we might have originally thought, for in the overall scale of the universe, everything is small, especially us. As cerebral individuals we do have the potential and the ability to seize control of our lives and to mold them into a shape that pleases us. The reality remains, however, that no short-cut or quick-fix to better health awaits us.

How Does Get a Life, America! Work?

If we begin with principles and philosophies, what follows? *Get a Life, America!* continues by providing direction. *Get a Life, America!* explains the process of achieving health and wellness.

First and foremost, *Get a Life, America!* presents **useful information** about health and wellness. I excavate and lay a foundation of scientifically based information in understandable language and concepts. My background in basic science and my enthusiasm to search the current literature, leads me to propose observations and conclusions. My experience in medicine, tempered with a preventive philosophy, positions me well to offer opinions and criticisms.

I keep an open ear and mind to new, alternative solutions, and to ideas presented by persons outside of the medical and research professions. These "lay" ideas may be among the best. Norman Cousins authored *Anatomy of an Illness*, an insightful book about the power of the mind in healing. He discovered the power of humor as an agent for healing. Watching old Laurel and Hardy movies in a hotel room (across the street from the hospital he just departed against medical advice), he laughed himself back to health from a serious illness.

Get a Life, America! continues and gives **reason** to the process of achieving better health. We are incessantly barraged by conflicting claims of what to do to make us fit or healthy. In fact, we are constantly being told what to do, health related or not. Parents told us what to do, teachers told us what to do, governments tell us what to do, but rarely in our lives does someone share with us the why. Without an understanding of the why, we are but robots, performing mindless tasks. Understanding the why facilitates our active management of our lives, thereby potentiating the successful implementation of the what. For this reason, the whys greasing the skids for the whats, I explain the thinking behind current recommendations for health and wellness.

"OK, great," you will say. "I have an idea of what to do and an understanding of why to do it, but **how** am I supposed to implement and integrate this stuff?" You're right, the process of implementation is critical. Without that process, we lose. Knowledge is valuable, but only precious if we know how to use it. We need an outline, a blueprint, a flow chart of how to introduce new thoughts

11

and behaviors into our lives. Bridging the gap between knowledge and action is difficult, time consuming, at times frustrating, but oh so valuable when accomplished. So, I am going to assist your bridging that gap by showing you the whats, whys and hows of accomplishing better health, of getting a life.

I introduce several plans, techniques, tricks and ideas for getting a life. By no means do I imply just one route, my route. I want you to take all of the information you can get, or that you need, then map your journey to *Get a Life!* I will help as much as I can, but in the end it is your job, your responsibility, and your gain.

I simplify complex concepts and provide novel ways to remember them. It is especially difficult to recall philosophies or techniques when your world crumbles around you. For instance, when you feel overwhelmed and outnumbered, do what the pioneers did, "Circle the Wagons" for protection. Remember that you are the boss of your own life and that "you are the CEO of your company." I will try to express ideas that are self-evident, but more so when you see them in print. In that regard, I hope this book may serve as a mirror for your self-observation.

Utilizing the principles of potentiation and synergy, your integration of healthy behaviors and attitudes results in a whole, greater than the sum of the parts. Certain behavioral and physical changes empower and facilitate others. For example, Dr. Dean Ornish documented that combining diet and exercise reduces the risk of recurrent heart disease. The real magic of his discovery lies in the individual's learning to adopt a new loving attitude. The addition of a new loving attitude to the foundation of diet and exercise evokes a reversal of the atherosclerotic disease process. The integration of modalities for health offers unknown potential.

Finally, I don't know everything, and I am not afraid to say, "I don't know," when I don't. However, health and wellness is my area of expertise and I am confident that you will find reliable and useful information in *Get a Life, America!* Although I might attempt to share information as a teacher, I will always reserve my seat as a student.

Investment House Illnesses

A few years ago, a small restaurant opened on Cape Cod. They called themselves, "Breakfast of Champions." No sooner had they poured their first cup of coffee than General Mills' lawyers threatened to shut them down if they didn't change their name, because everyone knows that the "breakfast of champions" is Wheaties. In similar fashion, the Disney Corporation warns, "Don't mess with the mouse." So I have to tell you this next story descriptively.

Do you remember the corpulent, raspy-voiced, venerable character actor, probably best known for his investment house commercial? "We make money the old fashioned way. We earn it," resounds the convincing closing line of the commercial. I contend that "Investment House Illness" defines most of the illness in our country.

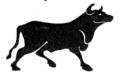

"We earn it!" Illness just doesn't happen. When we're ill, if we run life's movie-reel backward, and if we search it diligently, we will find a reason, a pathway, a continuum, leading to our illness. The body's natural state of existence, one of health and good function, eludes most of us. Although we possess innate defense mechanisms that have evolved over centuries to assure our survival, we build upon a foundation of ignorance, mistreat our bodies over time, and create an unnatural end result, sickness and poor health. Those elaborate and effective immune responses, physiologic filters and adaptive techniques that must be overwhelmed in order to produce illnesses, click past like mile markers as we race towards ill health.

Not necessarily an easy task to achieve ill health, to become chronically ill or to capture a terminal state, we Americans do it with a facility unmatched by any other country. Especially adept in the arenas of cardiovascular diseases and malignancies, we're tops. We earned our leading position in mortality and morbidity. Curiously, we seem rather proud of our accomplishment and of our ranking. Are we so preoccupied with being a "leader" or "number one" that we take pride in leading the world in deaths from heart disease?

Our focus is wrong. What we consider normal existence in the United States is quite abnormal physiologically. Our existence deviates significantly from the physiologic design and intention of our bodies. Designed to be physical animals, active, running, chasing and growing our food; with the advent of the modern industrialized society, we have become progressively sedentary. Our physiology has adapted to a less active lifestyle, creating a new "norm," a new homeostasis that carries with it increased risk of disease. If we were able to return to the original design intended homeostasis, the state more in synchrony with our physiology, then our disease risks, and indeed the incidence of disease would be far less.

Do we have illusions, or delusions, of immortality? Are we so ignorant and unaware that we allow our behaviors to taunt the specter of ill health and death? Yes, we are that ignorant, and yes, we do have delusions of immortality. We do until it may be too late, until the wake up call, the alarm that heralds our need for awareness. Can we not focus our energies on creating and maintaining good health with the same zeal and vigor that we earn our poor health? Certainly we can, but to do so will require a change in perspective.

That change is to view good health as desirable, worth working for, and entirely within the realm of our individual control. No, I am not a starry-eyed Pollyanna. Rather, I am a working realist. The unconscious, careless neglect, the abdication of responsibility for our well-being, the tenacious clinging to bad habits, the seeming unwillingness to change, the wanton disregard for health, the leading of stressful lives with blinders on, all take energy to sustain. I get tired just thinking about it. That same energy output, that requisite work, when applied consciously in the prospective direction of health would serve us much better.

Wouldn't you rather beam, "I earned my good health," than confess, "I earned my illness?" The choice is simple, and it is yours. The actual energy required is the same for each. All you have to do is to point your energy in the proper direction of health. I will show you the way. Then you may *Get a Life!* with America.

What I Learned in Writing Get a Life, America!

In spite of *Get a Life, America's!* grudging reluctance to allow itself to appear on paper and become entrapped between soft covers, it relinquished only after much coaxing, pleading and gnashing of teeth by its author. In the process, *Get a Life, America!* taught me lessons I had not anticipated.

I learned that changing one's self-perception is difficult, but not impossible. I resisted viewing myself as an author with the stubbornness of a mule. All I had ever been was a physician. It was all I had known. I had not explored worlds outside of my comfort zone, and I had certainly considered writing to be beyond my comfort zone. Persistence won out. I rented an office and went there every day to write. The repetitive practicing of my new endeavor catalyzed my evolution to an expanded self-image.

Another unanticipated lesson was my struggle with providing an answer to the question of how to create and maintain good health. I thought I would easily outline my ideas and principles, expand on them, offer them to you and, *voila, Get a Life!* Not quite! Without question, the how, the making a change, the doing, opens as the most intimidating and fearsome chasm to be bridged in the process of achieving our goals. Because of my literary naivete, it was also a huge hurdle to writing this book.

We can talk about doing something all day long, but sitting down and doing the requisite work is quite another story. I offer to you that the task ahead is not easy, but it is possible, and it is ultimately within your purview to accomplish. You will learn how to narrow the chasm as you *Get a Life!*

Oh, my, another surprise ambushed me along my journey – many people don't want to *Get a Life!* Maybe they don't know better health is a choice for them. Maybe they don't understand the benefits of good health.

The first time I had "finished" *Get a Life, America!*, I sent the manuscript off to a prominent New York literary agent. Enthusiastically interested, he called me to ask, "Hey, nice book, but how are you going to get those people who don't want to exercise to exercise?" Hmm, good question. Then, one morning at our local Einstein's coffee shop, an overweight patron sitting adjacent to me inquired of my work. When I shared that I taught people how to be healthy, he lowered his gaze to challenge me, "How are you going to motivate me to change to a healthier lifestyle?"

My reflex response was to tell this sedentary sack of potatoes that motivation is his job. But after daylong reflection, I realized and accepted that if I hold myself out as a teacher of healthy lifestyles, then motivation is my job.

Wrestling with the task of motivating people to change now consumes ninety-percent of my time. But it's a necessary ninety-percent. Motivating people to change requires enthusiasm, dedication, persistence, omnipresence, innovation, and any other tool we can find as we work to *Get a Life!* In short, we must sell the concept of *Get a Life, America!* like we're running for public office.

So, I present to you information about health and wellness, that I offer as a foundation for your getting a life. You may take control of your lives and stay healthy. I have tried to facilitate your use of the information, integrating the various principles of health and wellness for maximal gain. Again, I have not given you one pathway to *Get a Life!*, but have provided you the map for you to plan your journey to health, happiness and love, to *Get a life!* I want you to realize your ability to use information and create your healthy life. Not only in better health, but in the process, the doing, you will find great reward. *A votre sante!*

Oh, do you know what else I learned? I learned that I am just like everyone else in thinking I could accomplish changes quickly. Only in retrospect did I realize this. I now understand that my evolution from curmudgeon physician to teacher was long, sometimes painful, and quite arduous. In fact, my change continues with thousands of baby steps. But what a fun process and what a *great new life!*

Organization and Use of *Get a Life, America!*

Get a Life, America! begins by explaining the process of changing behaviors. This process provides the foundation for the remainder of the book.

Making changes in any or all of the Major League Players of Health and Wellness (those life practices, that when neglected or practiced poorly, turn on us, bite us in the backside and cause illness) relies on behavior modification. Presentation of each of the Major League Players of Health and Wellness follows in logical order, beginning with nutrition, then exercise, stress management, depression, lipids, weight and body composition management, and vitamins and minerals. A chapter on their integration ensues. Each of these players packs a powerful health punch, but when they play together, synergy evidences. Their product is greater than the sum of their talents. Everyone wins and no one loses. Finally, this book which began as *Get a Life!*, a book for individual health, addresses a program to improve the health of our nation, and we realize that together we can *Get a Life, America!*

I recommend that you scan *Get a Life, America!* before reading it. Pay attention to the Table of Contents for areas of your particular interest. Read it through one time, making notes of your "trouble spots." Then go back and focus on your individual concerns, whether they be nutrition, exercise or stress.

Although I think it's best, you don't have to read the book initially from beginning to end. Certainly, read through Chapter I, "A Change of Heart," and then you may proceed to your chapters of interest. Yes, any Major League Player of Health and Wellness can stand alone, but they perform better as a team.

Get a Life, America! provides a load of information, so take it slowly. I've tried to make it fun, to provide breaks in your reading, and to present punctuating reviews; all to assist your learning some life-enhancing, life-saving principles and practices.

I trust that I can provoke you to action. I want this book to make a positive difference in your life. If you have new ideas, differences of opinion, axes to grind, my mailing address appears at *Get a Life, America's!* end. Write to me.

Why wait for the end? Here's my address now. It's at the end, too.

Leonard R. Mees
c/o Sabec Publishing Company
P.O. Box 82545
Portland, OR 97282-0545

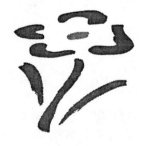

Chapter I

A Change of Heart

*"Beyond that glorious five second rage,
everything is choice."*

❖

*Elisabeth Kubler-Ross, MD,
internationally renowned thanatologist*

This chapter teaches the process of change. It's about learning to change how we live our lives, about choosing to change our unhealthy lifestyles. We begin by examining how behavior develops, proceed through the stages of behavior change, recognize stealthy adversaries to change, learn to hear wake-up calls for change, practice assertive behavior, reconcile the two-year stewardship of behavior change, and prevent the failure of our efforts to change. As in each chapter, the latter portions focus squarely on how you can change.

Without the knowledge of how to change, we're doomed to drone through our lives practicing repetitive, disease-producing, life-threatening behaviors. So let's *Get a Life!* and learn a few things about behavior modification.

Nicole, a 42 year-old sales representative, had lived her entire life under the ever-present, domineering control of her old-school Italian mother. Mom ruled the roost. This very capable, attractive, but emotionally blunted, 42 year-old woman had little freedom of expression, scarcely an idea that she could have her own thoughts and emotions. She began to realize that her developmental background hampered her interpersonal relationships. After a series of failed relationships, she desperately wanted to change. But how?

My friend David's car wasn't running well and he wanted to fix it, but similar to Nicole's dilemma, he didn't know how. He bought a manual on how to fix cars, read it, went to work on the car, and fixed it. That's what Nicole can do, learn how to fix her problem. Then she will *Get a Life!,* a wonderful, loving life, one full of emotions and self-expression.

❖

This chapter and this book are for her and for the many people like her.

❖

Behavior modification is learning a new skill. So is learning to be healthy. So is learning to be happy. So is learning to love. As *Get a Life, America!* is a book about learning new skills, moreover, it's about learning to change our hearts. As no one can deny the absolute value of learning, could anyone debate the veracity of learning to change our hearts?

The new skills that we learn will make our lives more enjoyable, productive and healthful. They will bring us health, happiness and love. They allow us to change our hearts, to *Get a Life!*

Why even discuss behavior modification if we are getting by in our lives doing the same things that have served us reasonably well in the past? One answer is that we may not be getting by, but remain unaware of that fact. Another answer is that by reviewing our present behaviors and by consciously questioning if those behaviors are serving us well, we may stimulate awareness. Then we may be able to choose better behaviors for better living.

I will address changes of a remediable nature, but emphasize changes of prospective potential. All of us are living parts of our lives poorly, and our lifestyles put us at health risk. I want us to learn to identify those risks, address them, and fix them before they cause disease, or worse.

Happily, some among us live very healthy lives. This book and chapter addresses you, too. It encourages you to seek new ideas, new behaviors and new experiences. None of our lives extends long enough to experience a fraction of the marvels and beauty awaiting us in our worlds. I encourage all of us to seek growth in our lives.

If you are satisfied with your present behaviors and coping mechanisms, that's fine, as long as you review them periodically, assuring yourself that they function as you choose. As you review, be mindful of what your behaviors are, why they developed and how they serve you.

How Does Behavior Develop?

A basic genetic template predetermines some of our behavior. Beyond that foundation the remainder of behavior must be learned, learned behaviors emerging immediately after birth. Although an infant cannot reason, it learns

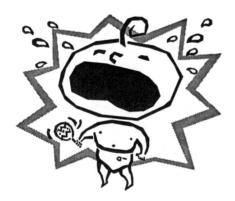

quickly that crying creates the most rapid route to a breast or bottle. Similarly, her parents reward her cooing, smiling and laughing with smiles and hugs. In this manner, an infant learns to perform "conditioned responses." Rewarding her responses conditions and strengthens her behaviors. Conditioning occurs through a combination of two methods, operant conditioning and stimulus-response conditioning.

Early learning follows the operant method, with random behaviors selectively rewarded. Feeding rewards crying, and a smile rewards a baby's giggling. Spitting out milk receives little or no reward (at least no smiling) and the behavior hopefully ceases. Random choices or behaviors are either supported and rewarded or not supported and ignored. The reward strengthens the behavior and allows it to continue, while behaviors extinguish without reinforcement.

A more direct method of teaching behavior, the stimulus-response-reward conditioning sequence attempts to produce a specific, desired behavior. Teaching a child to eat finger food, placing peas on her high chair tray and verbally encouraging her to take the peas with her hands to eat them, provide direct stimuli. If she responds correctly, she has performed the desired response. We give her a smile and praise as her rewards. Both methods of conditioning are effective, but other factors play a role in learning behaviors.

The individual's environment emerges as another important aspect of behavioral development. For an infant or a young child the family milieu assumes critical import. Her family is her world. All of her stimuli and rewards come from her immediate family. The voices she hears, the actions she mimics, the prejudices she witnesses, define her existence.

As she grows older and ventures out into society, her environment changes. Exposed to different behaviors, different stimuli, she receives different rewards. No longer with only one set of values to guide her, she faces seemingly limitless and conflicting social values. Fledged from the protection of her home nest, thrust into school at earlier and earlier ages, our young student meets the silent danger of peer pressure. Later she will experience the stressors of competition in society. Her world has changed, and she has been subjected to society's influences.

A child will most likely conform to the norms of the society in which she lives. She may become a South American beef-eater, an American who will work herself to a stress-induced heart attack, or a stoic Finn, impervious to pain. Wherever she happens to be born and reside, it is highly likely that she will unconsciously accept and adopt the local societal behavioral norms. Only through education and experience may an individual begin to question her normative behavior. She may then decide if she wishes to choose a different lifestyle, different behaviors and, indeed, a different self-identity.

Although plausible, changing behaviors offers considerable resistance because the automaticity of behavior is steel-trap strong. This automaticity serves us well to a point, as long as the behavior supports our direction and growth. When the behavior becomes counter-productive and detrimental, we have a problem. If we are unaware of the counter-productive nature of the behavior, our difficulties have grown exponentially. We become vulnerable to the phenomenon of the **generational compulsion to repeat.**

An important psychosocial phenomenon, the generational compulsion to repeat is the automatic, unconscious repetition of behaviors to which we were exposed as children. It is the reason that we are likely to repeat the behaviors of our parents, grandparents and great grandparents. The generational compulsion to repeat prompts daughters to marry their "fathers," sons to marry their "mothers," alcoholics to produce alcoholic children, prejudice to beget prejudice and bigotry to beget bigotry. It shapes our attitudes and expectations if we allow it to. It makes us narrow in our views, for we rarely stray far afield from familiar and comfortable experiences.

The good news is that we are not necessarily held hostage to the generational compulsion to repeat. We have choice, once we are aware of the specter of this monster. We may choose to seek worlds different from our own, attitudes different from those of our parents, and to expand our experiences by orders of magnitude.

The Process of Choosing to Change Behaviors

The psychologic sequence of events in behavior modification is a continuum from having the capacity to change, to awareness, to external motivation, to internal motivation, and to execution of the change. Each step must be completed before the next one may be undertaken. No shortcuts provide quick access to changing behaviors.

Having the **capacity** to change assumes a certain level of intelligence. Reasonable intelligence will suffice, for nothing about behavior modification is esoteric or lofty in principle. The ability to assess and comprehend information and to plan ahead are basic to having the capacity to change.

Awareness may be a different story. We may be so well defended psychologically from the pain and conflicts in our lives that we are unaware of our need to change. Many people live from crisis to crisis because they are not sensitive to their conflicts. If we learn to read our emotions, then we can determine our conflicts. Psychologic dissonance, an emotional itch that we just can't seem to scratch, becomes our alarm, our wake-up call. Awareness results from our answering the wake-up call.

External motivations, those signals from our environments heralding our need to change, readily avail themselves to us if we look. "Things aren't going well at the office." Why? "I am becoming argumentative with my spouse." Why? "I just had a heart attack." Why? "I don't enjoy making love like I used to." Why? "So, I never did enjoy it," says your mate. Oops, what a big externally motivating wake-up call! External motivations to change pepper our personal panoramas, but we will not become truly motivated until we take the external signals and make them our own. We must accept and acknowledge the reality of our circumstances.

The development of **internal motivation** increases the likelihood of our achieving behavior change. Attempting to leap from external motivation to execution proves futile. It fails because we don't yet "own" the problem. We must accept ownership of our dysfunctional behavior before we can successfully modify it. We must grasp the Certificate of Title to Behavior firmly in our hands before we can legitimately change the form of our behavior.

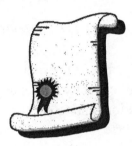

Acceptance and acknowledgement rise as integral parts of bringing the dysfunctional behavior into a personal and vulnerable realm. This critical step frequently causes emotional pain, but pain spurs us to change. Seeing ourselves clearly in a light that we do not like underscores the fact that the problem has surfaced well into our consciousness. Once we have the aberrant behavior clearly in our sights, identified as no one's other than our own, we may then proceed to implementing the change.

Without understanding the process of behavior modification, the perceived chasm between internal motivation and **execution** often looms wider and more fearsome than the Grand Canyon. Seemingly the most difficult step in the process of behavior change, this apparent schism may be narrowed by our realizing that the completion of one step facilitates the undertaking of the next.

The **execution** of a plan for behavior change demands an entirely conscious effort. "I have a problem. It is mine. I don't like it, and this is how I am going to change." We must develop a specific plan for implementing change. Planning takes considerable time and requires significant effort. We expect periodic failures as part of the process, but we must refuse to be imprisoned by them. Through practice we will achieve our desired end result – we'll *Get a Life!* with a new and better behavior.

It sounds rather easy doesn't it? Well, not so fast, let me warn you about a few potential bumps in your road to getting a life.

Stealthy Adversaries to Change

Have you ever wondered why we don't adopt new behaviors readily and easily? Many barriers to change baffle our smooth transition through the process. **Homeostasis**, the tendency to maintain the emotional and physical body in a functional state of balance doesn't accommodate changes readily. If our homeostasis is disturbed, whether internally (illnesses) or externally (environmental changes), our body chemistry responds with an attempt to restore the original balance. Our bodies fight rapid or large changes, and taken too far afield from our balance point, we die.

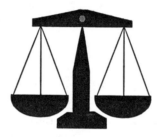

What else are we fighting? We fight a lifetime of learning that has created a steadfast **inertia**, a stable force mitigating against the probability of our changing. Traditions, "the way it has always been done," resist modification.

The ability to conceive new or novel solutions is rather rare. We fear the prospect of searching for new ideas. New ideas might invalidate beliefs we have held all of our lives. Doubts about ourselves and doubts about the future obstruct potential change. The deck is stacked against our making positive changes unless we choose to learn the process of making the changes, and then proceed to make those changes on a prospective conscious plane.

The **generational compulsion to repeat**, also a stealthy, subconscious adversary to our changing behaviors, regularly rears its ugly head. The only way to stop our mindless repetition of dysfunctional behaviors is to create awareness of the problem. We must slam a crow bar into the cog-wheels of this generational repetition and yell, "Stop!" "Look at yourselves!" "Wake up!"

Answering Our "Wake-up Calls"

Wake-up calls, alarms to stimulate our awareness of dysfunctional behaviors, ring for us daily. Do we or do we not answer our wake-up calls? Are we motivated to change our dysfunctional behaviors?

With motivation as the physical or emotional stimulus to performance, awareness becomes our motivation to change those behaviors. Once aware of our aberrant behaviors, we have lost any legitimate excuse not to change, and have begun to facilitate the prospective process of changing.

If wake-up calls ring daily, why would we not answer the call? Perhaps we receive some sort of manipulative gain from our dysfunctional behavior. Possibly we fear the unknown, the perceived threat of the realm of unfamiliar behaviors. Maybe we mantle ourselves in a cloak of ego defenses, clouding clear vision of our future. All functional reasons for behavioral blindness, why allow them to dictate and dominate our lives?

I suggest that we choose to answer our wake-up calls, to anticipate them, to search for them, and to welcome them into our lives. If we do not make that choice, we doom ourselves to emotional and behavioral stagnation. Having answered our wake-up calls, having become aware of behaviors that scream for change, we, as responsible people, will choose to proceed with change.

What are some areas in which you might consider modifying your behavior? How is your participation in and your contribution to work, exercise, nutrition, family, sex, recreation, sleep, personal relationships, community, and social service? Do you perceive the need to change? Are you aware?

Awareness may be achieved retrospectively, prospectively, or both. Retrospective cultivation of awareness includes information from family and friends (the MCI approach), physical illnesses, accident histories, sensing of dissonance (the un-scratchable emotional itch), and the taking and scoring of psychological tests. Retrospective awareness is an unfortunate necessity because we drone through our lives on auto-pilot, not regularly mindful of our existence. Prospective awareness begins with planting the seeds of mindfulness, for mindfulness is awareness. The common denominator to both, however, is our responsibility to open our eyes and look.

Friends and family provide valuable information about how we are functioning. We can ask them, hoping for an honest and assertive response. We can listen and sense any changes in their behavioral reactions to us. Have our relationships changed? If so, why? Are they telling us something, and we aren't listening? Do your friends call you less or avoid you? Often a signal of their discomfort in the presence of your unrecognized and unacknowledged depression, they respond to your depression by avoiding you.

Be sensitive to other clues. Is your mate less attractive, less giving, less sexual, less loving than formerly? You may unknowingly participate in a primary relationship downward spiral, each person perceiving a small decline in the level of the relationship, each responding defensively by incremental withdrawal. Dysfunctional communication begins, followed shortly by no communication. Our denial, inattention, and insensitivity earn such positions in our lives.

Pay attention to events in your life, for they are barometers of function, too. Have you been ill? Why? Are you working too hard? Do you perceive time to be inadequate? Are you having stressful relationships? Have you had headaches, abdominal pain, changes in bowel habits, stiff neck or fatigue? Whatever their origins, these physical symptoms warn of worse events to come. Have you been irritable, sad, lonely, depressed, angry, frustrated? Open your eyes and do some reconnaissance, some self-discovery. I want you to develop the ability to sense early alarms, and not by your insensitivity, to suffer bigger, louder ones like a heart attack or cancer. **Physical illness is always a wake-up call. Always, Always, Always!**

Have you had any accidents? They may not be purely accidental. The circumstances of your life may predispose you to accidents. I can laugh about this now, but at the time I was quite frustrated with an accident-prone period in my life. I was dealing quite poorly with an accumulation of personal stressors. Futilely attempting to "function" by denial, internalization, suppression and the concept that I could do it alone, I became accident-prone. Actually, I became auto accident-prone, not on the road, but in parking lots, at low speed, but still expensive. Two times in the parking lot of my own office I hit parked cars. Once in particular I looked and noted a car directly behind me and told myself, "Don't hit that car!" I promptly climbed into my car, put it into reverse and, CRUNCH. Only after remodeling the third car, and after considerable out-of-pocket repair costs, I finally admitted to myself that I had become overwhelmed by events in my life to a point of gross inattention. Can you imagine the insensitivity?

Internal clues to the need to change our behavior often come from psychologic **dissonance**, a seemingly inexplicable unsettled feeling, the emotional itch that we can't scratch. We may sense restlessness, ennui, emotional abrasiveness, unusual anger, or depression, all signs that something is out of balance in our psyche. While much of our behavior is subconscious and habitual, we must be alert for signals urging us to change. Dissonance occurs when we begin to have conflicts between automatic behaviors and the purpose they were to serve. When the dissonance reaches a threshold level, we become conscious of our behaviors.

When you experience dissonance, pay attention and look further. You may realize that your current patterns of behavior are not serving you well at all. Search for the reasons why you are feeling the dissonance. Search your immediate past, the past few days, weeks or months. What has changed in your life? Has your response to events in your life changed? If you can't identify anything in particular, try taking one of the screening surveys in *Get a Life, America!*

Pay attention to the results of the screening surveys. Some of the surveys are for depression, some are for stress, some are for indicating your satisfaction with your life, and some are exercise and eating surveys. All promote your awareness of how you are participating in your life.

I suggest that a better approach to achieving awareness is to routinely practice mindfulness on a daily basis. Mindfulness is not simply increasing your surveillance and alertness, although that will be a byproduct of your effort. Mindfulness is prospective living.

Begin your day with mindfulness meditation, a fifteen or twenty-minute sitting. Search, feel, think, ask, project, plan, sense, explore and be. Every day can begin with your own gift of a wake-up call from meditation.

Spot potential trouble before it occurs. The requisite modifications in your behavior will be of smaller magnitude, less arduous and less time consuming to accomplish. Practicing mindfulness meditation heightens our ability to perceive minute, yet critical, areas for needed modification. Through the daily practice of mindfulness, both in specific sittings for meditation and in conscious attention to our daily existence, one achieves a greater self-understanding. Through this routine practice, our need for change becomes glaringly obvious. I present the technique of mindfulness meditation in the chapter on stress and stress management ("Through the Eye of the Tiger," chapter IV). For more information on meditation, go to your local bookstore or library and explore the shelves.

We can motivate ourselves from a positive perspective in other ways, too. Jamie Lee Curtis became the target of tabloid criticism for "seeing a psychiatrist."

She responded that her visits were of her own choice and for positive growth, rather than for remediation. What a nice response and an excellent choice for her, prospective personal exploration. One of my mentors in psychiatry often suggested to me, "Everyone needs an hour on the couch each week, if only for a clearer vision of their future." It is good advice, whatever or wherever your couch happens to be.

Of course I recommend mindfulness, awareness, and regular periods of meditation for self-examination. That's my couch. Behavior modification isn't exclusively remedial, as we are responsible to explore for positive options. Reading and assertive communication are other useful tools to explore for new ideas and potential changes in our behaviors. Another of my mentors quoted, "Our choice to associate with worlds entirely different from our comfort zone results in quantum leaps of growth."

Three "Flavors" of Behavior

Before I proceed into the nuts and bolts of behavior change, I would like to introduce a very critical concept, one essential to our success in choosing a healthy lifestyle and in our considering changes. I call it one of the critical intangibles that increases our chances to have successful lives. I speak specifically of **assertive behavior and communication.**

Behavior is a form of communication, and it comes in a wide variety of forms including verbal communication, body language, how we present ourselves privately vs. publicly, and whether we are generous or selfish. In large part it is the manifestation of who we are.

We list three "flavors" of behavior on our menu of *Get a Life, America!* – aggressive, non-assertive (passive) and assertive. Let's review the three, from gutter to gourmet.

Aggressive behavior is destructive, combative, and paradoxical. It is frequently reflex, thoughtless and reactionary. Most certainly counterproductive, it is borne of insecurity and is ego defensive. It prevents dialogue, and in the mid to long run destroys communication. Aggressive behavior is inappropriate, and it will not serve you well. Don't employ it. Expressing yourself angrily or aggressively at the target of your frustration rarely changes the facts of the circumstance. When anger is no longer aimed at the target, it turns back inward and slowly destroys the individual. Enjoy the "five second rage" (per Dr. Kubler-Ross), then choose better responses.

Non-assertive or passive behavior is a manifestation of avoidance or escape. A means of being physically present but choosing not to participate, passive behavior accomplishes nothing other than allowing frustrations to grow, fester and then explode in an aggressive manner. How awful is that? What has been accomplished? Passive behavior is never appropriate. Silence or no behavior is acceptable only if you are formulating your plan for assertive behavior.

Assertive behavior is honest. It is always appropriate because it is direct, affirming, problem solving, enhancing and vulnerable. It is risky because of the obligatory vulnerability one must expose in order to practice assertive behavior. To behave assertively takes energy, for it is an uphill effort, requiring constant practice.

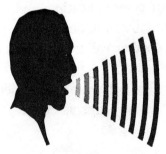

Assertive behavior is loving behavior, and it always sets the other person free. Loving behavior has the other person's best interest at heart. If we practice this principle, loving and considering the interests of others, our participation on this earth will be fuller and more complete.

How can we practice assertive behavior? We can be good listeners and good hearers, consequently becoming better information gatherers and understanders. We can be positive and build good foundations for ourselves. In being direct we gain reality-orienting feedback. Honesty provides a reflective mirror for others. Our loving teaches the world a new behavior.

Assertive behavior is the only behavior to which we aspire. As with all good things, developing assertive behavior takes time and practice.

The "Two-Year Stewardship" of Behavior Change

Let's assume that we position ourselves at the precipice of executing behavior change. We have the capacity, awareness, external and internal motivation. We're pumped, ready to go. "Let's get it on!" "Oh, by the way, how long is this going to take?" The entire process takes **two years, two years minimum, two years to make it your own, two years to** *Get a Life!* You do an internal Snoopy scream, "Aargghh! No, it can't be." It is.

Everything in our society races to some ill-defined destination. Fast food, fast cars, fast travel, two-week weight loss programs, instant credit, on the scene televising of wars brought to you "live in your living room," all underscore the rapid pace of our lives. "I want it now," is the battle cry of the millenium. Sorry, Charlie, it just doesn't work that way when it comes to good things. Behavior change is a good thing. I think that telling you honestly how long the process of behavior modification takes is one of the most powerful and important parts of this book.

Physical and emotional adaptations take time, lots of time. Weight loss, strength training, dietary modification, attitude adjustment and raising our consciousness all take time, and lots of effort. I trust that you have heard the admonition that "if it seems too good to be true, then it probably isn't true." So it is with pie-in-the-sky promises of quick weight loss, fast fitness programs or rapid accumulation of wealth. A sobering reality that I wish to share with you is that behavior change is good and it does take time.

When viewed in an evolutionary sense, the long time required for change is a very important species defense mechanism. Rapid changes kill us. Slow changes allow us to adapt and to evolve.

Adaptation is one good reason change takes so long. Adaptation, the gradual accommodation of an organism to changes in its environment, central to the process of evolution, is also an integral part of the concept of homeostasis. Homeostasis is a dynamic concept in that homeostasis changes, but it changes slowly. The slow and gentle process of adaptation allows us to reach a new homeostasis, a new comfort level, without the threat to our survival.

Adaptation is the perfect "lens" through which we may view changes in our bodies. We are constantly adapting to new environments. Changes in our diets, changes in our activity levels, changes in our peer groups are all changes in our environments. I prefer to view the body's responses to various environmental challenges like aerobic training, strength training, emotional stresses and nutritional excesses or insufficiencies as adaptations. The specific adaptations are the body's coping mechanisms for survival in a changing environment.

Weight loss is the body's adaptation to negative energy balance (inadequate available calories for current energy needs). Larger, stronger muscles is the body's adaptation to routine overload stimulus of the muscles. Increased numbers of mitochondria, improved cardiovascular efficiency, and increased red blood cell mass is the body's adaptation to aerobic training. All of these gradual changes occur to ensure organism's survival in a new and different environment.

If we allow adequate time for changes to occur in our lives, we increase our chances of making those changes valid. If we proceed too rapidly, we risk physical and emotional injury, and failure of our intent.

Watch Out for Recidivism!

Again, before we address the specifics of how to accomplish behavior change, I would like to mention the concept of **recidivism**. A "politically correct, 90's word," we offer recidivism as an excuse for failure, as if it were a mystical entity over which we have no control. By definition, recidivism refers to the lapsing back into previous behaviors, as a criminal who suffers recidivism and lapses into his former anti-social, criminal behaviors. Persons who have lost weight and then gain it all back have suffered recidivism.

Functionally, **recidivism results from ignorance**. If we experience recidivism, it means that we did not understand the process of behavior change, did not apply it correctly, or were in too great of a rush to complete a lengthy process. Periodic lapses are to be expected and are not recidivism, unless we allow the progressive process of behavior change to stop.

Recidivism also functionally relates to our **perception of control.** If we perceive that we are not in control of making the changes in our lives, that we are simply "following orders," rather than "commanding our own troops," then we are at high risk for recidivism. It is imperative that we understand the behavior change process and accept our individual responsibility for making the changes in our lives. In our practicing these two principles, we may avoid the pitfall of recidivism.

Now we can talk about **how** to change.

How Do We Accomplish Behavior Changes?

A World War II veteran, thirty-year smoker, and virtual non-exerciser, my father worked all his life as an electrical engineer for General Electric. A well-taught and practiced stress internalizer, every day he followed the same routine with emotional blinders adroitly placed. He had a family to support, and that was his consuming responsibility. He did it well, but as he found later in life, to his detriment.

In his early seventies, on the heels of a period of fatigue, he was diagnosed with angina pectoris (clogged coronary arteries). He only shared his diagnosis with me when I noticed some weight loss and questioned him about it. His weight loss had been purposeful, and I found out that this formerly sedentary individual had become a regular exerciser at a local health club.

He, like Damocles, had a sword over his head. It motivated his changing an unhealthy lifestyle to a more healthful one, and he did make healthful changes. Most people don't.

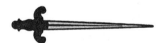

I offer his success, and it has been a success because his angina seems well controlled, as testament to the possibility that if my father can change, anyone can. You can. Here's how you can *Get a Life!*

First, check your attitudes and expectations

We are unlikely to achieve what we cannot conceive. Without a positive "can do" attitude and the associated expectation of success in *Getting a Life!*, it is quite certain that we are doomed to stagnation. What are **attitudes** and **expectations**? How do they make a difference in our lives? Can we choose our attitudes and expectations?

Attitude is our mental position or feeling with regard to a circumstance. Our attitude serves as a foundation for subsequent beliefs and actions about that situation. Consider that attitude determines behavior. Someone knocks at your door collecting money for the Save the Snails Foundation. Your attitude about charity might be in favor of charitable efforts and your attitude about snails could be equally positive. Therefore, you give $100. Alternatively, your attitude about charity could be positive, but negative about snails. You don't like escargots, so you give nothing. Your attitudes dictated your behavior.

Expectations compliment attitudes. An expectation considers something probable or certain. We may expect results, actions, behaviors, and goals. We may expect to get married, expect to have a child, expect to be healthy, expect to create our own business, expect to write a book. Expectations do not guarantee, but increase the likelihood of the result. Conversely, what I call negative expectations decrease the likelihood of an event occurring. Negative messages like, "I can't throw the ball, I can't love, I can't be loved," reasonably reassure that you will not throw, love, or be loved.

Attitudes and expectations facilitate the realization of our goals. Resistance and hurdles in our paths of progress become less onerous obstacles if our attitudes and expectations synchronize with our direction and goals.

Whatever our definition of success happens to be, we will more likely achieve success if our attitudes, expectations and goals are aligned. Our ability to change, to achieve legitimate behavior modification is predicated upon attitudes and expectations. If we do not have an attitude that agrees that change is good and desirable or have expectations that we do not consider change a reasonable possibility, then we simply aren't going to change.

It seems obvious that our attitudes and expectations affect our lives, but do our attitudes and expectations affect persons around us? You bet they do. We are all teachers, setting examples of successes, failures, good behaviors, not so good behaviors, how to do some things and how not to. We are on public view, like it or not. While our attitudes are usually on public display, our expectations may be a little less obvious to view. Over time, however, our attitudes and expectations become quite apparent and transparent to those around us. Our attitudes and expectations manifest in our behaviors. Through our behaviors we are strong and effective teachers of our children. We do understand that actions speak louder than words when teaching our children about life values. Therefore, we must carefully consider and choose our behaviors, attitudes and expectations that our children will see.

"What do you mean choose them well," you query? "I thought the stuff we learned as children – how we think and act – was cast in stone, and we can't choose or change." Attitudes and expectations are learned behaviors, learned throughout our lives. Learning is subject to modification and relearning. Yes, we may choose our attitudes and expectations.

Examine bigotry. Does growing up in a bigoted household demand that you continue in that tradition forever? No, bigotry is bad. It is within your purview to change your attitudes and expectations. Does growing up poor demand lifelong poverty? Certainly not, poverty hurts. One can learn to expect success. One can choose to change.

Behavior modification is not all or nothing, win or lose, black or white. It is a process, a sequence of baby steps, a progressive summation of the parts resulting in the whole. The process is long, but we may choose to see it as fun just as easily as we view it to be arduous. Remember, we get to pick our attitudes and expectations. Select a positive attitude and a "will-be-successful" expectation in your approach to behavior modification.

We begin the process by examining if we have the capacity to change. Our first concern is not awareness, not external motivation, not internal motivation and not execution. Do we have the capacity?

Capacity to change

I have always assumed that we have the innate capacity to change. However, some circumstances mitigate against our having the capacity to change. Frank stupidity is one, but thankfully that is very rare. Blatant refusal to change is hard to overcome, too.

Judicious application of ego defense mechanisms can mute our capacity to change. Denial, internalization, sublimation and projection all hide problems from our conscious vision. Do we have the capacity to remove our ego defense mechanisms? Yes, for it is by choice alone that we accomplish that task. But how do we choose to do that if we are unaware that we employ those defense mechanisms? It is rather simple. You have already begun by reading this book. *Get a Life, America!* facilitates discovery.

Ask yourself if you have the capacity – If you are at the point of asking the question, I can assure you that you do.

Create awareness of your roadblocks to change – Are your ego defense mechanisms protecting you from unbearable hurt? Ask yourself. If so, you may choose to proceed very slowly or choose to ask for professional help. Either is fine, but choose a forward direction.

Awareness of your need to change

"A problem, once recognized is half solved," quoted our first President, George Washington. Awareness is critical and powerful. Without awareness, we are bereft of choice.

How do we become aware of our need to change? Again, the answer is by active participation and choice. We discussed some principles of cultivating awareness in the section entitled, "What are Your Wake-Up Calls." Here are some additional methods to stimulate personal awareness.

Talk – Dialogue is one of the most powerful exploratory techniques available to us. Talking with different people about their experiences and sharing your experiences with them affords both people valuable insights. Seeking out people whose worlds are quite different than yours will expand your vision. You may see yourself from a new perspective. How do you find these people? Take a continuing education course at a university in a subject foreign to you. The room will be full of people from a "different world." Talk with them.

Talk with your friends. Talk with your family. Talk with members of your "first team." Talk occasionally with members of your "crisis team." "First and crisis teams" are presented in the chapter on stress management (Chapter IV). Bucket loads of discovery awaits you.

Ask – Periodically, pose these questions to chosen people, "How am I doing for you? Are we OK? Do you see in me a need to change?" It may seem unusual to ask such questions, but asking is a direct and assertive method of obtaining information. It is quite legitimate.

Write – Write letters. Write poetry. Write a short story. Keep a journal. Writing forces thinking and organization. It uncovers questions and information. Writing is a powerful tool for self-discovery. Whatever your chosen medium, get some words on paper.

Robert G. Allen proposed that "an idea not committed to paper remains merely a wish." While bonding words to paper increases the probability of our succeeding at whatever we choose, it also provides visual impact of the reality of our circumstances. Thoughts and dreams loom ethereal, words on paper are material.

Take a screening test – Take a personality profile test, a job preference test, a life satisfaction test, or a stress index test. The process of taking the test will begin to waken a general awareness in you. The resultant scoring of the test will provide you with visual impact of your need to change.

Think – What a simple means of stimulating awareness. Just think. Derek Bok accepted a faculty position at Stanford University after his tenure as president of Harvard University. Maintaining a modest office at Stanford, he begins each day there with one hour dedicated to thinking. Wow, how absolutely powerful! Let's take a lesson from him.

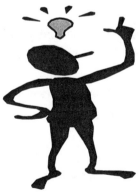

Meditate – I suggest routine meditation. Do it every day. Mindful, non-judgmental observation of your world can reveal hitherto unnoticed wonders. Meditation differs from thinking in that meditation is observation of what is. Thinking involves what was, what is and what may be. Meditation focuses on conscious awareness of the present.

Listen – Learn to listen. Sit in silence for a while and just listen to what is said. Listen to what is not said. Practice listening and you may become quite good at it. Careful listening to people, to Nature, and to events heightens our sensitivity and awareness.

Hear – Learn to hear. Hearing is listening with heart. Hearing is listening with understanding. Hearing is listening with love.

Sense dissonance – Put your antennae up and receive the subtle waves of dissonance. Do you feel different, upset, angry, bored, frustrated, fatigued, or "just not quite right?" That's dissonance. Search for the cause.

Please feel free to use any or all of the above methods to generate awareness about your need to change. Reminding yourself that behavior change is a process, and that it takes time, also creates awareness.

External motivation

External motivations, events in our lives that are out of our norm, signal the need for our attention to the causes of those events. Our charge is to sense their existence, then to search for the causes.

Examples of external motivators might be: 1) Your golf game has gone south. That could be a sign of overload or inattention in your life. 2) Your mate becomes less communicative. It could be that you have been too busy to keep up your end of the marriage. 3) Your energy took a vacation. You might be depressed or stressed.

How do you learn to translate the meaning of your external motivations? Treat the translation like a railroad crossing.

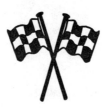

Stop – If you are so darned busy, you probably will not allow time to observe the occurrences in your life. Make time to take time. Go visit your "oasis" (presented in Chapter V, "Denial is Not Just a River in Egypt"). However you choose to do it, stop for a while.

Look – Look with clear vision. Focus on you life and your problems. See the big picture and all of the small details. Purposely view your life from different angles. How do you look from different angles, you ask? Simply project yourself into the mind of someone else. How would they see your life?

Listen – Pay attention. Don't deny. Don't modify. Hear the reality of what you see. Gather information by non-judgmental observation.

Internal motivation

Every step in the process of behavior change depends upon the successful completion of the previous steps. Now comes internal motivation, an emotionally challenging step. Internal motivation is accepting the circumstances and problems of your life as your own, admitting to yourself that you are the owner of the problems. They are threads of the very fabric that is you. How do you do such a potentially painful thing? Ask yourself which hurts more, living with the behavioral manifestations of your problems, or accepting the fact that you own them? You choose.

Let go – Release your death grip on your life. It is not going anywhere. It won't run away. Relax and just be.

Don't judge – Don't apply labels to anything. Nothing can be good, bad, important or insignificant. Practice non-judgmental observation.

Allow – Allow what you observe to exist within the realm of your life. It is there anyway, you may as well choose for it to be there.

Look and listen – Become as familiar with the circumstances and problems as possible. The more you see, know and understand, the better you can cope.

Accept ownership – Choose to take ownership of your life, your problems and your conflicts. Place your name squarely in the center of the Certificate of Title to your life.

Say yes – I can't hear you. Say it louder. Say yes, I accept and own my life, my circumstances and my problems. They are no one else's. Say yes, I can change what I wish to change. Practice saying yes.

Execution

Execution and implementation, these frightful concepts stand to stonewall us. We have no history, no basis for experience when we plan to change an old behavior to a new one. We venture into an ethereal unknown. Must we take a leap of faith? No, we have a number of choices available to us.

Articulate what you want to change – Identify and commit to paper what you want to change. Keep it simple. Don't make a long list. Long lists guarantee failure.

Identify and articulate the behavior you wish to adopt – Select your new behavior as if you were using a book of wallpaper samples. "This one is good. That one is ugly. This is OK. I really like this one. I'll take it." Write it down.

Or you may picture yourself weaving a new self-fabric, and you may select your individual threads for the fabric. Choose pretty threads. Record your choice.

Sign a contract – You have identified what you want to change. Now, write it down in the form of a contract and sign it. Ask a member of your daily "first team" to countersign it with you. If you do not commit your plan to paper, it remains merely a wish.

Review your attitudes and expectations – Reassure yourself that your have chosen a "can do" attitude consistent with the goal to be achieved. Are your attitude and goal synchronous, compatible? Are your expectations ready and in order, too? Ask these questions and double check.

Look for role models – No new behaviors exist in the world. The anticipated behavior is just new for us. Search for someone who may model your selected behavior and copy him or her. The process boils down to monkey see, monkey do. It can be child's play.

Select support systems – Where are your best support systems for behavior change, internal or external? Are you your own best fan or would someone else serve you better? Frequently, initial support gained externally is more valid than our own internal support. As we progress toward our goals, our internal validation becomes increasingly strong and effective.

Practice – Behavior modification is learning a new skill. Repetition of the desired behavior is the single most important and effective mechanism leading to successful behavior change.

Reward yourself for successes – Without reinforcement behavior extinguishes. Rewards may be internal, a quiet self given verbal acknowledgment of success. They may be external, like buying a new article of clothing for weight lost or a new art hanging in recognition of adopting better communication techniques.

Reinforcements (rewards) come in many varieties. Positive reinforcement is more effective than negative. Negative reinforcement may occasionally be necessary, but its effect dissipates quickly. Immediate reinforcement is more effective than delayed. We tend to forget quickly what the reinforcement is for, so it becomes valueless. Intermittent reinforcement is stronger than regular reinforcement. Material rewards saturate our expectations quickly, while social rewards are better for long term. Which would you rather have, a new dress or your husband's happiness and respect for your having lost weight, money or life-long friendship for having adopted assertive communication techniques?

Use your "first team" circle of social support – Choose a member of your first team for personal support. Call your chosen person at least weekly in the initial stages of your effort, then biweekly as you feel more control. If you slip a bit, go back to weekly calls. Ask your friend to call you periodically, because intermittent, unplanned rewards are very strong. Certainly, their call rewards your efforts as well as it affords social support. Share your efforts and aspirations with your working peers and ask not only for their help but also for their consideration in not sabotaging your progress.

Keep written records of your progress and review for trends – Written records provide feedback about how well you are doing. Review is important and takes only a moment.

Pictorial and graphic feedback is excellent, too. If you are losing weight, take a "before" picture and post it on the mirror in the bathroom. Every two months take another and place it in sequence. Obtain a full-length mirror and use the "naked-in-the-mirror" technique for motivating and supporting weight loss and strength training efforts.

Remind yourself that change is good and that it takes time – Short of winning a big lottery prize, few good things happen over night. Good things take time. It's worth spending the time.

Work in concert with the forces of Nature – I offer three concepts that will assist you in effecting your plan for behavior changes.

Nature abhors a vacuum. Create a vacuum and Nature will fill it. Mount St. Helens erupted in Oregon, killing plant and animal life for miles, creating a virtual wasteland, a "natural vacuum." Within one year, re-growth began "spontaneously." Monsoons regularly lay waste to large areas of Bangladesh, killing people and crops, destroying fertile farmlands. With the flooding and destruction comes the deposition of more fertile soil, ensuring future replenishment and re-growth. The natural order of the universe balances itself and maintains equanimity. Rapid change, unnatural and uncomfortable, creates a partial vacuum. When any vacuum is created, an attempt to balance or fill the void always follows.

If we create a void in our life, we sense discomfort and are immediately motivated to fill the emptiness. When we lose our life's partner, some are moved in short order to find a new partner. Normal and natural, choosing a new partner alleviates the pain of loneliness. If we have gone to the movie each and every Friday night for the past ten years, and then the movie house burns to the ground, will we sit alone idly doing nothing for three hours each subsequent Friday night? No, we fill that time with something else.

Habits and behaviors respond to the natural vacuum principle. If we eliminate a habit or behavior, creating a physical or behavioral void, we will replace it with an alternative. Consider smoking. If you stop smoking, what happens? A vacuum forms. The money that you spent will be used elsewhere. The time that you spent smoking can be used for talking, walking, reading, making love, chasing the dog; all good choices of alternate behaviors to fill a void created by the removal an unwanted behavior.

What if we were to cut fats and cholesterol from our diets? We will naturally fill that artificially created void with healthier replacements. Instead of sauces, red meats, cookies, cakes and pies, we may choose salads, vegetables, fruits and grains. Conversely, If we try to incorporate soups, salads and vegetables into a cholesterol and fat laden diet, difficulty confronts our integrating healthy foods into our diet. It becomes too crowded. Creating the emptiness demands substitutions.

What if we choose to eliminate anger from our daily emotional armamentarium? Oops, a void, what to fill it with? Maybe we could choose kindness and charity. Better yet, choose forgiveness. Let's choose to eliminate hate. What to substitute? Choose love. It's working, watch this:

Eliminate:	Choose:
Frustration	Peace
Depression	Happiness
Additives and sugars	Water and natural foods
Sedentary lifestyle	Activity
Denial and internalization	Expressive emotions

You get the idea, create a hole and it gets filled. The beauty of this little exercise is that you get to fill the hole with your choice. The elimination was conscious choice, so make the substitution consciously. Make it a good and conscious choice.

You may choose to employ **catalytic behaviors**. In the biochemical environment a catalyst is a compound, often a vitamin, that exerts a rate-controlling effect on a chemical reaction. Most catalysts potentiate and facilitate a change from one substance to another. I use the term catalytic behaviors in the same sense.

Catalytic behaviors are those that facilitate change from old to new behaviors, hopefully from dysfunctional behaviors to functional ones. The conscious insertion of a catalytic behavior often makes change possible when it was "impossible" before. The examples of catalytic behaviors that I will illustrate are simple, easy choices of behavior that allow a free flow of change to occur.

Let's say that your life has gotten out of control for the past few years. Circumstances, too busy, trying just to survive, wondering if you will survive, and you have gained weight; your life is a mess. These are factors and events, all combining to make your life painful and seemingly unmanageable. You step from the scales, look in the mirror and wretch at your weight and shape. How do you begin to lose the weight when the cyclone still swirls around you?

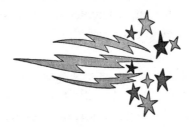

It is a tough question. The answer might be to begin changing your life by incorporating one catalytic behavior. Your catalytic behavior might be to monitor fat intake. Choose nothing more. Whenever you eat, simply ask yourself, "How many grams of fat are in this food?" Select a maximum number of fat grams you will allow yourself in a day. Target 30 grams in a day, 270 calories from fat in your daily intake. What benefits do you receive from the simple behavior of monitoring fat intake in grams?

You automatically become aware of what you are eating. Because you will choose from low fat content foods, your dietary mix will be healthier. You will choose more fruits, vegetables and grains, automatically, and you will eat less meat, less dairy, less sauces and less snacks. Cutting fat from your diet demands a healthier replacement. Weight loss will follow. Improved vigor, self-esteem and sense of control will come home wagging their tails behind them.

Exercise can be catalytic. Consider the same scenario, you are out of control. What else could you do? Choose another catalytic behavior. Start exercising. If you can't develop a full-blown program at the gym, then walk. Go outside and walk for 30 minutes. If it is raining, stay inside and walk in place. Just move your body. What happens? You begin to feel better physically and begin to consider that you can make choices and changes in your life. Success in one behavior choice begets sequential successes. It is empowering. Soon you will feel the beneficial effects from walking. Feeling better, you may be moved to begin dietary improvements. As you walk you might begin to appreciate the beauty surrounding you. You might even meet a new friend. The possibilities are legion.

The functional result of catalytic behaviors initiates awareness, awareness of what you are doing, awareness that you can and have chosen to change. What are some other catalytic behaviors? Keeping a journal, making a time management schedule, developing a hobby, doing nothing twice daily, taking news breaks, finding a mentor, becoming a mentor, hiring someone to do work that has become a burden to you, beginning to meditate, are all catalytic behaviors. The list of examples could go on endlessly. Open your eyes, be aware and choose.

Catalytic behaviors can break a cycle of stagnation, overload and futility. They may introduce you to any new direction you wish. You must make the initial effort and then keep your mind and eyes open for what opportunities will follow. Remember, we fear not only failure, but even more, the possibility of success. Be ready for success.

Your successes may be potentiated through the principle of **synergism.** Synergism refers to mutually supportive processes, often with the product being greater than the sum of the two parts of the process. For example, exercising decreases the incidence of disease. Good nutrition does also. Nutrition and exercise exist in a mutually supportive environment. Together, they decrease the incidence of disease more than the sum of each acting alone. They act synergistically.

Isn't Nature wonderful? She helps us fill voids in our lives. She allows the presence of one behavior to encourage the initiation of others. When two complimentary behaviors act in concert, She gives us the bonus benefit of synergism. Remember to work in concert with the forces of Nature. Create the behavior vacuum, fill the void with a catalytic behavior, and wait for synergism to compliment your efforts.

In conclusion

Behavior modification is not a total change or make over. It is modification. Take the good and build upon that foundation. Modify what isn't good. Please do not think that, "I am all bad. Nothing is right. I need to change entirely." Listen to Dr. Elizabeth Kubler-Ross who says, "It is OK to be you and it is OK to be what is OK with you."

You chose a role model that had qualities similar to those you wished to emulate. Your selected role model became a pictorial representation of your goal. As you progress and succeed, begin to consider the possibility of your becoming a role model for others

As you ponder your position as a role model, do you ask yourself, "Why even consider behavior changes, for it is so darn complicated and so much work?" One answer comes at least in recognition of how we expand our world. We expand our world by exposure. Normally, we seek people and experiences that validate our database. If we desire personal growth, we must consciously force ourselves to seek people, experiences and behaviors different from ours. Quantum leaps in growth and expansion come from associations with worlds and ideas totally outside of our own. Gaining access to a reality totally outside of our own is one way that we get answers and begin to change our behaviors.

Finally, wouldn't it be wonderful if societal norms were synchronous with healthy behavior? Wouldn't it be equally desirable if modern medicine's philosophy and expectations were aligned with our attitude about being able to choose health instead of earning illness? These changes will occur, I trust, but will evidence more rapidly if we can mobilize large numbers of people to support the change. Societal norms eventually will follow the choices of large numbers of individuals, and I sense that we are beginning to think about choosing healthy behaviors. Yes, we're thinking about getting a life!

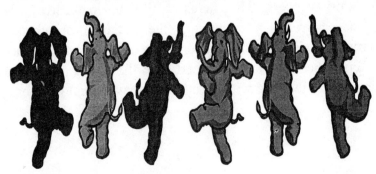

Chapter II

What's Eating You?

Your Survival Guide to the Russian Roulette of American Cuisine

*"If you can't be a vegetarian,
then eat a vegetarian."*

❖

*William Castelli, MD, Director,
Framingham Heart Study
(Recommending low-fat, low-cholesterol shellfish,
like clams, scallops and oysters,
the vegetarians of the sea)*

Nutrition, how boring! It's so boring that we don't teach it in medical school. Yet, our poor nutrition as a nation contributes mightily to our poor personal productivity, and to gargantuan expenditures for sick care. Our shameful nutrition habits are eating us alive!

In this chapter, we'll begin to learn how to take charge of our poor nutrition and make it good nutrition. We'll learn about "good nutrition," a little anatomy, some food fundamentals, supermarket shopping survival, the fundamentals of eating well at home, as well as how to survive the Russian Roulette of Restaurant Dining. We'll end with some good advice on how to eat healthfully on the run.

My friend and colleague, Annie Bell, MS, RD, lamented one evening, "You know Lennie, I studied nutrition formally for seven years. I work hard every day counseling people about nutrition. Still, I find little to no perceived value of or respect for my work by the medical community, and not much by my patients, either. Doesn't anyone realize the foundational importance of good nutrition? It seems that people are more interested in fad diets than good nutrition!"

I felt her frustration viscerally.

So I responded, "Annie, I toil 24/7 pioneering methods to teach about health and prevention. Ironically, nutrition, like health, is a tough-sell. But, if we think we have something of value for individuals and for society, we must stay the course. Remember to 'sell' our knowledge like we're running for public office. Create unique perspectives about your discipline, 'hooks,' if you will, then broadcast them with enthusiasm. Challenging, certainly, motivating people to adopt healthier behaviors is part of our charge as teachers. Let me tell you a story about how I was moved to begin my study of nutrition."

I began, "On a recent trip to Paris and southern France, awed by the omnipresence of beauty in art and Nature, I embraced my surroundings. The architecture, consumingly complex and delicate; bridges, ornamented with sculpture; parks, tastefully treed and flowered; museums, plentiful and peopled; the population, well dressed, thin and healthy, painted a palate so magnificent as to defy you to fall in love. Why resist?"

I confessed, "I fell in love with everything French, especially French women. Oh, yes, French women, they are so pretty, and so thin." I mused, "Why are French women skinnier than their American counterparts?"

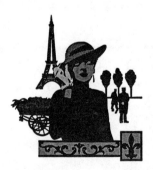

My study launched, I found the answer to lie in the "French paradox." French women weigh less than American women of the same height but eat just as much. One reason for the difference, according to epidemiologist Curtis Ellison of Boston University School of Medicine, is their appetite for snack foods. French women consume only 7% of their calories from snacks (largely fat) while

American women get 22% of their calories from snacks. Explanation of why the difference exists affords understanding, but sometimes more pleasure derives from simple observation.

On returning to the United States I sought information on food shopping and eating habits of Americans. When we consider that the American shopping cart top-five items by total volume of grocery store sales is: Coca Cola, Pepsi Cola, Kraft processed cheese, Campbell's soup, and Budweiser beer; we realize that we certainly have a big job to accomplish – changing the buying and eating habits of Americans.

Nutrition, like most aspects of our lives, is a matter of individual responsibility and choice. Limitless choices and combinations of foods provide fun, creative and rewarding culinary experiences. Short-term benefits of good nutrition include self-satisfaction, increased sensibility, and better physical and mental performance. Long-term benefits include better health, better job performance, and increased overall life productivity. While it is highly unlikely that anyone will assume the responsibility for our nutrition, it is most rewarding if we accept the responsibility and accomplish the task ourselves.

Will we actually accept the responsibility? A recent poll of the American Dietetic Association revealed that although 82% of the persons polled were concerned about their nutrition, only half of those polled said they were concerned enough to take some sort of action. Concern doesn't always translate into changing behaviors. I would like to encourage the half that said they would change to do so. At the same time, I would like to encourage the other half, those who indicated that they wouldn't change, to keep an open mind about changing in the future, to keep an open mind, at least, about learning what is good nutrition.

What is "Good Nutrition?"

"Experts" differ in their opinions about what constitutes "good nutrition," so I will give you my answer. Good nutrition consists of a diet composed of a variety of foods, providing 65% (or more) of calories from complex carbohydrates, 15% of calories from proteins and 20% (or less) of calories from fats, with no more than one-third of the fats being saturated. High in fiber with substantial water volume, a good diet provides vitamins and minerals well in excess of the RDA's. Good nutrition emphasizes complex carbohydrates, and concentrates on successfully meeting my recommendation of supplying a minimum of seven servings of fruits and vegetables per day. Food sources include grains, pastas, fruits, vegetables, low fat dairy products, fish and poultry.

Good nutrition provides the requisite fuels, catalysts (vitamins), volume and water needed for the chemical conversion of food to energy. That conversion of food to energy begins in the upper part of the digestive tract, as soon as we put the food into our mouth.

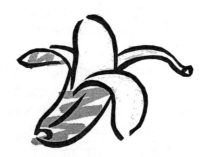

Anatomy of the Digestive Tract

We ingest food through the **mouth**, where some absorption of simple sugars occurs. No other nutrients are processed here. Saliva is mixed with the food and it passes through the **esophagus** into the **stomach** where the breakdown process begins in earnest. No absorption or processing occurs in the esophagus.

The stomach secretes hydrochloric acid and intrinsic factor, and continues the mechanical destruction of the food. Hydrochloric acid helps to break down macronutrients while intrinsic factor facilitates the absorption of vitamin B-12. The **pylorus**, the last portion of the stomach, locates immediately before the **duodenum**, the first portion of the small intestine.

Two important ducts enter the duodenum, one from the **gall bladder** and one from the pancreas. The gall bladder stores bile acids produced in the **liver** and the **pancreas** produces insulin and lipolytic enzymes. Bile acids and lipolytic enzymes break down fats, while insulin effects glucose storage in the liver. Early fat metabolism takes place in the first portion of the **small intestine,** where fat is absorbed in the form of triglycerides through the intestinal villi.

All subsequent absorption of nutrients takes place in the approximately 23 feet of small intestine. Carbohydrates, broken down into smaller units of glucose, are absorbed as this 6-carbon chain. Proteins, broken down into amino acids, are similarly absorbed. By the time the conglomeration of nutrient and waste product reaches the **large intestine,** the only remaining function is to reabsorb water from the intestinal contents. Thus, the large intestine stores waste product and preserves water for the body by reabsorbing it from the stool. Once absorbed into the blood stream, the varying fuels may be processed to energy.

Fundamentals of Food

Food, which supplies energy, primarily consists of three elements – carbon, oxygen and hydrogen. Carbohydrates and fats are essentially composed of these three elements, while proteins are composed of carbon, oxygen and hydrogen, plus nitrogen and sulfur. All energy-supplying foods are either carbohydrates, fats, proteins or a combination of the three. Vitamins and minerals, although critical in the metabolic process, supply no energy for work.

We shall examine the three basic food energy sources – carbohydrates, proteins and fats. Fiber and water, although not energy sources, will be discussed because of their integral importance in nutrition. Let's begin with the most important energy source, carbohydrates.

Carbohydrates

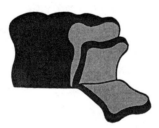

Carbohydrates are organic compounds made of carbon, hydrogen, and oxygen. The basic building block of carbohydrates is the six-carbon sugar, glucose. Complex carbohydrates, the starches, are all constructed of multiple units of the 6-carbon basic building block, just as proteins are made of amino acids and fats are made of free fatty acids.

Simple sugars, those consisting of one 6-carbon unit, are monosaccharides. When two monosaccharides are joined, a disaccharide results. Table sugar (sucrose), a common disaccharide, results from the union of one unit of glucose and one unit of fructose. A polysaccharide is a multiple 6-carbon unit structure or complex carbohydrate. Polysaccharides occurring in plants are starches, and in animals, glycogen. Starches and glycogen are the storage form of carbohydrate energy.

These complex carbohydrates contain from 300 to 1000 simple 6-carbon units linked together to form the larger structure. It is these large, complex structures, the complex carbohydrate's, that should be the staples of our diets.

Animal reserves of glycogen are relatively small compared to plant stores of starch, therefore, the plant kingdom, as opposed to animal sources, provides the major dietary supply of complex carbohydrate. Through the digestive process all complex carbohydrates are broken down progressively to disaccharides, then to monosaccharides, and finally to glucose. It is this 6-C unit of glucose that is used in the metabolic process to produce energy.

Consumption of complex carbohydrate, contrasted to eating simple sugars, is critical for two reasons. First, complex carbohydrate is broken down slowly to glucose, allowing a more gradual absorption of glucose into the blood stream. This gradual absorption prevents wide swings in blood glucose levels. The attendant "sugar highs" and "sugar lows" associated with concentrated sugar intake may be avoided, and insulin secretion remains less chaotic with complex carbohydrate ingestion. Second, simple sugars have "empty calories" compared to complex carbohydrates. Additional nutrients like proteins, vitamins, and minerals do not exist in simple sugars. Complex carbohydrates like rice and potatoes are wonderful sources of glucose, but also provide vitamins, protein, and minerals. Fruits, in addition to fructose, supply water and fiber. As we can readily see, food sources of complex carbohydrates provide a myriad of nutritional benefits.

As wonderful as complex carbohydrates may be, hidden dangers lurk in the shadows of manufactured sources of carbohydrates. Most natural carbohydrates (starches) are fat-free and contain some protein, but manufactured sources of carbohydrate are another story entirely. Consider that while candy bars, those sweet cavity-producing sensations, contain about 25% fat by weight, more than 50% of their calories come from fat. The carbohydrate provided arrives in the form of simple sugar, and little fiber is present. Few nutritional benefits accrue from this high fat, high sugar combo; but make the carbohydrate complex, and benefits do accrue.

Complex carbohydrates are wonderful for a weight loss diet because carbohydrate provides only 4 calories per gram compared to 9 calories per gram of fat. Complex carbohydrates frequently occur in combination with high fiber and high water content in foods, water and fiber combining to produce a zero-calorie satiety effect of gastric filling.

Recent studies have shown that excess calories in the form of complex carbohydrates require 25% of that figure to metabolize the conversion of excess carbohydrate to storage as fat. Only 75% of extra carbohydrate calories end up as adipose tissue, as stored fat. By comparison, excess calories from fat require only 3% of that figure to metabolize their storage as fat. This metabolic advantage leans very much in our favor, and we shall gladly accept the gift.

How much carbohydrate should we eat? Eat as much as possible (within the limits of total calories). No down side risk is inherent in the consumption of complex carbohydrates. Current recommendations from the experts suggest that 65% of the calories in our diets come from carbohydrates. I suggest making 65% the minimum intake of carbohydrate, for the more carbohydrate you eat, the less fat you will consume. Assuming that you select a variety of carbohydrate sources, your protein requirement will inherently be covered.

Great sources of carbohydrate are: all vegetables, cereals, rice, pasta, nuts, seeds, grains, and legumes. What is a legume, you query? Dried beans are categorized as legumes (vegetables that come in a pod) and include beans, peas, lentils, soybeans and peanuts. Legumes are a nutrition bargain. Remember variety of carbohydrates for the added benefits of adequate protein, vitamins and minerals.

Proteins

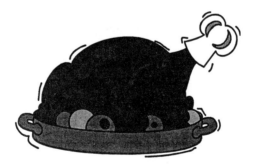

Proteins are the building blocks of our bodies, with protein supplying 20% of the body weight. Muscle, bone, cartilage, connective tissue, skin, and some body fluids are all made in part from proteins. Protein, essential for growth, repair and formation of new body tissues, is an important regulatory agent for body processes since enzymes and many hormones are proteins. Antibodies and other components of the immune system are also protein based.

Proteins are organic compounds made up of smaller units called amino acids. Proteins and amino acids are unique in that they contain nitrogen and sulfur in addition to the usual carbon, oxygen, and hydrogen of fats and carbohydrates. Twenty-two separate amino acids, under genetic control, are connected by peptide linkages to form proteins. Not only the number of amino acids, but the sequence of linkage, determines the particular protein formed. Thirteen of the amino acids can be manufactured by the body, nine can not be. The nine which can not be synthesized by the body must be eaten in our diets and are called **essential amino acids**. Without the essential amino acids our bodies could not function. Therefore, dietary protein is not optional.

Protein food sources vary with respect to their ability to supply amino acids. Some supply more or all of the nine essential amino acids, while some do not. We make an important distinction between **complete proteins** (containing all nine essential amino acids) and **incomplete proteins** (lacking at least one of the essential amino acids). In general, animal sources of protein are more complete than plant sources.

A conundrum arises. Animal source proteins are often in combination with dangerous and unwanted fat, but they are complete. Vegetable source proteins are without fat, but are usually incomplete. What to do? Limit animal intake sources and eat "complimentary" vegetable proteins. Combinations of vegetables, each vegetable deficient in one or another of the nine essential amino acids, will in total supply a complete compliment of amino acids. One excellent example is the meal pattern that evolved in South American countries, that of rice and beans. The combination supplies all nine essential amino acids.

Other example combinations to form a complete protein are:

Peanut butter on whole wheat bread
Rice cakes with peanut butter
Corn tortillas with pinto beans   **Remember items on
Rice and kidney bean casserole   this list when searching
Chile with whole wheat bread   for non-meat sources of
Spaghetti with tomato-meat sauce   protein.
Cereal with low fat milk
Vegetable-clam chowder

Protein Sources and Amounts in Common Foods

Food	Portion	Protein (g)
Beans	1/2 cup	6-8
Beef	1/4 pound	20-28
Beef bologna	1 ounce	3
Cheese	1 ounce	7
Chicken	3 ounces	21-28
Chili	1 cup	20
Corn	1/2 cup	3
Cottage cheese	1/2 cup	15
Fish	4 ounces	25-30
Hamburger	1/4 pound	20
Milk	1 cup	9
Peanut butter	1 tbsp.	4
Pizza	1 slice	10
Scallops	3.5 ounces	18
Tuna	3.5 ounces	28
Yogurt	8 ounces	12

Protein availability is listed in the chart above, but how much protein do we really need? For adults the minimum requirement is 0.8 grams per kilogram of body weight. A simple calculation will express your individual need in calories or grams (2.2 pounds per kilogram). For most people, this equates to 8 or 9% of total calorie intake, a very modest requirement. Most Americans average 12-14%, with some as high as 20%. **My recommendation of 15%** more than adequately covers the metabolic requirement. No harm comes from consuming up to 20% as long as it is not combined largely with fat. Excessively high protein consumption, however, can be hazardous to the kidneys and the liver. Protein requirements are higher for pregnant and lactating women, children during growth years, and athletes on a weight loss diet.

The need for dietary protein arises from the fact that muscles and other protein tissues are in a constant state of flux, normally at equilibrium. The breakdown and reconstruction rate of tissues is 1-2% per day. The products of the breakdown process are primarily proteins; 80% of the breakdown product is used for resynthesis while 20% is excreted. Since there is no storage of protein, daily intake is essential. The 8-9% of daily calories supplies that need nicely.

If 8-9% protein intake is adequate for restoring structural needs, and we eat 15% protein, are the extra calories used as fuel? Is protein an energy source? Sure it is, 4 calories per gram, the same as carbohydrates. Because carbohydrates and fats are so readily available and are more easily metabolized for fuel, they are used primarily. Excess protein calories are mostly converted to and stored as fat. Only in a starvation condition is protein a major fuel source, then the protein comes from muscle breakdown.

Fats

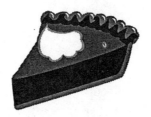

Like carbohydrates, fats are composed of carbon, hydrogen, and oxygen, but in differing ratios and structures. Fats contain much less oxygen in their molecules than carbohydrates, making them a much more concentrated energy source. Fat produces 9 calories per gram when the body metabolizes it.

The basic framework of fat is called glycerol (a 3-carbon chain), to which three free fatty acids are attached. The product of their union becomes a triglyceride. Free fatty acids are grouped into three families, saturated, monounsaturated, and polyunsaturated. Saturated free fatty acids have a hydrogen attached to every available carbon atom in the molecule. Animal fats are high in saturated fats, as are the tropical oils (palm and coconut). If one hydrogen is missing, the free fatty acid is called monounsaturated. Avocados and olive oils are good examples of monounsaturated free fatty acids. If two or more hydrogens are missing, the molecule becomes polyunsaturated. Most vegetable oils, including safflower, sunflower, and fish oils are polyunsaturated.

The critical importance of this distinction lies in the fact that saturated free fatty acids promote the generation of cholesterol by the liver, and hence raise our risk of hardening of the arteries and of all of the associated arterial disease processes. For this reason we must assiduously avoid consuming saturated fats.

Some portion of fat in our diets is necessary, but too much can be disastrous. Excessive intake of fat can lead to obesity and to associated diseases like diabetes mellitus, hypertension, strokes, and heart attacks. Cancer risk is higher in high-fat intake diets – specifically, colon, lung, and bladder cancer. Some researchers consider prostate cancer to be among the risks of a high fat diet.

Most fats are a mixture of saturated, monounsaturated, and polyunsaturated fats in varying ratios. It is important to limit or eliminate saturated fats. If you consume fats at all, aim for the polyunsaturated ones. **Avoid the tropical oils** (palm and coconut) and **use the flower oils** (safflower and sunflower). Animal products are almost guaranteed to be high in saturated fats. Stay away! In general, the more liquid a fat at room temperature, the less saturated the fat.

What about margarines made of vegetable oils? For appearances and utility at room temperature they have been hydrogenated, immediately defeating the purpose of using unsaturated vegetable oil fats. Hydrogenation increases the saturation and creates a less desirable fat product. What is the solution? Don't use margarine. Have a bagel with jam or toast with jelly.

Our bodies can manufacture saturated fatty acids, but not certain important polyunsaturated ones. For this reason we must consume these essential fatty acids in our diets. They are necessary for cell membrane synthesis, cholesterol metabolism, and hormone synthesis.

What other function does fat perform in the body? All cells contain fat in some form, and it plays various and crucial roles. In addition to its synthetic role, it may serve as an energy store, or it may bind the fat-soluble vitamins, A, D, E, and K.

In summary, some fats are necessary, while most of the fats we eat are not necessary. Eliminating fats or choosing polyunsaturated ones remains a critical factor for the health of our blood vessels and related organs. By eliminating or minimizing fats in our diets, we do not become nutritionally deprived or deficient. In fact, we gain something that we had not anticipated. We have created a partial void or vacuum in our diets that will naturally be filled with healthier foods. Fill the void with complex carbohydrates.

Fiber

What a marvelous substance, fiber. It has no nutritive value, is not essential for life or growth, but provides varied and useful benefits to the digestive process. For example, fiber binds cholesterol and lowers serum cholesterol in the process. Fiber protects us from colon cancer. It allows us to eat greater quantities of food, to feel satisfied, but not to ingest too many calories.

Fiber comes in two forms, water-insoluble and water-soluble. Water-insoluble fiber is found in whole-wheat products, wheat bran and the skins of fruits and vegetables. Water-soluble fiber is found in fruits, vegetables, beans and oats.

Insoluble fiber attracts and binds water in the intestinal tract, creating a softer and bulkier stool. It improves transit time through the intestine, thus relieving constipation and lessening the chance of diverticular formation. It decreases the time of toxin exposure to the intestine, toxins that may be carcinogenic. Soluble fiber, like oat bran, has been proven to bind cholesterol, thereby decreasing cholesterol absorption, thus lowering total serum cholesterol. This effect, although real, remains rather small. It is, however, one of the additive efforts in controlling cholesterol.

Fiber, soluble or insoluble, is a wonderful adjunct to a weight loss program. Because of its bulk, fiber allows us to feel full without consuming as many calories as we might with lower volume to calorie ratio foods, i.e., calorie dense foods. Foods with fiber require more chewing and exit the stomach more slowly, extending our eating process. The longer we take to eat and the fuller we feel, the less we apt are to over-eat.

What are good fiber sources for a variety of fiber intake? Remember whole grain breads, cereals, pasta, brown rice, fruits and vegetables, and legumes. This list sounds suspiciously like the one for complex carbohydrates.

Water

Often taken for granted and certainly overlooked by most, water is the most essential compound to support life. Without it we die. In short supply to the body, dehydration, our cellular function and performance suffers. Fluid in blood transports glucose to working muscles and carries away metabolic waste products. Fluid in cells maintains their turgor (the pressure within the cell) and cellular architecture, while providing a transport medium for nutrient transport across cell membranes. Sweat dissipates heat through evaporative cooling of the skin. Without adequate water intake, all of these processes are inhibited. In severe dehydration, irreversible kidney damage can occur. If not treated with dialysis, metabolic waste products build up in the body, eventually poisoning organ systems including the brain. Death often results. It may sound rather extreme, but that's how important water is.

Given that water is critical, how much do we need? The current recommendation is 8 glasses of water per day, minimum. What is the reasoning behind the eight glasses per day recommendation? A general rule of thumb is to consume one quart of water for every 1,000 calories of energy expense. If a glass is eight ounces, then eight glasses of water makes two quarts. That corresponds nicely to an energy expense of 2,000 calories, the average energy expense for most of us. Enough water for a mildly active person, very active people obviously need more. The prudent water consumer will stay ahead of his metabolic water needs.

Why can't we depend on thirst to guide fluid intake? Cerebral recognition of thirst lags behind actual hydration status. Increasing serum sodium concentration, which results from water loss from the serum, triggers the sensation of thirst. By the time the brain recognizes thirst, we are already at a considerable water debt. In an exercising person, or in a hot environment, by the time the brain senses thirst the individual may have lost 1% of his body weight in sweat. Continued water loss without replacement, which may result in a 2% body weight loss, will reduce work capacity by 10-15%.

Children and seniors, notably, have respectively poorly developed and insensitive thirst recognition abilities. For that reason, seniors and children must think ahead, anticipate hydration needs, and drink even when they don't sense thirst.

How do we know if we are adequately hydrated? Let's think ahead about drinking, stay ahead on water, and observe our urine. Light colored urine and frequent urination are reassuring signs that we maintain a good state of hydration.

What about water and exercise? Assuming that our hydration is routinely adequate, we should drink 1-2 cups of water 5-15 minutes before exercise, then consume one cup of water every 15-20 minutes during exercise. Sweat losses total 2 cups of water for every 300 calories expended during exercise. If we exercise at the rate of 600 calories per hour (10 cal/min), we need water replacement of 4 cups. The one cup every fifteen minutes suggestion nicely meets that requirement. Exercise in hotter environments or at greater intensity obviously requires more water in total, but the two cups for each 300 calories spent remains an excellent guide.

With a basic knowledge of the chemistry of food, our next step towards good nutrition becomes buying foods that meet our definition of good nutrition. The difficulty of that task, challenging to the pedestrian shopper, is compounded by the wide varieties of foods available at our supermarkets.

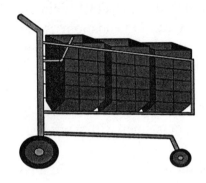

Supermarket Shopping Survival

What's a supermarket? It's a business, and as such, has profits as its primary goal. Unfortunately, our good nutrition sits low on the priority list of most supermarkets. If good nutrition happens to sell, then supermarkets will support it, but what sells tops their priority list. The evolution of supermarkets from the old-fashioned mom and pop grocery store to the current one-stop shopping extravaganzas; those with entertainment, quasi-cultural centers, hardware departments, and full-service pharmacies seems a positive event. The positivity reveals itself more economic than functional. Most supermarkets provide layouts and products chosen only after careful market research. What sells stays, what doesn't sell doesn't stay.

Supermarket managers place items strategically. On sale or featured items find themselves displayed at the end of aisles. Dumps and freestanding bins hold new or special products. Holiday or seasonal displays are placed so obnoxiously as to risk injury by tripping over them. Tasting islands or stations are manned by persons who appear as if they just stepped out of their own kitchens to serve the shopper a special delight. Check out aisles and counter displays teem with items for impulse buyers.

While price incentives, dazzling displays, freebies, coupons, and other marketing tricks do attract customers, we are evolving towards a smarter breed of shopper, one who is "nutrition aware." This awareness is underscored by the 1993 marketplace report, which cited:

- increased sales of calorie and portion controlled frozen foods
- increased sales of low calorie sauces and dressings
- increased sales of salt substitutes
- increased sales of fresh and frozen fish and poultry and fresh vegetables
- a decline in beef sales
- **BUT,** skyrocketing sales of premium ice creams.

I am not sure that we as consumers are truly aware, educated or able to make good market choices. I think we are still subject to excellent marketing techniques. To help in our efforts to become better shoppers and to successfully pass through the marketing maze, let me suggest a few guiding principles:

➢ **Go to the supermarket one time to educate yourself** – Walk through, with a notebook, observe and note, but buy nothing. Educate yourself about the layout, philosophy, and pitfalls of the store. Learn to avoid your vulnerable aisles.

➢ **Always go to the supermarket with a prepared list** – Having a list eliminates the danger of impulse buying. With list in hand, your trip will be more expedient.

➢ **Five aisles are always worth visiting, concentrate on them:**

- fruits and vegetables
- breads
- poultry
- dairy
- cereals and grains

➢ **Buy storage items in large quantities** – Stored properly, they will keep 6 months or longer.

> **Never go to the store hungry** – A hungry shopper loses all reason and becomes a hapless victim of advertising.

> **Envision yourself on a carbohydrate hunt** – Make the purpose of your visit to the supermarket to find and buy as many good sources of complex carbohydrates as possible.

> **Read labels** – Make label reading an integral part of your ongoing nutritional education.

Unfortunately, the desired departments are usually located at opposite ends of the store or located sporadically throughout the store. The seemingly chaotic arrangement forces you to walk through the entire store to find what you want. No surprise is it? This is a difficult environment in which to survive nutritionally. But we're going to try. Let's begin by taking a moment to review food labels so that we may be wiser shoppers.

Food Labeling

Food content labeling has evolved considerably since the FDA first established nutritional labeling guidelines in 1938. Until recent years food labeling consisted of a list of ingredients, the order based on the weight of each ingredient, not the volume or caloric contribution. From the mid to late 1980's food labeling elevated to provide increasing nutritional information. At the millenium food labels contain the following information:

1. Serving size and number of servings per package
2. Calories per serving and total calories
3. Protein content in grams
4. Carbohydrate content in grams
5. Fat content in grams
6. Number of calories from fat, occasionally the % of calories from fat
7. % of USRDA for components, including vitamins and minerals
8. Cholesterol, occasionally
9. % of daily requirements, based on a 2,000 calorie diet
10. Some give saturated fat content

Unfortunately, no labeling standardization exists; thus labeling may differ from package to package. The lack of standardization creates confusion among consumers, but the current labeling is certainly better than having no information at all. Let's examine a sample label from a fictitious food.

Wonder Chow From a Cow

Serving size 1 cup	Servings per package 4
Calories per serving 150	Calories from fat 90
Protein 4 gm	Cholesterol 60 mg
Carbohydrate 11 gm	Sodium 100mg
Fat 10 gm	

Vitamins and minerals	% daily USRDA
A	20
B-2	10
D	25
B-6	5

This label provides reasonable information. Through simple division, 90 fat calories per 150 total calories, we can readily see that Wonder Chow is high in fat – 60% of total calories come from fat. The label discloses no fiber information. Cholesterol and sodium seem to be acceptable. Some protein and some carbohydrate are present, but not much. Vitamin content is unimpressive. Are we going to buy this product? No, based on the high fat content alone, it's not a good choice.

Obviously, some product labeling is better than others, but we, as gullible consumers, are more likely to be influenced by a large-print "low-fat" declaration on a label than by actually taking the time to compute calories from fat. Even if we were to compute the fat content at 35% of calories, we would probably still buy the product because the label declared it to be "low-fat." Irresponsible manufacturers and gullible consumers – what a marriage!

Vulnerable consumers must need protection, don't we? Need it or not, we have it. Attempting to defend us, the protectors of our food supply, FDA, USDA, EPA, and BATF, have defined certain terms commonly used and abused in marketing. Unfortunately, these definitions change with time, but for now, be aware of the following when purchasing foods:

- **Low sodium** – maximum of 140 mg per serving.
- **High** – must have at least 10% more of particular nutrient than comparable products.
- **Fortified or enriched** – must have 10% greater of the stated fortified agent than similar products.
- **Sugar free** – does not contain sucrose (table sugar), but can contain other calorie rich sweeteners like honey, corn syrup, or fructose.
- **Reduced calorie** – must have one third less calories than a similar product (for meat 25% less calories), often accomplished by adding water.
- **Low calorie** – must have no more than 40 calories per serving or 0.4 cal/gm.
- **No added salt** – no additional sodium was added in the process, but the product could be naturally high in sodium or a sodium containing preservative could be added (potentially very misleading).
- **Prime, choice, and select** – in meats, according to fat content, the higher the fat content, the better the grade, and the worse the nutrition risk.

What a jungle, the food industry, and what latitude for abuse! Marketing hype can lead to consumer blindness in a myopic shopping population who falls prey to the hawking of "new," "100%," "fiber rich," "no cholesterol," and "free inside" claims in large red print on the front of the packages. While not outright lies, these claims are attention-getters that work remarkable well. These advertising claims may be in part true, but the products often have a significant down-side like high sugar content, multiple additives, or high sodium. Sports drinks advertise "more carbos" while in actuality it's simple sugars that they contain. Not errant advertising, it's just misleading advertising. Certain words are great motivators to purchase, like "rich," as in "calcium rich" and "fiber rich." Other advertising words are more subtle like "fresh," "nature," and "old-fashioned." **We as consumers simply must be aware that the bold labels on the front of packages trumpet a marketing fanfare, while the small-print labels on the back of the package quietly present nutritional information.**

If we find labels misleading and confusing, we're going to feel like a mouse in a maze when we venture into the inner sanctum of supermarket shopping. But, we have to eat, so let's be smart monkeys in the supermarket jungle.

A Guided Tour Through the Maze

Let's now take a thoughtful trip through a supermarket, prepared with list in hand, but with the simian curiosity needed to become an informed consumer. Where shall we begin?

Fruits and Vegetables – This should be one of our favorite sections in the supermarket. Always start here. Shoppers tend to buy more in the departments where they start to shop. Healthy, bright, colorful, and usually spacious, it just feels good. A winning area, you are apt to see the healthiest people in this section. Look to satisfy nutrition needs like vitamins (A, B's, C), fiber, calcium, iron and potassium. Fats are virtually non-existent here.

When buying fruit think of your fruit bowl at home. What's appealing?

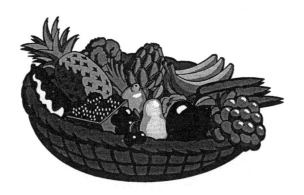

What do you like to have at hand for a snack? I suggest that you over-buy a little on fruits and vegetables under the theory that we eat what we have at hand. Buy fruits that can stand out at room temperature. Fruits hidden in the refrigerator are less likely to be eaten routinely or spontaneously. Apples, pears, bananas, grapes, berries, and cherries are great nutrition and great snack food. Unfortunately, a week normally defines the upper limit on non-refrigerated fruit. That's OK, eat the fruit and buy more.

Vegetables are equally appealing. Physically attractive in color and texture, a veritable cornucopia awaits you. Purchase a variety of vegetables twice weekly to assure freshness and good nutrition value, as vegetables are prone to lose nutrients quickly and easily. Avoid precut vegetables because nutrients are lost by cutting. Buy fresh, not canned, vegetables since nutrients leech into the packing fluid. A reasonable substitute for fresh, frozen vegetables retain much of their nutritive value. In general, the darker the vegetable the greater the nutritive value.

Legumes – Dried peas, beans, and lentils, legumes are a nutrition bargain. As such they are often not prominently displayed, often with poor selection available. Some of the more nutritionally conscious, responsible markets (some do exist) devote significant space to these items along with a grand variety of rice and whole grains. Their high protein content makes legumes an excellent meat substitute. Stored in dark, airtight containers, legumes have a prodigiously long shelf-life. High in fiber, iron, zinc, magnesium, phosphorous, and B vitamins, they are a superior source of complex carbohydrates.

As we recall, plant proteins are incomplete, lacking certain amino acids. Legumes if eaten on a regular basis need to be supplemented by a "complementary" food source that will complete the protein. Rice, whole grain wheat, nuts, and seeds are rich in the two amino acids that legumes lack.

Tofu – Dr. Dean Ornish is a tofu devotee. A fine source of protein, although rather tasteless, tofu can be included for its nutritive value in vegetable dishes. If we search diligently, we may find tofu hiding in the vegetable department.

Breads – Fun, just like fruits and vegetables, bread beckons your taste buds. I advise buying whole grain flours and making your own bread using your newly purchased bread maker. By making your own bread, you have complete control of the ingredients. Warm fresh bread, impossible to beat, low in cholesterol and fat, deserves a prominent position on your table. And, because it's fresh and warm, it never needs butter. If you must purchase, buy whole grain breads with 2 or more grams of fiber per slice. The fiber content should be readily available on the label.

Cereals – Cereals, one of our best fiber sources, an excellent complex carbohydrate source, provide some protein, but precious little fat. Vitamins readily available in most cereals include vitamins B's and E, while some cereals are fortified with vitamins A and D, vitamins not usually found in cereals. Some seemingly nutritious cereals have a hidden downside. Sugar and sodium content can be high, and granola type cereals may have high fat content due to added nuts and oils. Often those oils are tropical. With prior warning we can avoid these subtle pitfalls and garner excellent nutritive value from the cereal section.

Pasta – Oh boy, pasta, one of my favorite foods, and a ready source of complex carbohydrates, has no fat. High in protein and a good fiber source if made with whole grains, pasta provides some of the B vitamins. The danger with pasta is never with the pasta, but with the choice of sauce. It often contains enormous amounts of fat. Cream-based sauces, like an Alfredo, ooze fat, while vegetable sauces offer little fat. Read the sauce labels to select a lower fat sauce.

Rice – Certainly, a winner all the way, rice feeds the world. Pass by the white, processed rice, and select whole-grain brown rice instead. Buy and eat great quantities of rice. Very versatile, it contains fiber, protein, and complex carbohydrates.

Soups – Soups purchased in the supermarket pose some potential risks. Many contain significant amounts of fat and salt. Read the labels. Better yet, make your own soups as part of your weekend cookfest.

Vegetable oils – Know two or three and know to avoid the tropical oils. Safflower and sunflower oils are the best choices. Remember that oils are still fats, so minimize their use.

Meats – Here beef, poultry, and fish are offered in plentiful supply. Wouldn't it be wonderful if the supermarket would post a large sign over their display that reads, "Meat as a garnish?" You can still take that sign with you mentally to the store, reminding yourself as you shop, "Meat as a garnish." Meat doesn't have to be a staple of our diets, and heart attacks and strokes don't have to be part of our medical history.

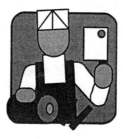

Just as with milk products, meat lists fat content as a percentage of weight. **"Seven percent fat" ground beef provides 45% of it's calories from fat.** Meat, a good protein source, but not the only one, is a source of iron and B vitamins. My best advice is to eliminate red meats from your diet. Aside from the fat content and the attendant risk from that fat, it is known, but not well publicized, that red meat eating countries (Brazil and other South American countries) have exceedingly high colon cancer rates.

Be aware of freshness in buying meat, for meat serves as an excellent bacterial culture medium. Salmonella is a well-known inhabitant of poultry products. Check the "sell by" date, and use your nose to sniff for freshness. Buying meat is a crapshoot, actually. It is a long way from the farmyard to your dinner table, with loads of stops in between, lots of places for meat to become infected with bacteria or otherwise contaminated in un-refrigerated conditions. I have personally known meat department employees who routinely repackage meat that has passed the "sell by" date, updating the packaging label on the meat. The investigative reporting team on *20/20* found a grocery chain that dipped old fish in bleach to neutralize the odor and then resold the fish as fresh. Watch out, danger lurks in this jungle.

I am obviously circumspect about the idea of meat, from the industry to the attendant health risks. It's unrealistic to think we would eliminate meat from our diets, but I certainly suggest minimizing our consumption. When you do buy meat, unpack it immediately upon returning home, smell it, repack it and either freeze or cook it. I would not have meat refrigerated unfrozen for more than 24-48 hours once purchased.

What about prepared and sliced meats? Again, avoid beef and red meats. Sliced turkey or chicken breast are reasonable items. They are white meats, with fewer calories and fat than dark meat, but still rather high in per unit cost.

Consider fish and shellfish, great sources of nutrition and culinary delight, if you can get them fresh. High in protein, relatively low in fat and containing omega-3 fatty acids, they are winners all around. Always skin fish before cooking because most of the fat in fish rests in the subcutaneous (under the skin) layer, as it does with poultry. Shellfish, which was once labeled as high in cholesterol, is now known not to be high in cholesterol. What was originally and mistakenly analyzed as cholesterol was actually a composite of several different sterols. Interestingly, these sterols are now known to inhibit cholesterol absorption. And, finally, it is so easy to use shellfish as a garnish.

Fresh is the word when it comes to buying fish or shellfish. Bacteria grow rapidly and can be transferred easily in the handling process from fish to fish to shellfish and vice versa. I am a bit of a fresh fish snob, having lived for twenty years in a coastal fishing community. If you live inland, be sure to ask your supplier where the fish came from, how long since it was caught and how it was handled in transport. For lobsters and crabs, buy only live ones and eat them immediately after cooking.

Canned fish is another source to consider. Tuna, sardines, and salmon present good protein and vitamin opportunities but can be risky in high sodium content and high fat content if packed in oil. Always buy tuna packed in water. Packing tuna in oil can increase fat content by 200 to 500 percent, compared to water canning processes. Fish with bones remaining, like sardines or salmon also offer the added benefit of providing reasonable amounts of calcium.

Dairy products – The dairy section, including milk, cheese, yogurt, and eggs and is a great spot to find sources of protein, vitamin A, the B vitamins and calcium. The danger of excess fat lurks here, but the purchase of low-fat products protects you from this killer. In the defatting process of milk much of the vitamin A is lost because vitamin A is fat-soluble. Vitamin A is replaced (fortified) after the defatting process. Most milk is also fortified with vitamin D, which is fat-soluble and lost in the defatting process. Milk and milk products supply 75% of the calcium in the American diet. One cup of 1%-milk contains 300 mg of calcium, one third of the RDA.

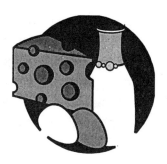

Check labels! Buy milk well before the "sell by" date and select the latest "sell by" date among the supply. Pick the milk from the back of the refrigerator because it's cooler there. Purchase milk or any refrigerated products last in your shopping trip so that it has less time to remain un-refrigerated. Reassure yourself that the 1%-fat milk, or preferably skim-milk, has been fortified with vitamins A and D. Remember, the 1% figure is 1% by weight, not by calories. **One-percent milk actually presents 20% of its total calories as fat calories.**

Watch out for dairy substitutes. Their fat can be riskier than the fat in dairy products, for they are frequently made with palm and coconut oils, the tropical oils. Remember yogurt, plain, low fat yogurt. It's a great alternative dairy product, an alternative with which you can create many delicious dishes.

Eggs are a good source of protein and vitamin A, but a precarious source of cholesterol. My advice is to avoid eggs. Too many other good, healthy foods are available for our enjoyment, than to risk raising our cholesterol by eating eggs. If you need eggs for cooking, choose cholesterol-free egg substitutes.

Our shopping cart brims over with great food. Now lets go home and cook up some really delicious, nutritious, and attractive meals. *Bon appetit!*

Eating at Home

One-third or more of meals eaten in America are eaten away from home, mostly in restaurants, some at schools, and many from brown bags at work. That means two-thirds of meals are eaten at home, and that's a load of meals. Due to our busy schedules we frequently can't avoid eating out, but with mindful preplanning we have great choice about where we eat.

Eating at home offers variety, affords us better control of our nutrition, generates family socialization, provides fun, allows creativity, and is less expensive by far than eating out. Eating meals outside of the home conservatively costs an extra ten dollars per day, $3,650 per year. Is that possible? With economy and good nutrition in mind, we should plan to eat more of our meals at home.

I always suggest beginning with principles when approaching large complex issues. Healthy eating at home can be a large, complex undertaking, but by beginning in this manner, with principles, we simplify the task.

Keep a few principles in mind as you consider how and with what to stock your kitchen:

- What you have at hand will dictate what you eat. It is entirely under your control.
- Variety is easy to achieve and modification is an adjunct to variety.
- Think carbohydrates.
- Think food value.
- Think of meat as a garnish.
- Think low fat.
- Think ahead and cook ahead. Plan social weekend cookfests.

Essential food items to keep on hand at all times in a healthy kitchen include:

- Brown rice – with bran intact
- Whole grain flours – for fiber and B vitamins
- Legumes – Peas, beans, lentils (low fat protein source, B vitamins, iron, calcium)
- Vegetable oils – sunflower, safflower, or corn (avoid tropical oils)
- Vinegar and lemon juice – great for salad dressings and vegetables
- Herbs and seasonings – avoids salt and adds variety
- A modest variety of wines – for cooking and for drinking while cooking

Essential kitchen tools make life so much more enjoyable and easier:

- Bread maker
- Microwave
- Vegetable steamer
- Food processor
- Good set of knives
- Large and small cutting boards
- Wok
- Skimmer, strainer
- Heavy gauge pots and pans
- Kitchen scale

Keep some of these principles of food storage in mind, too:

- Frozen foods should be stored at 0 degrees F.
- Dried foods should be stored in airtight containers and kept from light.
- Vegetables should be refrigerated and used soon.
- Fruits should be kept is a shaded area in a cool environment.
- Meats should be refrigerated in a cooler part of the refrigerator, kept refrigerated no more than two days, frozen immediately if needed for long term.

Kitchen tips

They abound in magazines, cookbooks, and in conversation. Here are some selected tips particularly applicable to the healthy cook's kitchen:

- Make soups and chilies, for they are healthy, easy to make, and store well.
- Think salads, be creative.
- Think of raw vegetables as appetizers, with low-fat dip.
- Develop your own list of favorite menus.
- Make your own salad dressings.
- Use lemon juice and vinegar on vegetables and salads.
- Learn to season and spice.
- Keep vegetables whole until ready to cook, thus preserving water-soluble vitamins.
- Cook vegetables with skin on to prevent vitamin loss.
- Save the liquid of canned vegetables for soups, for they are nutrient rich.
- Use chicken broth or tomato juice to cook vegetables.
- Remember the calcium content of leafy green vegetables as a milk substitute.
- Combine iron rich foods with vitamin C containing foods, thus enhancing iron absorption.
- Eat baked potatoes with the skin on, thereby increasing the fiber.
- Bananas are a good source of fiber to add to cereal.
- Consider fruit as a staple.
- Light food on a dark plate gives the appearance of more food.
- Fill your plate two-thirds full with carbohydrates.
- Trim fat and skin from meats before cooking.
- Use paper towels to absorb fat from meats after cooking.
- Use greater portions of vegetables in stuffing.
- Use yogurt instead of eggs in the breading of chicken.
- Light meat has less fat and fewer calories than dark meat.
- Use egg whites rather than whole eggs whenever possible.
- Make home pizzas with low-fat cheese, no oils, and fresh vegetables.
- Yogurt substitutes for mayonnaise and sour cream.
- Make your own hummus as a dip.
- Low-fat cottage cheese is versatile and can be used for many dips.
- Cook with non-stick vegetable spray instead of oils.
- Replace some of the flour in recipes with oat bran.

- Avoid ice creams, especially designer ones; use low-fat frozen yogurt at 22 cal/oz.
- Drink more water than juices; cut juice strength and calories with water or sparkling water.
- Make meal preparation a social event and involve the family members.
- Cook ahead for the week on a weekend day.

With forethought, eating at home can become an exciting nutritional and social endeavor.

How to establish good eating habits at home

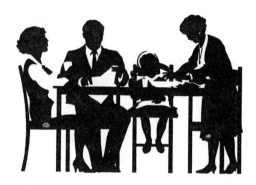

Having developed a lot of information about good nutrition, we will now put that education on our plates in the form of delicious, nutritious home cooked meals. Here is an easy method to ensure good home eating. The following suggestions fall into common denominators of the execution part of behavior change. They include the principles of committing to paper, drawing up a specific plan, signing a contract, asking for help, using support teams, practicing and rewarding.

Remember 65% carbohydrate, 20% fat, 15% protein – This is your basic framework. It should be foremost in your memory when you think about eating. The percentages refer to percent of calories from carbohydrate, fat and protein (NOT percentages by weight).

Keep a food diary – Keep a record of everything you eat for a two to four week period. At the end of that time, calculate the composition of your diet. How many calories did you consume? What was the distribution of the calories in percentages of fat, carbohydrate and protein? Are you surprised? Disgusted?

Compute your calorie requirement – Use the formula in the chapter on weight management (Chapter VII, "Eating to Live") to calculate your daily caloric needs. Apply the 65% carbohydrates, 15% protein and 20% fat ratio to approximate how much of each food type you will need. Performing the calculations reinforces your learning experience.

Choose how you want to spend your calories – Do you prefer larger breakfasts? Would you prefer that all of your meals be of equal caloric value? It's your choice. Would you prefer to graze? That's fine, too.

Focus on complex carbohydrates – Complex carbohydrates are the staple of your diet. Minimize fats and be conscious where your proteins are. Remember these choices: all vegetables, cereals, rice, pasta, nuts, seeds, grains, and legumes.

Eat a minimum of seven servings of fruits and vegetables per day – By accomplishing this task, you will naturally avoid eating fatty foods that you might have consumed had you not eaten the fruits and vegetables.

Involve the whole family for support – Make good home nutrition a group effort. That way no one will sabotage your good intentions. Ask family members to support your nutrition behavior change, especially in the beginning.

Design meals that fit the component ratio – Keep your selected meals written on 3 X 5 cards, available to any member of the family who might be cooking. Design the following for rotation:

Five breakfasts   Include the food analysis
Ten lunches   on the recipe card
Twenty dinners

Snacks should be thoughtful and low calorie – Be sure to allow for the additional calories in your overall calorie allotment.

Know how many calories you are consuming in each meal – Have a decent perception of the caloric value of everything you eat. Don't surprise yourself by finding out that your dinner just provided 1500 calories. That could be 75% of your daily allowance.

Try an all vegetable and fruit meal – Pay particular attention to how you feel afterwards, especially compared to how you normally feel after a heavy meat-laden meal. It's a rather interesting, eye opening experience.

Practice the art of recipe modification – Obviously, some recipes will be easier to modify than others. With a positive outlook the basic guidelines are easy as pie to master. Begin by reading the list of ingredients. Ask yourself what purpose each ingredient serves. Red-flag any food items that you are trying to avoid or that you know are inherently bad for you. With each red-flagged item use one of the following methods to modify its presence in the recipe:

Elimination – If the ingredient isn't essential, eliminate it. For instance, mushrooms are often sautéed in butter and wine. The butter simply isn't necessary. Eliminate it and use the wine only. Pasta recipes often call for salt and oil in the water. Neither is necessary.

Reduction – Whoever writes the recipes in cookbooks must own stock in the ingredient companies. Many of the ingredients are added with a heavy hand. In many dessert recipes, sugar content could be cut by half at least. Skillet meals calling for oil in the pan over-estimate the amount needed. Nonstick pans all but eliminate the need for oil. Remember the philosophy of meat as a garnish. The amount of meat in many dishes can be substantially reduced.

Substitution – Always look for a more healthful ingredient. Low-fat yogurt should lead your list of potential substitutes. It can double for sour cream in salad dressings and dips, and it serves as a topping for baked potatoes. Margarine, lower in saturated fat than butter, still contains calories and fat. Use it sparingly.

Substitution applies to cooking methods as well as to ingredients. Steam vegetables. Never cook them in butter or oil. Bake, poach or grill meats and fish. Use wine, water or broth for poaching. Never fry meats.

Use meats sparingly. When you choose to eat meat, always trim the fat carefully before cooking. Similarly, remove the skin from poultry prior to cooking. High in protein, low in fat, fish is a great meat choice. Remember, though, that the fat in a fish, like poultry, is just beneath its skin. Remove that layer before cooking.

Substitute herbs, spices, lemon juice, citrus peels, garlic, vinegar and various onion products for salt and oils. Cookbooks usually have sections on uses of herbs and spices. With a little practice, you will find yourself quite adept at seasoning.

With Americans hooked on simple carbohydrates (sugars), making substitutes for sugar becomes mandatory. Unsweetened fruit purees make fine replacements for high-sugar jams and jellies. Replacing the usual syrup, purees provide a great topping on pancakes and waffles. Certain vegetables like onions, carrots and sweet peppers lend sweetness to sauces, stews and salads.

Be alert for hidden sugars. *Beaucoup* sugar hides in catsup, salad dressings and mayonnaise. If you insist on using those condiments, make your own.

Tricks of presentation – Consider the color and size of your dinnerware. Light food on a dark plate gives the illusion of a larger portion. Vary sets of dinnerware for a change of pace. Decorative garnishes add visual impact. Flowers on the table create a festive atmosphere. It's all so fun and healthy.

Practice makes perfect – The longer you practice your healthy home dining, the better you become at making healthy dining routine. As your new behavior establishes a foundation in your daily routine, you may look for other healthy behaviors to adopt.

Reward yourself for success – By choosing to eat more healthfully at home, you deserve congratulations. One reward comes automatically with the behavior change, and that's better health. I suggest that you give yourself other rewards, too. How about buying some new attractive dinnerware?

Providing good nutrition at home requires thought, planning and practice. That same thought, planning and practice will serve you well when you choose to eat away from your home.

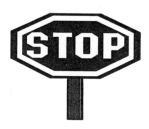

Take a break. So far in this chapter on nutrition we've covered a lot. Let's review:

➤ America practices dismal nutrition habits. We can and must do better
➤ Good nutrition encompasses a diet of 65% carbohydrate, 15% protein and 20% fat, with fiber, water, and adequate vitamins and minerals.
➤ Supermarket shopping is a hazardous jungle, but we can survive quite well in the aisles of: fruits and vegetables, breads, poultry, dairy, and cereals and grains.
➤ Practice reading food labels.
➤ Eat mindfully at home. It's fun, easy, and inexpensive.
➤ Design your meal cards for home dining.

Eating Outside of the Home

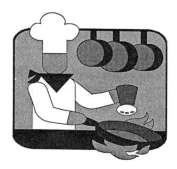

A huge industry, the restaurant business grows with the population, with the American trend towards dining out, and with the expansion of our economy. As the economy expands, discretionary income per capita increases, thereby allowing increasing numbers of people to spend money dining out. The amount of money spent on dining out seems obscene and unwarranted, but remains a fact of American culture.

Why do we eat at restaurants instead of cooking and eating at home? From business lunches to boredom, the reasons are many. Convenience of eating out, the most often cited reason, frees the diner from the necessity of shopping, cooking, and cleaning up. Lives are busy, and many people trade time and convenience for increased cost and loss of nutritional control. Restaurant dining has become part of the entertainment industry, with many restaurants realizing that atmosphere, presentation and conversation are as important as the taste of the food. For some, dining out is part of their job, entertaining prospective clients. Where better to "sell" yourself and your product than in a restaurant over a fine glass of wine and a sumptuous lunch or dinner.

Variety, the average American's solution to boredom, is an oft-offered reason for dining out. Most households select from a maximum of ten different dinners for their meals. For many, ten is too high. Over the course of a year, they will eat the same meal at least 36.5 times. Variety becomes a necessity in the face of non-creative repetition.

Why do we settle on restaurant dining for variety? Restaurants are readily available, and most of us haven't the experience of making other creative choices. We repeat familiar behaviors.

The economy of restaurant dining is familiar, but baffling. Consumers spend dining-dollars reflexly and mindlessly. A restaurant meal for two of $60 receives little forethought and attention, but a purchase of a $60 dress often meets careful thought, consideration and guilt. The difference in thinking lies in the contrasts of mindlessness in dining and the mindfulness of purchasing material goods.

Restaurateurs are businessmen, not babysitters or nutritional therapists. They're mindful of profits, mindful of selling as much as possible of what their clientele desires. Unfortunately, their clientele still wants high-fat foods. Some public request (as opposed to demand) is surfacing for healthier foods. In response to the request, the restaurant industry has acquiesced and presented some "healthy choices selections" on their menus. At best, the "healthy choice selections" donate merely polite lip service to the public request. When many of those items are analyzed, the fat content remains above 30%, often above 40%, with significant calorie content. Are they healthy? No, but it is still better than 60% fat content of some restaurant dishes.

Are better solutions available? Yes, but restaurants that serve a menu satisfying my nutritional recommendations are as rare as hens' teeth. One of my favorite solutions to the dining dilemma is to establish restaurants that cook and serve exclusively 20% fat (or less) meals.

How do we survive the restaurant dining dilemma?

Given that my utopian restaurant doesn't exist on every street corner, how do we wind our way through the maze that defines restaurant dining? Practicing mindfulness and awareness will solve half of the problem. Without mindfulness and awareness, we are bereft of choice.

Let's do a bit of home schooling before we venture out into the hazards of the restaurant world. In the form of good versus evil, allow me to present choices available to you at each meal.

	Choose (good)	**Avoid (evil)**
Breakfast	Whole grain cereals with skimmed milk, whole-wheat toast, bagels, waffles with fruit toppings	Eggs, bacon, sausage, muffins, donuts, croissants, pastries, fried foods, and especially granolas
Lunch	Salads with fresh greens, fruit, chick-peas, beans, lemon juice or vinegar dressings	Marinated vegetables, eggs, cheese, creamy dressings, cole slaw, meat salads made with mayonnaise
	Broth type soups like minestrone and chicken noodle, lentil or bean	Cream soups like New England clam chowder
	Entrées like soup and salad, baked seafood, lean turkey breast sandwich	Liver, duck, red meats, poultry with skin left in place, sauces, sandwiches with mayonnaise
Dinner	Pasta, rice and vegetables, baked fishes or white meat poultry, steamed vegetables and baked potatoes	Red meats, liver, duck, sauces, foods cooked in butter, hollandaise, sauces on vegetables
Dessert	Fresh fruit, sorbet, or sherbet	Cakes, ice cream, pies, cookies

Before we mindlessly venture into the restaurant milieu, we must ask ourselves if we truly want to and need to dine out. Other good choices are available to us.

Eat at home – This is the single best solution to the Russian Roulette of Restaurant Dining. Do you really need to or want to eat out? All of the control and responsibility for good nutrition remains with you. Eating at home is often a matter of choice, so choose home more often.

Brown bag it – If lunches or other meals at work are mandatory due to time or distance restrictions, brown bagging becomes a great choice. Good nutrition remains within your control. Low-fat sandwiches, salads and fruits are brown bag staples. If you have a time restriction for lunch at work, brown bagging is right for you. No one enjoys rushing to a restaurant, eating with one eye on your watch and urging the waitress to bring the check so you can return to work with anxiety-provoked gastritis.

Lets now assume and accept that restaurant dining is your choice or necessity. How do you survive? Here are some suggestions to assist you when you are eating outside of your domain.

Select user friendly restaurants – Frequent restaurants that in your experience have proven their mettle with respect to ease of procuring good nutrition. Restaurant dining is supposed to be pleasurable. You do not want to sit and calculate fat content of foods or grill a waiter about how food is prepared. Menu choices of low-fat, high-fiber, high-carbohydrate items should be clearly labeled and easily ordered. I suggest that anything a restaurant advertises as a "healthy choice selection" should meet the 20% fat requirement, and provide ample fiber and carbohydrate.

If the restaurant does not have readily identified "healthy choice selections," I would expect them to accommodate requests. The attitude of management and staff is critical. If they are pro-health, your dining experience will be positive.

Look at a menu before accepting a seat – A quick scan of the menu before making your decision to dine will provide information about the availability of and attitude about good nutrition in that restaurant. If the menu contains primarily red meat dishes, heavily sauced items, and no simple baked fishes or the like, it's probably going to be a tooth-pulling contest to get what you desire. Go somewhere else.

Have a seat of the pants nutrition sense when you dine – Know what is high-fat and what is not. Red meats, duck, sauces, creamy salad dressings are all high-fat items. Baked and poached white fishes, vegetables, potatoes (without sauces, butter or sour cream) and salads with lemon juice or vinegar as dressings are not high in fat. Gravitate to those choices.

Be assertive in your ordering – Be assertive, not aggressive or argumentative. If you don't see what you want on the menu, order specific *a la carte* items that may not be on the menu. For instance, you might order a raw or moderately steamed vegetable tray for an appetizer, with lemon juice for dipping. The main course might be: Baked fish, steamed broccoli, and a baked potato (low-fat yogurt on the side). Dessert? None. Have black coffee or an aperitif. Enjoy your company. If the restaurant cannot accommodate such a simple request, ask for a salad with lemon juice for dressing and a baked potato. Enjoy your meal, and then never return to that restaurant again.

Modify and substitute, but don't be a nuisance about it – Try to follow a pathway of minimal resistance. Modify your order with consideration of the kitchen, what you sense they can and can't do. Remember, dining is fun, not a competition. If a fish dish comes with sauce, ask that the sauce be omitted or served on the side. Baked potatoes are always the best potato choice, as opposed to *au gratin*, country or whatever melange they serve. Salad dressings are always lemon juice or vinegar on the side. Coffee? Learn to drink it black. Cream has loads of fat calories that we just don't need. Dessert? I would suggest that you pass, but if you must have dessert, order one dessert and three or four forks, then share. All you really need is a taste to satisfy your curiosity.

Consider an appetizer and soup as your meal – A couple of choices might be: 1) a soup and salad or 2) steamed vegetables with a bowl of lentil or barley-based soup to follow. What could be easier and healthier? Fat and calories remain low while fiber, volume and enjoyment soar.

Choose ethnic restaurants – Select from among a myriad of ethnic restaurants like Chinese, Italian, or Indian. These are cultures whose cuisine, in general, is much healthier than our American cuisine. Their dishes are lower in fat, use meat as a garnish, and offer high percentages of complex carbohydrates. Choosing from their menu on average will produce a healthier plate. Unfortunately, we don't always know the composition of many of their dishes, so it becomes another game of nutritional Russian Roulette. Rely on your nutritional sense and experience to guide you through.

Go for broke and eat like a mindless pig – This is actually a good learning experience. Eat poorly, high fat and lots of it. Stuff yourself. Then pay attention to how you feel for the next three or four hours. Most likely you will be sluggish, bloated and irritable. Abdominal cramping will follow, and if you chose creamed sauces, perhaps some quality bathroom time will be in order. It is a unique learning experience.

Eat at a restaurant that serves an exclusively healthful menu – Where do you find them? You don't, because they don't exist. They should, however. I have felt for a number of years that a healthful restaurant would be a viable business, especially considering the trend towards awareness of health management and the steady growth of the restaurant industry.

With a mindful approach, we may succeed quite well in the dining dilemma. Thought, planning and practice are again important to our surviving the Russian Roulette of Restaurant Dining.

Tips for Quick and Healthy Eating

Thought, planning and practice are equally applicable to our nutrition on the run. Just because we might be busy is no reason to abdicate our responsibility for good nutrition. Here are a few ideas that we may use when we are on the run.

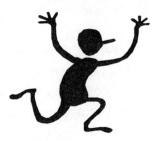

❖ **Eat a high fiber cereal for breakfast** – You will likely eat less fat and cholesterol during the remainder of the day. High fiber cereals are those that provide at least 4 grams of fiber per serving.

❖ **Soften margarine at room temperature** – If you choose to use some sort of fatty spread on your bread, you likely use only one quarter of the amount of warm margarine as you would cold margarine. Avoid butter.

❖ **Use fruit preserves, jam or an unsweetened fruit puree as a spread for toast or bagel** – You will save about 4 grams of fat (36 calories) for every pat of margarine you don't use.

❖ **Use skim milk** – Although whole milk is but 4% fat, the 4% figure is the weight of the fat, not the calories from fat. Approximately **50% of the calories in whole milk come from fat.** Two-percent milk provides 35% of its calories from fat. One-percent milk delivers 20% fat calories, while skim milk has only 5% of its calories as fat.

❖ **Drink fresh orange juice** – Fresh orange juice has more vitamin C than the same amount made from frozen concentrate. Better yet, eat a fresh orange.

❖ **Instant breakfast is better than no breakfast at all** – Of course it's better to eat a decent breakfast, but on those occasions when you're unavoidably rushed, a breakfast drink of complex carbohydrate and protein will suffice.

❖ **Steer clear of muffins** – Even muffins with loads of oat bran can weigh nearly half a pound and contain up to 600 calories. They're usually loaded with fat and sugar.

❖ **Avoid prepared pasta dishes** – Usually made with high-fat content mayonnaise and tropical oils, these are very high in calories and fat.

❖ **Declare one day in your week to be a vegetarian day** – You will increase your intake of fiber, vitamin A, and vitamin C. Meal preparation becomes simple. You don't have to worry about completing proteins or considering what meat to provide. Adequate protein is available every other day of the week. If you choose to do it more often, remember complementary vegetable sources of proteins.

❖ **Try a low-fat tuna salad** – Combine water-packed tuna with two tablespoons of red wine vinegar and chopped onions to taste. Don't even think of mayonnaise.

❖ **Use low-sodium broth** – Make a hearty meal by adding vegetables and chunks of turkey breast to the broth. Add herbs and spices to taste.

❖ **Be wise at the salad bar** – Avoid high-fat and high-calorie dressings. Skip the ham and bacon bits. Use vinegar or lemon juice only as your dressing. Choose spinach or leaf lettuce, beans, beets, cucumbers, tomatoes, green peppers and carrots.

❖ **Choose baked potatoes** – They are delicious with a few drops of olive oil, soy sauce, yogurt or an herb and spice blend.

❖ **Oven baked chicken without a trace of added fat** – Rub skinless chicken breasts with prepared mustard and then coat them with yellow cornmeal. Bake as you would normally.

❖ **Make your own pizza** – Buy a prepared pizza shell and add your own toppings. I find tomato, mushrooms and low-fat cheese pizza to be terrific. My daughters complain when there is none left over in the refrigerator.

❖ **Microwave an apple for dessert** – Keep the doctor away! Peel the top third to allow moisture to escape. Cook for three minutes. Top with maple syrup flavored yogurt and cinnamon.

❖ **Never eat out of the container** – You will eat much more than you had planned.

❖ **Brush your teeth** – When struck with an irresistible food craving, brush your teeth. The taste of toothpaste will offset your desire for food.

❖ **Microwave fresh vegetables as a snack** – You will preserve the vitamin content and provide yourself with a quick, low-calorie solution to your immediacy for food.

We have addressed a lot of issues about nutrition, from the chemistry of foods, to shopping, to eating at home, to dining out, to eating on the run. It is a large volume to digest. If you feel overwhelmed, remember to eat it like an elephant, one bite at a time.

Recipes

By no means do I intend that *Get a Life, America!* should be a "cookbook" in any sense of the word. The following recipes are included to demonstrate that you may find tasty dishes which satisfy the following requirements:

1) Relatively low in calories
2) No more than 20% of calories from fat
3) Easy to prepare
4) Adequate protein
5) Substantial fiber
6) Significant quantities of complex carbohydrates

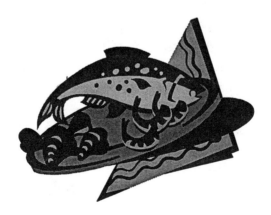

Curried Turkey Salad

In most turkey salads, the turkey is well-masked by tons of mayonnaise. Here, sliced vegetables and fruits compliment the turkey in a low-fat dressing. You may enjoy the principal ingredients of the salad without a mayonnaise disguise.

1/2 cup fat-free mayonnaise
1/2 cup plain low-fat yogurt
1/4 cup buttermilk
1/4 cup chopped chutney
1 1/2 teaspoons curry powder
1/8 teaspoon ground ginger
3 cups skinless, cooked turkey breast, cut into 1-inch cubes
One 16 ounce can of pineapple chunks, drained
1 cup thinly sliced celery
1/4 cup thinly sliced scallions
1/2 cup frozen green peas, thawed
1 tart green apple, peel on, diced
1 head of Boston lettuce
2 ounces snow peas, blanched
1/2 cup finely shaved carrot
1/4 cup chopped, dried cranberries

1. Combine the mayonnaise, yogurt, buttermilk, chutney, curry powder and ginger into a small bowl. Set it aside.
2. In a large bowl combine the turkey, pineapple, celery, scallions, peas, apple, carrots and cranberries. Add the salad dressing and toss. Refrigerate for later.
3. For serving, place a bed of lettuce on a clear glass plate. Spoon the salad on top. Garnish with snow peas.

Nutritional information:			
Servings	4		
Calories	380	Cholesterol	102 mg
Total fat	2 gm	Fiber	5 gm
Saturated fat	0.7 gm	**% fat cal**	**5%**

Oriental Pasta with Snow Peas and Peppers

This is a simple vegetable and pasta dish made special by the use of soy, garlic, and ginger. Phenomenally low in fat, the pasta supplies the protein.

> 1/2 pound snow peas
> 1 red bell pepper
> 1 yellow bell pepper
> 2 cups broccoli florets
> 1 pound linguine
> 1/4 cup low-sodium chicken stock
> 2 tablespoons reduced-sodium soy sauce
> 2 tablespoons lemon juice
> 1 tablespoon vegetable oil
> 2 tablespoons minced fresh ginger
> 1 garlic clove, minced

1. Bring a large pot of water to a boil.
2. String and cut the snow peas diagonally. Dice the bell peppers
3. Blanch the snow peas for 30 seconds, then cool immediately. Blanch the broccoli florets for 3 minutes, then cool immediately. The peppers remain raw.
4. Cook the linguine for 10 minutes.
5. Make the dressing by combining the stock, soy sauce, lemon juice, oil, ginger and garlic in a bowl.
6. Serve on a dark plate. Place the linguine first, followed by the dressing, and top with the snow peas, broccoli and peppers.

Nutritional information:

Servings	4		
Calories	400	Cholesterol	trace
Total fat	5 gm	Fiber	3 gm
Saturated fat	0.7 gm	**% fat cal**	**11%**

Spinach Lasagna

Skim milk mozzarella and low-fat cottage cheese are the reasons that this meatless lasagna remains low in total fat. Delicious and very low in cholesterol, this spinach lasagna wins praise from your family.

> 1/2 pound fresh mushrooms, sliced
> 2 garlic cloves, crushed
> 1 cup chopped onion
> Two 16 ounce cans tomato puree
> 1 tablespoon dried basil
> 2 teaspoons dried oregano
> 2 tablespoons chopped fresh parsley
> 1/4 teaspoon salt
> 1/4 teaspoon freshly ground pepper
> 1/4 teaspoon red pepper flakes
> One 10-ounce package of whole-wheat lasagna noodles
> Two bags of fresh spinach
> 1 tablespoon olive oil
> Pinch of freshly grated nutmeg
> 2 cups low-fat cottage cheese (1%)
> 2 tablespoons low-fat milk (1%)
> 2 ounces part skim mozzarella cheese, shredded
> 2 tablespoons grated Parmesan cheese

1. Bring a large saucepan of water to a boil.
2. Combine the mushrooms, garlic and all but 2 tablespoons of the onion in a large non-stick skillet. Cover and cook over a medium heat, until the vegetables soften (about five minutes).
3. Add the tomato puree to the skillet. Stir in the basil, oregano, parsley, a pinch of salt and pepper, and the red pepper flakes. Cover and simmer for 30 minutes.
4. Cook the lasagna noodles according to directions.
5. Preheat the oven to 350 degrees.
6. Dice the fresh spinach. Cook the remaining onion in oil in a non-stick skillet until slightly softened. Add the spinach and cook until the liquid

evaporates. Add the remaining salt and pepper and the nutmeg. Remove the skillet from the heat.

7. Blend the cottage cheese and milk until smooth.
8. Using a 9 x 13 baking pan, spread a little tomato sauce in the bottom of the pan. Layer the noodles, tomato sauce, cottage cheese, spinach and mozzarella successively, with the top layer being noodles, tomato sauce and Parmesan cheese. Cover with aluminum foil and bake for 50 to 60 minutes, removing the cover for the last ten minutes. Allow the lasagna to stand for 10 minutes before serving.

Nutritional information:

Servings	6		
Calories	380	Cholesterol	10 gm
Total fat	6 gm	Fiber	6 gm
Saturated fat	2 gm	**% fat cal**	**14%**

Chicken Baked in Parchment

Parchment paper
4 boneless skinless chicken breast halves (4 ounces each)
1 cup matchstick size carrot strips
1 cup matchstick size zucchini strips
1/2 cup snow peas
1/2 cup thinly sliced red bell peppers
2 1/4 cups low-salt chicken broth, divided
2 tablespoons all-purpose flour
2 garlic cloves, minced
1/2 teaspoon dried thyme leaves
1/4 teaspoon salt
1/4 teaspoon ground nutmeg
1/4 teaspoon ground black pepper
1 package (6 ounces) wheat pilaf mix

1. Preheat oven to 375 degrees. Cut parchment paper into four 10-inch squares. Place 1 chicken breast in the center of each parchment; arrange carrots, zucchini, peas and bell pepper around the chicken.
2. Combine 1/2 cup of chicken broth and flour in a small saucepan. Add garlic, thyme, salt, nutmeg, and black pepper. Bring to a boil over high heat, stirring constantly. When thickened, reduce heat to low and simmer for one minute. Spoon mixture over the chicken and vegetables.
3. Fold over parchment, artfully, and place in a 10 x 15 inch baking pan. Bake for 25 to 30 minutes.
4. Place remaining broth into a saucepan and bring it to a boil. Stir in pilaf mix (discard spice packet). Reduce heat and simmer for 15 minutes or until broth is absorbed.
5. Arrange parchment packets on plates and serve with the pilaf.

Nutrition information:

Servings	4		
Calories	320	Cholesterol	58 mg
Total fat	3 gm	Protein	28 gm
Saturated fat	1 gm	Fiber	3 gm
Carbohydrate	41 gm	**% fat cal**	**9 %**

Mandarin Orange Chicken

1 pound boneless skinless chicken breasts
1/8 teaspoon salt
1/8 teaspoon ground black pepper
Nonstick cooking spray
1/2 cup finely chopped onion
1/2 cup orange juice
2 teaspoons minced fresh ginger
1 teaspoon sugar
1/4 cup cold water
2 teaspoons cornstarch
1 can (11 ounces) mandarin orange segments, drained
2 to 3 tablespoons finely chopped fresh cilantro
2 cups hot, cooked white rice

1. Preheat broiler.
2. Pound chicken to ¼-inch thinness using two pieces of waxed paper and a mallet.
3. Spray broiler rack with cooking spray. Place chicken on rack, 4 inches from heat. Broil, turning occasionally, for 14 to 16 minutes. Sprinkle with pepper and salt.
4. Spray medium saucepan with cooking spray and heat. Add onions and cook for 5 minutes. Add orange juice, ginger and sugar. Bring to a boil over high heat.
5. Combine water and cornstarch in a small bowl, then add to the juice mixture, stirring until thickened. Boil for one minute, stirring occasionally. Finally, add the orange segments and cilantro.
6. Serve the chicken over rice and top with sauce. Garnish with additional cilantro.

Nutritional information:

Servings	4		
Calories	310	Cholesterol	58 mg
Total fat	3 gm	Protein	25 gm
Saturated fat	1 gm	Fiber	2 gm
Carbohydrate	43 gm	**% fat cal**	**9%**

Zesty Lentil Stew

Dried legumes such as lentils, beans and black-eyed peas are good sources of iron, thiamine, riboflavin niacin, potassium and phosphorous.

1 cup dried lentils
2 cups chopped peeled potatoes
1 can (14 1/2 ounces) low-salt chicken broth
1 2/3 cups water
1 1/2 cups chopped, seeded tomatoes
1 can (11 1/2 ounces) no-salt-added spicy vegetable juice cocktail
1 cup chopped onion
1/2 cup chopped carrot
1/2 cup chopped celery
2 tablespoons chopped fresh basil or 2 tablespoons dried basil leaves
2 tablespoons chopped fresh oregano or 2 tablespoons dried oregano leaves
1 to 2 tablespoons finely chopped jalapeno pepper
1/4 teaspoon salt

1. Rinse lentils under cold water and drain.
2. Combine lentils, potatoes, chicken broth, water tomatoes, vegetable juice cocktail, onion, carrot, celery, basil, oregano, jalapeno and salt in a 3-quart saucepan. Bring to a boil over high heat. Reduce to a medium-low heat and cook for 45 minutes, stirring occasionally. Lentils should become tender.
3. Serve in generous sized soup bowl with sesame crisps.

Nutrition information			
Servings	4		
Calories	370	Cholesterol	0 mg
Total fat	1 gm	Protein	19 gm
Saturated fat	0 mg	Fiber	7 gm
Carbohydrate	72 gm	**% fat cal**	**3%**

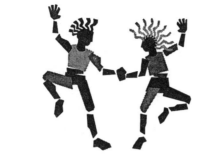

Use it or Lose it!

Better to hunt in fields, for health unbought,
Than fee the doctor for a nauseous draught.
The wise, for cure, on exercise depend
God never made his work for man to mend.

❖

John Dryden
1631-1700

Arguably, the most sedentary nation on earth, America earns a large part its trillion dollar sick care bill sitting mindlessly on our sofas, channel-changers in hand, TV dinners on our laps, watching Susan Lucci, Erica, of *All my Children*, lose another bid for an Emmy. Flash – she just won! In this chapter we'll examine individual and national costs of our sloth-like existence, reasons why we don't exercise, and the benefits of exercising. We'll reveal key points about muscle structure and function; then we'll learn about stretching, strength training, and aerobic exercise. We'll learn how to do it all ourselves. Perhaps most important, I'll give you some tricks for motivation and help you to *Get a Life, America!*

The scientific literature splits at the seams with studies documenting the sedentary lifestyles of Americans. Fifty-percent of us do no exercise at all, forty-percent exercise once a week, and less than ten-percent do enough exercise to

91

nieve aerobic benefit. Even more discouraging is our trend towards less exercise, not more. Sadly, we're losing it, not using it!

Healthy People 2000, the government's program to improve our national health, set a goal to have sixty-percent of Americans exercising by the year 2000. We failed to meet that deadline, as evidenced by the most recent statistics, which continue to document that less than ten-percent of our population performs meaningful exercise, and herald our getting fatter as a result of sedentary lives.

The United States Public Health Service uncovered a thirty-year trend towards obesity in our children. USPHS attributes this obesity problem to television and inactivity. With physical activity patterns developing in childhood, the risk for lifelong obesity is established early in our lives. Alarmingly, obesity as a child and as an adolescent looms as a greater predictor of adult cardiovascular disease than adult obesity.

The USPHS recommends solving the problem by: 1) counseling children about exercise 2) contacting parents and telling them to tell their kids to exercise 3) having health care professionals tell kids to exercise and 4) encouraging the American Medical Association to counsel its members about exercise in children. Since when does telling anyone what to do work?

We must show them. Parents, teachers, professionals, service organizations (police, fire, clergy), and business people must assume the position of exercise role models for our children. Assuming we accept our responsibility to be exercise role models, most of us lack knowledge about what to model.

After conducting considerable research, exercise physiologists of the 1980's recommended that individuals exercise vigorously for twenty to thirty minutes at least three times per week. Although a good recommendation, we have not heeded the exercise gurus' recommendations of the1980's because that advice was too demanding for a nation of people with no legacy of exercise. Many of us became discouraged from exercising at all.

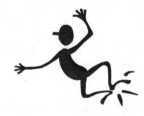

Hallelujah! Good news hovers on the horizon. Recent research has documented that the greatest health benefit is gained by simply becoming active. Researchers have defined five levels of activity from sedentary to very active. The change from sedentary to level one of activity bestows the greatest health benefit in terms of disease prevention. More good news rose from the same study, the exercise does not have to be continuous for an individual to receive health benefits. All of the exercise that you do in a day is additive.

Meaningful research came from a Stanford University study by Paffenbarger, who followed the exercise habits of 17,000 Harvard alumni for ten years. He found life-lengthening benefits from exercise, benefits accruing in an incremental and progressive fashion from using 700 calories to 2000 calories per week in addition to the participant's baseline normal activity. Spending an extra 2000 calories per week earned the participant an additional 2.5 years of life. No additional benefit accrued from energy expenditures greater than 2000 calories per week. This is great news, for now we can confidently encourage exercising for a better life, and for a longer one, too.

If we produce a nation of longer lived people, our average age will increase. An older population carries risks and responsibilities. The risks are deterioration illnesses of aging, and the responsibilities are to prevent those diseases and to care for them should they occur. I contend that each of us is individually responsible to our society for maintaining our health and preventing diseases.

Thus, the primary reason to exercise is for ourselves, to live **better** each day. The secondary reason is to live **longer**. The tertiary reason is to meet our **social responsibility** to maintain our individual health, lest we should become an unnecessary burden on society. No one has promised us a tomorrow, but if we are fortunate enough to be granted tomorrows, we should greet those tomorrows with health, fitness and wellness.

Health, Fitness and Wellness

Health is the absence of disease. Fitness is the body's adaptation to increased demands of exercise and encompasses both aerobic and muscular fitness. Aerobic fitness is the ability to take in, transport and utilize oxygen. Muscular fitness includes strength, flexibility and endurance. Health benefits incrementally from fitness, while fitness is predicated upon a healthy body. One hand washes the other. Wellness is a higher state of grace of health, achieved through active practice of the principles presented in *Get a Life, America!*

At birth we are granted miraculous physiology, and with rare exceptions, we are granted health. Whether we remain static and simply manage to maintain the function of our physiology, whether we abuse our bodies and earn illnesses, or whether we take control of our health and build it to wellness, is our choice. I recommend the latter.

I also recommend exercising vigorously, because a definite advantage accrues at higher levels of exercise. Paffenbarger's study proved that fact. One can have health without fitness, but an undeniable advantage is granted to health with fitness.

Why Don't We Exercise?

Although we understand that exercise benefits everyone who participates, fewer than 10% of Americans do any meaningful exercise, exercise of sufficient intensity, duration and frequency to effect an aerobic training response. Even fewer people perform strength-training exercises. Why?

The most common excuse from our national "slug patrol" is lack of time. We are simply too busy, busy with work, busy with family, busy drinking beer, busy watching television. To benefit from exercise, all one must do is enough exercise to spend 700 to 2,000 calories per week. At 10 cal/minute the time requirement ranges from 70 minutes to 200 minutes, about one hour to three hours per week. Thus, the time excuse for not exercising is common but flimsy, easy to offer and quite superficial.

Another reason for not exercising is that the individual does not enjoy exercise. Perhaps they did not enjoy the humiliation of high school gym class, but who can deny the exhilaration, well-being and satisfaction gained from a walk with a friend. People who don't enjoy exercise have never achieved a sufficient level of activity that allows them to feel better.

Many people don't have an exercise legacy. Their parents didn't exercise, and the individuals never exercised as children. They have no foundation upon which to build.

Conveniences dictate our lives in the modern world. We no longer plow fields with horses or walk ten miles to town. We drive to work, park as close to the building as possible, and take the elevator to our offices. Lawn mowers are self-propelled and ride-on styles. Golf courses urge golfers to use motorized carts for expediency.

Money is a problem, too. Exercise costs money, doesn't it? Plush gyms, country clubs, and lavish outfits for tennis and golf all cost money. We will spend money on dining out before spending on a health club. What misplaced priorities!

No valid excuse exists for not exercising. I suspect ignorance looms as the greatest impediment to exercise. Most people don't know much about it and are intimidated by the thought of exercising. We must change that perception. **If we don't make the time for exercise, then surely we will have to allow time for illness.**

Benefits and Risks of Exercise

Retired Episcopal Bishop Nelson Burroughs walked daily from his home overlooking Pleasant Bay and the Atlantic Ocean in Chatham on Cape Cod into town to get his mail at the post office. Sporting his trademark red felt hat, he was a walking landmark of the Chatham landscape. About one mile each way, his pedestrian trip sat solidly in his schedule.

Once or twice a year Bishop Burroughs would come by my office just to make sure he was "OK" to travel to England. No big deal you say? The last time I gave Bishop Burroughs his medical passport for travel, he was 92 years old. Bishop Burroughs' habit of walking served him well physically and emotionally. He loved it and he loved the people he met on his journeys. And he *Got a Life!* for a lifetime.

Next time you visit the city, take some time to look at the people around you. How many appear healthy? How many look happy? How many are overweight? It is rather discouraging isn't it? Disease, depression and obesity are omnipresent and obvious. Many of those people, if not most, don't realize just how bad they feel. Their lives and existences are their norms. If only we could reach out, take them by the hand and ease them into exercise, we could show them a whole array of benefits from exercise. What are those benefits, you ask? Allow me to list what we know:

- loss of weight
- loss of body fat
- increase of muscle mass
- better appearance
- better posture
- less back pain
- better digestion and colon function
- lowered blood pressure
- increased sense of health and well-being
- better pulmonary function
- better circulation to compromised areas
- stronger heart
- more efficient oxygen use
- increased endurance
- decreased resting pulse rate
- quicker recovery from exercise
- stress reduction
- adjunct to behavior modification of any kind
- ego and self-confidence support
- better participation in sports and the game of life
- bridging of the generation gap (exercising people of all ages have the common bond of exercising)
- socialization
- education, learning as you exercise (learning about your body, learning about physiology)
- getting in touch with your body
- better sexuality
- less illness, better immunity
- decreased risk of certain cancers
- slowing of the aging process
- adjunct to prevention of diseases
- decreased cardiovascular disease (CVD) risk
- stronger bones and ligaments
- more energy and less fatigue
- better fat metabolism
- emotional stability, more positive outlook
- improved efficiency of handling of glucose

- setting an example for others, a role model for our children
- healthier babies from pregnant women
- improved lipid profile
- increased metabolic rate

After reading that list, it seems that exercise solves the world's problems. It may just be a very good start.

> Mrs. Marcus, wife of a wealthy New York businessman, could have afforded a chauffeured limousine to drive her around town. Healthfully thin, muscularly strong, obviously enthusiastic, she, like Bishop Burroughs, served as a good role model for walking as a life-long exercise. Any day, short of one with blowing rain or snow, found her walking five or more miles to the grocery store and back to her home. A few years younger than the Bishop, Mrs. Marcus, in her early seventies, helps to assure her graceful transition into her older years.

Bishop Burroughs and Mrs. Marcus are no different than you or me. We can all get out, walk, and *Get a Life!*

What is the downside? What are the risks of exercising? There aren't many. Injuries can occur, but they are less likely in a fit person. Overuse injuries have been the bread-and-butter work of busy sports medicine doctors, but a moderate, common sense approach to exercise can prevent overuse injuries. Underlying disease is a legitimate concern, and that is why it is sensible to evaluate your health risk potential before starting a program. Although the risk of heart attacks and sudden death is small, it happens on occasion, and it is a real attention-getter. For that reason I am a proponent of maximum treadmill testing for sedentary individuals over forty who wish to start exercising.

Addictive and compulsive behavior is always a risk, and certainly is when applied to exercise. Excessive exercise can result in the cessation of menstruation, osteoporosis, stress fractures, immune deficiency, mood disturbances, and even shortened life expectancy. These extremes can be viewed as a disease state in themselves. A moderate, thoughtful, sensitive approach to exercise negates most all risks of exercise. We will be better able to avoid the extremes and to integrate exercise into our lives if we have a decent understanding of how exercise works.

Muscle Structure and Physiology

Muscle, the major biochemical machine in the body, converts chemical energy into mechanical energy by the process called metabolism. Marvelous muscle, the largest single tissue in the human body, makes up 25% of body mass at birth, up to 50% in the developed adult, and somewhat less than 30% in the aged adult. Thousands of muscle cells, all under the voluntary control of the nervous system, unify to form our skeletal muscle system. One nerve may supply its impulse to hundreds of muscle fibers, those muscle fibers and the supplying nerve comprising a motor unit. The motor unit concept is important in our understanding the efficiency of muscle function.

Muscle Fiber Types

Skeletal muscle cells differ in structure and function. Relatively recent research has demonstrated two (and probably three) distinctly different skeletal muscle cell types. For functional simplicity we shall focus on two types: **type I (slow twitch) and type II (fast twitch).** The type I fibers are red because they contain numerous mitochondria (small structures within the muscle cells specific for aerobic metabolism). Their metabolism is aerobic, and they maintain relatively sustained contractions. The type II fibers are white because they contain few mitochondria. They derive their energy from anaerobic metabolism and exhibit relatively short duration of contractions.

The third type of fiber is type IIA, a fast twitch fiber, capable of aerobic metabolism. This fiber is a crossbreed and may represent a potential transition fiber from one type to another. Although it is currently held among the scientific research community that the ratio of type I to type II fibers is under genetic control and established at birth, some researchers consider the possibility that significant training stimulus may generate the cross over of fiber types.

What we do know, however, is that all of the muscle fibers within a motor unit are of the same type. Of course, that makes sense, because if we are running a 100-yard dash, we want to recruit fast twitch fibers as efficiently as possible. One motor nerve impulse can cause hundreds of fast twitch fibers to contract. Conversely, if we were running a marathon, we would like to efficiently and selectively recruit the slow twitch fibers for our purpose. Slow twitch motor units provide nicely for that function. Aside from the neurologic efficiency, functional metabolic efficiency is manifested in the two cell types.

Metabolism

Within the cells of each type of motor unit, the method of energy production differs. **Anaerobic metabolism is the processing of fuel to energy in the absence of oxygen.** It is rapid, but, inefficient, yielding only **2 ATPs** (adenosine tri-phosphate) per molecule of glucose. ATP is the "energy currency" of metabolism. Glucose is the only fuel that can be metabolized anaerobically. Anaerobic metabolism occurs in fast twitch (type II) muscle fibers, providing for immediate, short duration energy needs. Anaerobic metabolism is limited by modest fuel availability, as well as by the rapid build-up of the metabolic waste products of lactic acid and carbon dioxide.

An important parameter of exercise is the anaerobic threshold (or lactic acid threshold), the point beyond which exercise cannot continue because of waste product accumulation. We sense the anaerobic threshold as muscle discomfort and fatigue with associated "air hunger."

Examples of exercise requiring anaerobic metabolism are lifting heavy weights to exhaustion, chopping down a tree as rapidly as you can, and running from the saber-toothed tiger in cave-man days. Another less obvious example is during the immediate post heart attack period, when blood supply to the heart muscle is interrupted and hence, no oxygen is available to the myocardium (heart muscle). Metabolism in the heart muscle, which is normally aerobic, becomes anaerobic. Rapid production and accumulation of waste products augments the precipitous damage to the heart muscle. Anaerobic metabolism may also be viewed as an evolutionary adaptation at the cellular level to produce energy when no oxygen is available.

Aerobic metabolism is the processing of fuels to energy in the presence of, and with the use of oxygen. Aerobic metabolism occurs in slow twitch (type I) muscle fibers, within the mitochondria. Slower to produce energy, much more efficient than anaerobic metabolism, it yields **38 ATPs** per molecule of glucose (a nineteen-fold improvement over anaerobic energy production). No accumulation of exercise-limiting waste products occurs; it produces only carbon dioxide and water as its by-products. It is limited only by oxygen availability and fuel depletion. Aerobic metabolism has the advantage of using all three basic fuels in the process, but **fat is the primary fuel.**

Examples of exercise requiring aerobic metabolism are running a marathon, normal heart muscle contraction, long bike riding, conducting a symphony, or running the cave-man's prey to exhaustion. Aerobic metabolism is an evolutionary adaptation to allow energy production over long periods of time.

Whenever we're active, we produce energy through both aerobic and anaerobic pathways. The intensity of the energy expenditure determines the ratio of aerobic to anaerobic metabolism. Rapid and intense work demands anaerobic production, slow and low-intensity work requests aerobic production.

Let's move now from the physiology and structure of muscles to the subject of muscular fitness. Muscular fitness encompasses flexibility, strength and aerobic capacity.

Stretching, Flexibility and Our Bodies' Responses

We should stretch routinely. Stretching improves physical performance, prevents injuries, aids in muscle relaxation, helps to rehabilitate injuries and promotes body awareness.

Stretching, a key adjunct to exercising, improves flexibility and increases muscle length. Flexibility is the range of movement of a joint or group of joints. Stretching increases and maintains flexibility by ensuring the pliability of the connective tissue around the joints, and by lengthening muscles and their tendons. Physiologic studies demonstrate that a lengthened muscle exerts a greater force of contraction than a shortened muscle. The increased strength associated with lengthened muscles always favors us, no matter what our activity. The stronger we are, the better we perform.

Stretching in anticipation of exercising is best performed on warm muscles, because warm muscles stretch more easily. Before exercising warm up for about five minutes, to a point of mild perspiration, then stretch.

Stretching isn't to be done exclusively with exercise. You may stretch any time you wish, but especially in the morning when you arise. Stretch for tension relief. Stretch after sitting or standing for long periods or simply when you feel stiff.

Stretching is best done on a daily basis, once or many times during the day. With the daily practice of stretching, you will notice a discernible difference in three to four weeks. Stiffness will be a nuisance of the past, and the range of motion of your joints will be markedly improved. Your potential for injury during exercise will be much less. Certainly less apt to injure yourself in strength-training, in competitive athletics or in aerobic exercise, you as a routine stretcher will also be less likely to suffer serious injury if you happen to slip and fall.

If you are unfortunate enough to have injured yourself, your rehabilitation from the injury may be aided with a stretching program. Recent research has demonstrated that stretching and massage integrate in healing injuries.

Stretch, on occasion, simply to meet your body. Pay attention to your neck as you flex forward or extend backward. Notice the tone of the muscles in your legs and buttocks as you flex forward. Become aware of how your body feels. Being sensitive to how your body feels will guide you well in your practicing an exercise program. It will serve you well in your deciding if you need to modify your life.

Stretching bestows many wonderful benefits. I suggest that you try it in conjunction with a meditation sitting. You will marvel at the results. Try stretching your upper body while you walk. It's a great technique to stimulate awareness and coordination.

The specifics of how to stretch are presented briefly in the How to Implement Your Stretching Program section. If you have greater interest in stretching, I would refer you to the book, *Stretching*, by Bob Anderson.

The natural progression from stretching invites a more active endeavor. Let's examine strength training, the processes by which our muscles may become stronger.

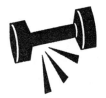

Strength-Training and Our Bodies' Responses

A strength-training effect on skeletal muscle is the increase in strength gained by the muscle in response to an overload of work for that particular muscle. Strength is the maximum force that can be exerted in a single voluntary contraction of a number of muscle fibers. The more fibers recruited, the greater the strength of muscle contraction.

Strength in skeletal muscle is achieved by training the fast twitch, type II, muscle fibers. Larger and quicker to fatigue, they generate more force on contraction than the slow twitch, type I, fibers. **Endurance of skeletal muscle comes through training the slow twitch, type I, fibers.**

The strength-training stimulus increases muscle fiber size. The increase in size results from the increased production and accumulation of the contractile proteins, actin and myosin. The increase in the protein availability translates to tougher connective tissue, to greater contractile efficiency and to less sensitivity to inhibitors of contraction. Normally, the increase in muscle strength results from increased fiber size, but a maximal training stimulus may produce an increased number of muscle fibers.

Some individuals have the mistaken concept that exercise transforms fat cells to muscle cells. This thinking is fallacious, for the transformation of fat to muscle, or the transformation of muscle to fat, never occurs. Muscles get larger or smaller depending upon the demands placed on the muscle.

What is the necessary stimulus to achieve a strength training effect? Strength in skeletal muscle increases when tension is applied to a muscle over sufficient duration and frequency. Physiologic research has demonstrated that the optimal tension to exert for a strength-training effect is two-thirds of the muscle's maximum force.

This tension or weight may be determined in two ways: 1) With well-warmed and stretched muscles, lift the maximum amount of weight possible with the muscle in question. This defines your maximum. 2) Through trial and error, determine a weight that allows you to perform a maximum of ten repetitions with the muscle to be trained. The injury potential is much less with the second technique, and this weight equates to two-thirds of your maximum.

Duration has been found to be optimal at three sets of from two to ten contractions. Repetitions of greater than ten begin to recruit slow twitch fibers, the endurance fibers. Frequency of training should be every other day to allow for recovery of the fatigued muscle. **A simple strength training formula to remember is: 2/3 of maximum force, 3 sets of 2-10 reps (repetitions), every other day.** When you can do more than ten repetitions, increase the weight. While it is true that some elite lifters and body builders do many more sets, three sets give quite an adequate strength training stimulus.

Most of us are not Olympic weight lifters or body builders, but we can all benefit from increasing our strength and maintaining it. Please do not feel that you must adhere strictly to the 2/3, 3 (2-10), every other day formula. It is a guideline for optimal results. If you feel like doing only one set, a lower weight, more sets, whatever, at least do something on a regular basis. The adaptive abilities of our bodies are so miraculous that our muscles will respond to most overload training.

Caution must be advised about over-training, however, because over-training increases the risk of injury and slows the progress of the strength-training response. Fast twitch fibers generally require longer to recover from an overload stimulus than do the slow twitch fibers. Always allow at least 24 and preferable 48 hours for recovery from a vigorous strength-training workout. Let's now discuss the training of the slow twitch muscle fibers.

Aerobic Exercise and Our Bodies' Responses

The aerobic training effect is marvelous and complex. It involves many body systems and produces multiple wellness benefits. How can training our bodies to use oxygen more efficiently in the process of producing energy translate into wellness benefits?

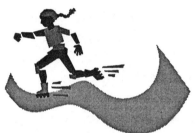

Wellness benefits accrue from the physiologic adaptations to the long duration, relatively low (under the anaerobic threshold) intensity exercise that is aerobic. Oxygen is taken from the atmosphere, transported through the lungs, into the blood stream via the heart, then to the muscles where it is incorporated into the metabolic processing of fuels for energy. **Formerly referred to as cardiovascular exercise, we now speak of aerobic exercise,** with the understanding that much of the adaptive processes of aerobic exercise occur primarily within the muscle.

The aerobic training effect is the body's adaptation or adjustment to an overload of work, to longer duration and more intense exercise over a period of weeks to months. The metabolic rate and oxygen consumption of muscles are elevated and sustained long enough to overload the aerobic enzyme system. The primary site of adaptation is in the skeletal muscle (mitochondrion), with secondary sites of adaptation in the respiratory system, heart and circulation, nervous system, endocrine system, body composition, bones, ligaments and tendons.

Within the muscles aerobic enzymes increase as well as do the number and size of the mitochondria. Consequently, the muscle cell is better able to use fat (the primary aerobic fuel source) as a fuel. This is critically important. The development of more mitochondria with greater branching is the primary adaptation of aerobic training effect. All other adaptations are subsequent to this one.

Pulmonary adaptation includes increased respiratory volume and better gas exchange with the blood. Fewer breaths are needed to supply the greater oxygen demand. Blood volume increases as red blood cells and hemoglobin increase, making the blood a more efficient transporter of oxygen. The heart and circulation respond with a decreased resting heart rate, an increased stroke volume (the amount pumped with each beat), an increased chamber volume (but no significant increase in heart muscle thickness), and a summarily increased total cardiac output.

Blood is redistributed from organs to muscles. The nervous system responds with increased efficiency and economy of motion. Hormonal response is manifested by adrenal gland enlargement, releasing more epinephrine. Epinephrine potentiates the release of fat (free fatty acids) from adipose tissue, even in the presence of lactic acid produced from anaerobic metabolism. Normally, lactic acid inhibits the release of free fatty acids from fat cells. Body composition changes to favor muscle over fat, and as a result, tendons, bones, and ligaments strengthen.

What phenomenal enzymatic, biochemical, cellular and physiologic adaptations to something so simple as increasing aerobic exercise of the body! Even more amazing, these adaptations equate with better health, less disease and longer life.

Aerobic exercise is unique in other ways, too. A significant difference between anaerobic exercise and aerobic exercise lies in their relative efficiency of energy use. **Aerobic exercise is far more energy efficient than anaerobic exercise.** Worth repeating, aerobic metabolism yields 38 ATP, the measure of "energy currency," per molecule of glucose compared to 2 ATP from the anaerobic processes. Each molecule of glucose metabolized via the aerobic process produces nineteen times more energy than if the same molecule were metabolized anaerobically.

Another difference between the two types of exercise is found in the fuels selected to provide the energy for each type. Aerobic exercise uses both fat and carbohydrate (and protein if carbohydrate and fat are unavailable) as fuels with a progressive increase in the carbohydrate/fat ratio as exercise intensifies. With intense exercise (anaerobic exercise) the fuel is primarily carbohydrate. With prolonged exercise (aerobic exercise), the fuel is primarily fat. Figure 2 demonstrates this relationship.

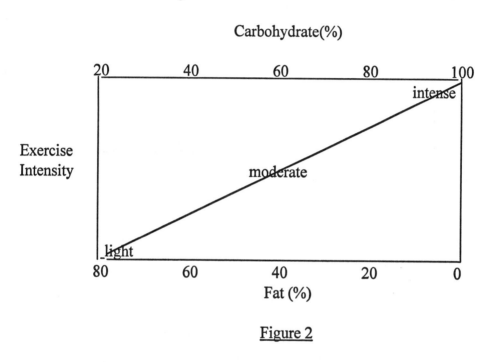

Figure 2

Relationship between exercise intensity and fuels used.

Fuel for work is stored throughout our bodies. As we have just seen, the fuel we select depends upon the intensity of the exercise. Some fuel exists in greater supply than others. We are relatively limited in carbohydrate stores, but have a generous supply of available fat. Figure 3 delineates the comparative availability of fuels in a 150-pound man.

Available Energy Sources		
Source	**Supply**	**Energy (cal)**
ATP	small amounts in muscle	5
Carbohydrate		
Muscle glycogen	15 gm (per kg of muscle)	1,200 (est.)
Liver glycogen	80 gm	320
Blood glucose	4 gm	16
Fat	adipose tissue	50,000-100,000

<u>Figure 3</u>

The following observations may be made from this data:

1) Muscle glycogen supplies only enough energy to run ten miles, assuming you could utilize glycogen exclusively.
2) Fat sources of energy supply 40 to 80 times more energy than does carbohydrate.
3) Blood glucose supplies precious little energy (its main energy destination is the brain, which uses glucose exclusively for its energy).
4) The amount of free ATP won't last more than thirty-seconds of a fast walk.

When energy stores are depleted by exercise, replenishment occurs in a specific sequence. Blood glucose is always maintained for the brain. Muscle glycogen is restored next, followed by liver glycogen. Fat stores are replenished last, and it is important to remember that **excess calories are always stored, and they are stored as fat.**

From storage to the mobilization and usage of fuels, the aerobic training effect is indeed miraculous, affecting so many body systems and providing wellness benefits. With continued practice of aerobic exercise, we will achieve increased levels of aerobic fitness.

Aerobic Fitness

Aerobic fitness is in part determined by genetic predisposition, but is highly subject to a training effect. Aerobic fitness (or lack of it) is measured by VO2 max; the maximum volume of oxygen an individual can consume at peak sustained exercise. VO2 max is specific for an individual and represents his aerobic (oxygen use) capacity. Heredity accounts for about 40% of aerobic capacity, leaving a potential increase of 60% through training efforts.

Determination of the VO2 max unfortunately requires a lab setting with treadmill, EKG and oxygen uptake analyzer. Because direct measurement of VO2 max is impossible outside of the laboratory, heart rate, which corresponds linearly to VO2 max, is used instead. The heart rate becomes an external indicator, a speedometer, if you will, of metabolic activity (VO2 max).

Determining Your Heart Rate

Maximum heart rate, which corresponds to 100% VO2 max, is calculated from the simple formula: **220 - age = max HR.** For example, the maximum heart rate of a 50 year old person is 220 - 50 = 170. If this person were exercising at an intensity of 70% of his maximum heart rate (heart rate of 119), he would also be exercising at 70% of his VO2 max.

Heart rate can be monitored by electronic means during exercise or by taking your own pulse. An alternate method of determining heart rate is the **Borg scale of perceived exertion**. On a scale from six to twenty, six being absolute rest and twenty being peak exertion, an individual's numeric estimation of exertion times ten corresponds surprisingly well to heart rate. For example, an individual exercising on a treadmill that senses exertion of 16 on the scale of 20 is probably running a heart rate of 160. This procedure and scale eliminates the necessity of taking your pulse while exercising. And as you immerse yourself into your exercise program and become increasingly sensitive to your body, you will be able to estimate your heart rate simply by your perception of exertion.

Achieving the Aerobic Training Effect

The aerobic training effect is muscle specific. Only the specific muscles trained will respond with an aerobic training effect. Running uses slightly different muscles than cycling uses. Swimming uses different muscles entirely. Aerobic training for swimming will not bestow an aerobic training effect for running, cycling or walking. To achieve an aerobic training effect in a specific activity, we must train in that specific activity.

Theoretically, any single muscle fiber can achieve the aerobic training effect of increasing mitochondrial surface area for increased aerobic metabolism of fuels. If we wish to achieve the aerobic training effect (adaptation) for the entire body, we must recruit and train large numbers of muscle fibers. Only through the exercising of large numbers of muscle fibers can we significantly increase the body's oxygen demands. With approximately 50% of the body's total muscle mass located in the hips and thighs, the **optimal aerobic training benefit is achieved by working the muscles of the hips and thighs.**

For an aerobic training effect to occur, one must exercise in the **aerobic training zone** for sufficient duration and with sufficient regularity. The training zone lies between the training threshold and the anaerobic threshold. The training threshold is the minimum work level to produce a training effect, generally a workload to generate 60% of the maximum heart rate. The anaerobic threshold is the upper limit of energy expense above which no aerobic benefits accrue, and all metabolism becomes anaerobic. The anaerobic threshold heart rate is approximately 95% of the maximum heart rate. The **aerobic training zone, therefore, is 60% to 95% of the maximum heart rate,** with the **most efficient aerobic training effect in the 70% - 80% of maximum heart rate range (Figure 4).**

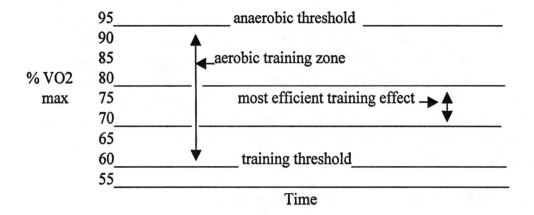

Figure 4

To illustrate the very important concept of the aerobic training zone, let's take Beth to the gym. She is 50 years-old and wishes to achieve an aerobic training effect. We will have her walk on the treadmill for her aerobic exercise. Understanding that her heart rate is a measure of her exercise intensity, what should her heart rate be to achieve her goal?

➤ Her maximum heart rate is calculated from:

$$220 - 50 \text{ (age)} = 170$$

➤ Her aerobic training zone is 60% to 95% of the maximum heart rate of 170:

$$170 \times 60\% = 102$$
$$170 \times 95\% = 161$$

➤ Her aerobic training zone lies between 102 and 161. The most efficient part of the zone lies between 70% and 80% of her maximum heart rate.

➤ Her most efficient training zone lies between:

$$170 \times 70\% = 119$$
$$170 \times 80\% = 136$$

At what intensity should Beth be exercising? She should exercise at an intensity that produces a heart rate of 119 to 136 beats per minute. Exercising in her training zone optimizes Beth's quest to become aerobically fit.

The FIT Principle

The total aerobic effect is a product of frequency, intensity and time spent performing aerobic exercise, a concept known as the **FIT principle** (frequency, intensity and time). FIT training within the aerobic training zone offers wide latitude for aerobic training effect from minimal to maximal, and it offers latitude for individual variations in fitness levels.

Frequency of exercise is essential. Low-fit individuals should exercise two to three times per week, and high-fit individuals may exercise up to six or more times per week. Generally, however, allow at least 24 yours to recover between exercise efforts. Untrained persons may need 48 hours to recover.

The minimum **intensity** necessary to achieve an aerobic training effect is exercising at a calorie rate usage of 7.5 cal/min. Walking a 15 minute mile satisfies this intensity requirement. Any activity achieving a heart rate of 60% of your predicted maximum also satisfies the charge. Below that level minimal aerobic training effect is achieved. Above it, benefits accrue in relation to the exercise intensity up to the anaerobic threshold. In short, the harder you work, the greater your gain.

Assuming constant intensity of exercise, **time** of exercise may be expressed in calories used. Depending upon the fitness level of the individual, different duration of exercise is necessary to achieve an aerobic training effect. A low-fit individual will benefit from a 100 calorie aerobic effort while a medium-fit individual needs 200 – 400 calories per workout to benefit, and a high-fit individual needs 400 – 600 calories per workout for significant aerobic training effect. No additional aerobic benefit is gained by workouts of greater than 600 calories. Aerobic efforts in excess of 600 calories obviously use additional calories, if that is one of your goals. So, duration is important, a greater duration being necessary for the fitter individual to achieve additional benefit. This does not mean that you have to continue working longer and harder as you become fitter. One can maintain at any level.

Maintenance at whatever level you choose is available with two to three times per week workouts at the same intensity and duration that allowed you to reach your plateau. A word of caution is in order. Short-term detraining, the loss of your aerobic training effect, occurs rapidly. Estimates vary from a 10% per week decline in aerobic fitness to half of the aerobic training effect abating in 4.5 to 9.4 days. Recovering to previous levels of fitness requires eight weeks of training. This is a strong argument for regularity of exercise. Use it or lose it.

The rate of gain in aerobic fitness varies and depends upon the participation principle, the more training, the greater the rate of gain. The decline in aerobic fitness over the long term is better defined. Aerobic fitness normally declines with age at an 8-10% per decade rate. **Remaining active can delay the decline to 4% per decade and training can cut it to 2% per decade.**

When we increase our exercise output to levels that provide health and wellness benefits, we must review our nutrition status. Are we supplying enough of the right kinds of fuel for our activities?

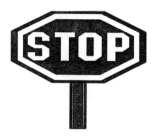

Take a break! We're overloading with information. Let's review:

➤ Americans are sedentary, and we pay a high health price for that fact.
➤ We have too many excuses for not exercising, none of which is valid.
➤ Benefits of exercise are unarguable.
➤ Two distinctly different muscle fiber types respond to different stimuli.
➤ Aerobic metabolism is nineteen times more efficient than is anaerobic.
➤ Stretch warm muscles.
➤ Strength training formula; 2/3 of maximum force, 3 sets of 2 – 12 reps, every other day.
➤ The primary site of aerobic adaptation is the mitochondrion of the skeletal muscle.
➤ The most efficient aerobic training zone is 70% - 80% of maximum heart rate.
➤ Remember to be FIT for your aerobic exercise: frequency, intensity, time.
➤ Excess calories are always stored as fat.

Nutrition Specifics

Dietary requirements for an athlete differ very little in composition from what is considered optimal for the non-athlete. The 20% fat (or less), 15% protein and 65% carbohydrate distribution is still ideal, however, athletes need more calories because of increased energy expenditures. Athletes do not need a greater percentage of protein in their diets, since we will eat more total protein with our greater total caloric intake. Doubling of the protein percentage is recommended only for an athlete on a weight loss diet.

Exercise performance is best on a high carbohydrate diet. Performance decreases as fat intake increases. Post exercise glycogen replacement in muscle, optimal with a high carbohydrate diet, is inhibited by fat intake.

What is the best fluid for hydration during exercise? Either water or a light carbohydrate solution (less than 6%) is adequate. Concentrated carbohydrate solutions inhibit absorption, while mild sodium and electrolyte concentrations enhance and maintain water absorption. Cool fluids stimulate stomach contraction and enhance the movement of the fluid into the intestines where absorption occurs.

Hydration (water intake) is important to the individual at rest and becomes increasingly critical as exercise intensity escalates. One quart of water is needed for each 1,000 calories burned in the metabolic process. As with the resting individual, adequate hydration in the athlete can be monitored by observation of urine color and frequency. Light color of urine and frequent urination is consistent with good hydration.

Water, electrolyte and fuel needs differ between recreational and competitive athletes. Exercise of less than 30 minutes, a 2-mile walk or a 3-mile jog, has no excess fluid or fuel requirements. Exercise of 1-3 hours with excess sweating, losing up to 2-3% of body weight in sweat, requires water replacement during the effort, and will benefit from calorie replacement. A five set tennis final at the U.S. Open will often take four or more hours to complete. Players drink routinely at changeover, and many players use calorie supplements.

Drinking 1-2 cups of water fifteen minutes before exercising will enhance fat metabolism and spare muscle glycogen during exercise. As a rule of thumb, plan to drink one cup of fluid for each 15-20 minutes of extended exercise. Water is fine for exercise duration of less than one hour, but for longer efforts replacement of fuel is desirable with 120-240 cal per hour of a 5% carbohydrate drink.

After exercising, replace water according to weight lost in sweating (weigh yourself before and after exercise), and optimize muscle glycogen replacement with 50 grams of carbohydrate every two hours. I drink water before and during exercise, but my favorite post-workout drink is a 32-ounce bottle of Gatorade, containing 200 calories (50 grams of carbohydrate) in a 5.5% solution by weight. Muscle glycogen replenishment rate, normally 5% per hour, may be increased to 7% per hour by using the 50 grams of carbohydrate every two hours technique. I recommend four or five of the 50-gram feedings.

Another reason that I drink Gatorade as a replacement fluid is the urine conservation property of light carbohydrate solutions. Water alone will stimulate urine production, a potentially undesirable effect when we are trying to replace those lost fluids.

Aside from general nutritional considerations in exercise, environmental conditions affect specific water and electrolyte (sodium, potassium and chloride) concerns. We know that hot environs promote greater fluid and electrolyte losses from sweating, and we know that those losses must be replaced. What are some other environmental conditions that deserve our attention?

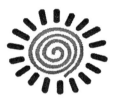

Exercise and the Environment

Normally, we do not give much thought to our environment when exercising because conditions are usually benign enough for us to ignore environmental considerations. Heat, humidity, cold, altitude, wind, clothing and pollution all have direct bearing on body temperature regulation, oxygen supply and energy demands. Anticipation of these environmental variables can prevent frustration, heat injury, frost bite, and altitude sickness.

Temperature regulation is essential for an exercising individual. Heat produced with exercise must be dissipated to protect the integrity of the body organs, especially the brain. The normal temperature regulatory mechanisms are evaporative cooling by sweating and direct heat exchange from the skin to the air. Both are aided by vasodilatation (relaxation of the blood vessels) for added efficiency of cooling. The core body temperature of an exerciser can easily reach 102-104 degrees F. Higher temperatures become increasingly dangerous. In cases of heat stroke, sustained temperatures of 107 degrees F may produce irreversible central nervous system damage or even death.

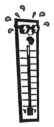

Exercising in high temperatures can be dangerous because of the narrowing temperature differential between the outside ambient air and the internal body temperature, that differential being crucial to heat dissipation from the body. Exercising in 70 degree F environment affords greater cooling capacity than exercising in 100 degree F heat. We can still exercise in hot environments, but these compensatory efforts should be employed: 1) drinking excess fluids with electrolytes 2) planning shorter duration and less intense exercise 3) wearing loose, breathable clothing and 4) exercising in the shade or with a breeze.

Humidity is critical, too. The drier the air the more rapid the evaporation of sweat, hence the better cooling effect. The combination of heat and humidity can be lethal to the exerciser because cooling efficiency is compromised. Although the trained athlete can accommodate this potentially lethal combination better than the untrained athlete, I recommend exercising indoors, exercising early in the morning, or exercising later in the evening in hot and humid conditions. Hydration, always important, is crucial in this environment.

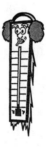

Exercising in the cold has its own set of concerns. Energy demands are greater in the cold, and if there is wind, the demands are greater still. In freezing temperatures frostbite is a concern. Fingers and toes are especially vulnerable, but exposure of the face to cold and wind makes it equally vulnerable. Do not go for a long jaunt in freezing temperatures and run out of energy. In your long walk home you may become frost bitten (or worse). Heat loss from the body occurs rapidly because of the vast temperature differential between the body and the air. As well, the increased evaporation from the skin in windy conditions adds to the cooling efficiency. Anticipate these dangers by dressing and exercising appropriately.

Dress in layers, with one of the newer "wicking" materials next to your skin. These materials remove moisture from the skin, preventing unwanted cooling in a cold environment. Cover your head and face, because a great percentage of body heat is lost there. Wear gloves, too. If it is too cold outside, exercise inside. If you do choose to exercise in the cold, stretch thoroughly. Cold muscles tend to be short muscles and are consequently at a high potential for injury.

Your choice of where you exercise decreases your risk for exercise related illness. As altitude increases, oxygen decreases. At 15,000 feet of altitude the oxygen concentration approximates half that at sea level; at 10,000 feet, about two-thirds; and at 5,000 feet, about four-fifths. Commonly, we hike or run at altitudes between 5,000 and 10,000 feet. Rocky Mountain skiing averages 12,000 to 14,000 feet in altitude. People who normally live at those lofty altitudes have adapted physiologically to the lower oxygen availability, but those of us coming from sea level to higher elevations may experience shortness of breath, nausea, and dizziness with exercise, classic altitude sickness.

Common in the Rockies, altitude sickness responds to time and gradual resumption of exercise. Our bodies require about three weeks to make good adjustments to a higher elevation, or about one week for each 1,000 feet above 5,000 feet. Persistent shortness of breath, however, may signal occult congestive heart failure, a legitimate medical concern, for which immediate medical treatment may be necessary.

Pollution hangs as a common concern in urban areas. Not only does it displace available oxygen, it carries a very real health risk of causing emphysema, lung cancer, prostate cancer, and cardiovascular disease in long term exposures. In the short term, exercising becomes difficult and uncomfortable in the midst of automobile or industrial pollution. Find city parks for exercise, as you will be less likely to inhale a full concentration of pollutants as you might if you exercised near congested traffic areas. Pollution in cities intensifies when temperature inversions occur. Watch your local weather to learn when the temperature inversions are present. Exercise indoors on those days.

Anticipate. If conditions are extreme, think ahead, and plan ahead. Heat, humidity, and altitude are thieves of temperature control and oxygen. Acting in concert, they are a deadly trio.

Special Considerations for Special Groups

Children

Children are the single most important group of people who should begin exercising, for people who exercise as children will most likely exercise throughout their lives. We establish our life-long habits and behaviors in childhood, and we must cement good habits early in our development, rather than change poor habits later in life.

We must teach our children the joy and freedom of physical movement. I would like to see young children avoid the constraints of competition and planned exercise. A child runs naturally. Encourage it. Play with your children; chase after them; let them chase you and catch you. Kick a ball around with them. Toss it to them. A child learns the joy of activity, coordination, balance and speed in these play activities.

I am not a proponent of weight training or specific aerobic exercises for children. Structured programs can be burdensome. If you offer your child one advantage about exercise, make it his or her realization that physical activity is fun.

Women

Anabolic steroids aside, a woman's muscularity and aerobic potential are genetically and hormonally controlled. Women often concern themselves about "bulking up" if they train with weights, but that occurrence is highly unlikely due to their genetic limitations and lack of anabolic (muscle-building) hormones. Testosterone, a hormone required for muscle growth, stays at relatively low levels in women, another reason women do not tend toward muscularity. Genetics determines how muscular a woman can get, she determines how muscular she will get.

Women have excellent aerobic capacity, and they have the ability to increase that capacity through training. The biggest obstacle to improved aerobic fitness for most women to hurdle is the perception that they are somehow limited by the very fact of their womanhood. No such limitation exists. The implication of limitation may have originated in our time-honored comparisons of men and women. Why do we persist in comparing men and women? Men are men and women are women. Their differences make each sex unique and wonderful.

Seniors

Seniors deserve very special consideration, in that so much can be done to forestall physiologic aging and to improve physical fitness. Exercise in seniors produces results. The muscle mass already lost by aging and disuse can be reversed if older people begin to exercise, whenever they begin (seventies, eighties or nineties). The physiology of muscle remains constant over a lifetime.

Muscles always respond to overload training with increased mass and strength. Bone density probably is unaffected by exercise in older ages, but increased muscle strength from exercising can prevent falls. Viewed prospectively, **the "normal" decline in muscle mass that occurs with aging can be slowed and nearly stopped if an individual exercises throughout his life.**

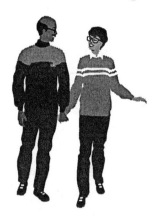

What are the advantages of exercising in our senior years? Seniors will maintain or regain independence, increase their balance, prevent or stabilize osteoporosis, prevent falls, and ameliorate depression and loneliness. Greater opportunities to socialize and foster integration among age-groups results from a healthier senior population. We will have independent, productive seniors, who can take pride in themselves by not burdening their families or society for their care. All of that results from exercise? Yes! The exercising senior may continue to be a positive contributor to our society.

Children, women, and seniors, oft-neglected groups in our society, shouldn't be. Vast untapped potential lies within the members of these groups.

We have discussed a lot of concepts and conundrums to this point. Now it is time to put our exercise knowledge to work.

How to Implement Your Exercise Program

As we learned when we approached changes in our nutrition, we shall select methods rooted in the common denominators of the behavior modification process.

Motivate yourself – How do we stimulate and encourage ourselves to exercise? For some it is easy, but not for others. Learning about exercise and realizing that it is truly beneficial, and that we do not have to be world-class athletes to gain from exercising is a good beginning. If we exercise, we feel better, physically and emotionally. Hard to convince non-exercisers may have to trust me until they can show themselves this truth. The best motivation to exercise is to realize that you are doing something good for yourself.

It's not selfish to want to feel good. Others around you will benefit from your improvement. If we cannot allow ourselves to exercise for ourselves, perhaps we can permit others to encourage us, to motivate us to exercise. Don't be passive and wait half a lifetime for a loved one to encourage you to exercise. Ask her to motivate you. That's right! If you can't motivate yourself, realize that fact, then ask a friend to help.

Choose your attitude – Ask yourself about your present attitude regarding exercise. If it's positive, that's great. You win. If, however, your attitude ebbs to neutral or negative, you have a little homework to do. Attitudes, like everything else in life, are ours for the choosing. I suggest that you search your soul, talk with your mentor, and then calmly choose a positive attitude about exercise.

Choose your expectations – What are your expectations? We generally achieve what we expect to achieve. If you think that you will not stick with exercise, you probably won't. Conversely, if you think you will, you will. Realistic expectations are critical. Write down what you expectation of yourself with respect to your exercise effort. Keep that notation in your notebook. Describe whether you expect to increase strength, increase aerobic capacity, lose weight, become a movie star (remember realistic), or be better able to have fun with your children.

I am fifty-three years old and enjoy tennis, snow skiing, water skiing, river rafting, mountain hiking and roller-blading with my adult children. I expect to have the same enjoyment with my grandchildren.

Choose your physical activity – Choose a physical activity you like, or one that seems intriguing. Exercise must be enjoyable, or you will not continue long at all. Create a list of all the physical activities you would consider: walking, biking, swimming, canoeing, weight training, tennis, and golf. They all count. Put a star by your favorites.

Consider your nutrition – Normally, dietary protein of 15% of total calories should be sufficient unless you are on a weight loss diet, then double the protein intake. Optimal energy comes in the form of a diet high in complex carbohydrates, high in fiber, and low in fat.

Create your exercise schedule – Now look at your weekly schedule. Yes, write it out, twenty-four hour days including sleeping. Is there any free, wasted or "could use it better" time? If so, block it out for yourself. Is your schedule totally full? You may think so, but I doubt it. Take time and make time. Do you watch TV? How long do you spend on meal preparation, eating and cleaning up? Eliminate TV and let the dishes sit. This is important. It is high priority.

Next, write a weekly schedule with your exercise periods written in ink. Allow or create at least three periods of one-half to one hour for exercise for each week. Take your principal calendar and for the coming two months (your committed period), write **EXERCISE** in bold marker across the entire face of each page.

Take your picture – This is the "before" photograph. Place it prominently in your daily planner, in your wallet, on the bathroom mirror, or on your nightstand.

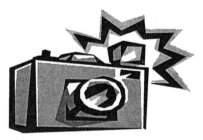

Sign a contract – Finally, write a contract to exercise. Sign it. Date it. Ask family members to witness and sign it, too. Now you may begin. Start slowly because you are in this for the long run (pun, pun).

Commit to a two-month exercise period – I want you to commit to a two-month effort and begin to exercise. Realize that improvement will be slow. It will be at least two weeks before you notice any discernible differences.

Record your workouts – Chart your workouts when you do them, or note your activity, but only review weekly or biweekly. Periodic review enlightens, usually demonstrates progress, but also points out weaknesses or mistakes. Don't frustrate yourself with daily review. If you feel compelled to weigh yourself, do it only every other week.

Reward yourself – Offer yourself rewards at review time, if you did something particularly well in an activity, or if you exceeded your weekly expectation. Rewards are great, like new clothing (it will fit better), a special lunch out (you are already a better calorie burner), or a special evening with your lover (yes, you are better there, too).

Make your exercise social – The social nature of exercise catalyzes success. Take advantage of that fact. Exercise with a friend, at a gym, or in a park. As you integrate socialization with exercise, you will find socialization augmenting your individual exercise efforts.

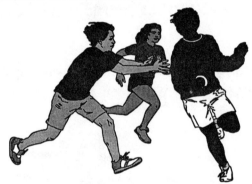

Be in touch with your body and mind – After two weeks you will begin to sense differences in how you look and feel. Pay particular attention to how your body feels. Be in touch with and aware of your body. Are you enjoying yourself? Is it fun? Do you need a change? If so, make the change.

Exercise where your body happens to be – If you choose not to exercise at a gym, then exercise where ever you are, home, office, or in the woods. Do some abdominal crunches while watching TV at home, perform push-ups in your office for a short break, or pick a challenging trail in the woods to hike. Remember, it all adds up; every exercise you perform crediting your activity account.

Practice awareness – Be aware of the motion and feel of your body as you exercise. Feel the arc of your strength-training exercise. Know your breathing. Be aware of your heel as it strikes the ground. You may meditate while you exercise.

Review, modify and communicate – Try a new sport, a different workout, a different locale. Put up reminders in prominent places around the house about your commitment and successes. Are there classes available that you might enjoy or benefit from? Talk with your friends or mate about your successes, failures, or problems. The solutions are usually self-evident when you verbalize. Ventilate. Tell people that you are exercising. It is surprising how many positive responses you will receive. Enlist people who are receptive and ask for their support. These efforts reinforce a wonderful behavior change that you are making.

Expect success – About four to six weeks into your commitment of eight weeks you will begin to sense success. You will have experienced physical and emotional improvement. Nothing succeeds like success. It's powerful. "I am doing it. I did it. I wasn't really sure that I could, but step by step, I did." An early congratulations is in order. Self-confidence and self-image are bolstered. Begin to see yourself as a role model for exercise. Your friends, family and peers will have watched you succeed (and I assure you that they do watch). Your success influences those around you, for they might consider that they can succeed as you have.

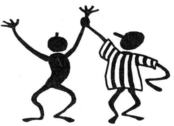

Sign a new contract – At the completion of your eight-week contract, you have a choice. You may return to pre-exercise slothfulness or sign another contract. I want you to sign another contract. You do, too. Repeat the original procedure and sign for sixteen weeks this time. Do all of the original planning, examination and review. It's the second contract that will begin to solidify your behavior change. During this second period, exercise will come more easily and naturally. It becomes part of your life. One step at a time, behavior modification is a long process.

Trick yourself if you feel stale or unmotivated – What do you do if you begin to feel stale and your enthusiasm wanes? Remember variety, fun, socialization, and realistic expectations. There's nothing wrong with taking a few rest-days off as long as you positively choose to do so. Assure yourself that you are not passively drifting away from your program. Remember rewards, too. Victory celebrations are great. Trick yourself. Bait and switch. If you don't feel like exercising at your scheduled time, go to your exercise locale anyway with the idea of doing just a light workout. After you have started, you will probably do more than you had planned.

Expect plateaus – Plateaus are to be expected. Both physical and mental, each is very real. Please don't be intimidated or discouraged by the normal occurrence of plateaus. Allow their existence and then proceed toward your goal.

Develop an active lifestyle – Finally, combine physical activity into your daily schedule. Walk the stairs; park at the far end of the parking lot and walk to your destination; walk to lunch. All of the energy that we spend accrues to our credit.

Develop a social conscience – Now that you have experienced success with your own exercise program, perhaps you would consider the larger picture with me for a moment. We must begin to change the social perception of exercise from exclusive to inclusive. Exercise must become easily accessible, socially acceptable, and desirable.

Service organizations like Rotary, Lions, and Kiwanis can donate their time and effort to implement on-going exercise programs for all ages, youths to seniors. Municipalities can make their parks more user-friendly, a place for exercise and socialization, with inexpensive fitness trails and good lighting for nighttime use. Advertise the new ideas and programs on public service TV channels, in newspapers, and through voluntary speaking engagements. Volunteers can go door to door with a personal invitation to join the fun. What great exercise for the volunteer to walk about town and meet new people. Police departments could reap great public relations rewards if they were to become active in encouraging and facilitating exercise in the community. The possibilities are limitless, and once initiated, will be self-stimulating and self-sustaining.

I ask you as individuals to take part in this effort because it is a good thing to do, and everyone wins. I have done it successfully on my own local level. We must integrate and involve ourselves into the process of improving our national health. By doing so, we will become strong threads in the fabric of our national health.

Enough editorializing, we must get back to specifics. Let's stretch.

Writing Your Own Stretching Prescription

Observe animals – We can learn a lot by watching animals. So instinctively aware of it's body, the big cat waking from his nap, takes a long, slow, purposeful stretch. Our Siberian Husky greets me at the door with a long, front-quarter extension and a low Husky growl-howl. Animals only move quickly to capture their food, usually after instinctively stretching and warming their muscles.

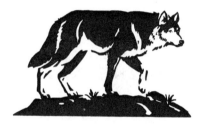

Stretch warm muscles – Break a mild sweat by warming up gently, then stretch. Warm muscles stretch more easily and with less injury potential.

Stretch statically – Don't do ballistic stretches. Ballistic, or bouncing stretches, have a high potential for injury and actually cause shortening of the muscle. Stretches should be gradual, purposeful, and held for a period of thirty seconds.

Don't cause pain – Stretches should never be done to the point of discomfort. If you ever sense pain, it indicates the initiation of the stretch reflex, a muscle-shortening phenomenon.

Be aware of the muscles that you are stretching – Know which muscle you stretch. If it's your quadriceps, know that. If it's your hamstrings, know that, too. Explore and experiment with your body, and learn what stretches are best for your needs. Discover how to best stretch your biceps, how to stretch your back, how to stretch your hands and feet. Don't rush, stretching educates you about yourself.

I prefer not to provide a cookbook style litany of specific stretches. I want you to experiment and discover. Take the time, for the benefits are legion. If you truly have no foundation for stretching, allow me to describe a few simple ones.

1) Neck stretch – Tilt your head to your right, keeping both shoulders down. Placing your right hand on the left side of your head, gently pull your head down toward your right shoulder. Switch sides and repeat. Hold each stretch for 30 seconds. Do a similar stretch forward and backward, being cautious not to extend your head too far aft.

2) Arm stretch – With arms fully extended, grasp the corner of a wall with your right hand. Gently apply a stretch to the front of your arm by rotating your torso slowly to the left. Stretch the other arm similarly. To stretch the back of your arm, flex fully at your elbow, then pull your flexed upper arm across the front of your torso with the opposite hand. Repeat for the other side.

3) Back stretch – Sit on a chair or bench and slowly bend straight forward, then forward to the left and forward to the right. Compliment this stretch by rotating your torso left and right, holding the stretch at the end of each rotation.

4) Thigh stretch (for quadriceps) – Place your left hand against a wall for balance, grasp your right ankle with your right hand, gently pulling your right heel toward your buttocks. Switch sides and repeat.

5) Thigh stretch (for hamstrings) – Lie on your back with both knees bent. With your right leg fully extended, grasp behind your right thigh and pull up and back toward your chest. Switch legs and repeat.

6) Calf stretch – Stand on the tread of a stair, supported only by your forefoot. Slowly allow your heels to sink beneath the level of the tread. Lean forward for additional stretch if desired.

7) Hip stretch – Step one foot up on the seat of a chair while keeping the other foot firmly planted on the ground. Allow your body to lean forward over the foot on the chair. Hold for 30 seconds, then switch to the other leg.

8) Outer thigh stretch – Lying on your left side, flex your right knee and hip, allowing your thigh to approach the ground with the pull of gravity. Hold for 30 seconds, then switch sides and legs.

9) Inner thigh stretch – Sit on the floor and bring your feet together as close to your groin as comfortable. Gently push your knees toward the floor, stretching the inner thighs.

These represent but a few of the many stretches you may enjoy. Use them as a basis for developing your stretching routine.

Writing Your Own Strength Training Prescription

Employ proper technique – Begin your program slowly, with weights that you can handle. Do not over-do and injure yourself early. Warm up for five minutes until you begin to sweat, then stretch thoroughly. Recall that warm muscles stretch better. Use a spotter for safety and companionship.

Remember, high resistance, low repetitions increases strength (fast twitch fibers) and low resistance, high repetitions increases endurance (slow twitch fibers). **No single exercise or machine trains both fibers simultaneously.**

Breathing and form combine as you perform strength training exercises. Exhale on the contraction phase; inhale on the release phase. Exercise through the full range of motion of each joint. Always exercise in control and slowly. I recommend a slow, "seven count rep."

1. Contraction phase - "One one-thousand, two one-thousand" (counting seconds)
2. Squeeze - "Three one-thousand, four one-thousand"
3. Release phase - "Five one-thousand, six one-thousand, seven one-thousand"

Work the larger, proximal muscles (those muscles nearest the trunk of the body) first, followed by the peripheral ones. The reason: exercising of the larger muscles usually involves concomitant use of the peripheral smaller ones. Early fatigue of the smaller muscles will limit your efforts to work the larger muscles. Allow recovery time between sets of the same muscle groups as you work out, either by a brief rest period or by alternating opposing muscle groups (e.g., alternate biceps and triceps, or alternate arms and legs).

An alternative to the classic rest periods between sets involves the incorporation of "drop sets." "Drop sets" refers to the practice of immediately following a set of one exercise by another set of the same exercise with a lowered weight. The muscle, already fatigued, becomes progressively fatigued with a lower weight, and the risk of injury decreases because of the lowered weight. I prefer and advise rest periods between sets, but the incorporation of "drop sets" provides variety for your program.

Have realistic expectations – Expect progress at a rate of 1-3% increase in strength per week, and expect to experience plateaus.

Consider frequency – Strength training is best accomplished with at least three sessions per week. As you progress, you may wish to increase the frequency, but always allow adequate time for your muscles to recover. To maintain strength, working out with resistance training two times per week will afford long term maintenance. Once weekly workouts will only maintain strength for six weeks.

Your strength training formula – We have defined the optimal strength-training schedule of 2/3 max, 2 – 10 reps (3 sets), every other day.

Proposed framework – I would like to offer you a skeletal framework upon which you may build your personal strength program. Remember to exercise proximal muscles first, and to alternate opposing muscle groups as well as to alternate arm and leg exercises. The alternation allows time for recovery of the immediately exercised muscle group. This example sequence of exercises incorporates the above principles.

1) Lat pull downs (back and biceps)
2) Chest press (chest and triceps)
3) Leg extensions (quadriceps, front of the thighs)
4) Leg curls (hamstring muscles, back of the thighs)
5) Deltoid raises (deltoids, shoulders)
6) Leg adductors (inner thigh)
7) Leg abductors (outer thigh)
8) Pectoralis flexors (chest flexors)

9) Biceps curls (upper arm, front)
10) Triceps extensions (upper arm, back)
11) Calf raises (lower leg, back)
12) Resisted toe raises (lower leg, front)
13) Abdominals (abs)
14) Back extensions (long back muscles)

Any health club in the country will have the equipment to perform and an explanation of how to perform these fourteen exercises. Three sets of 2 – 10 repetitions and you are done. Early on, do one set and progress to two, then go to three. Once you are well into your muscular training effort, do more if you wish.

This sequence of fourteen exercises works nearly all of the body's muscles and takes not more than fifteen minutes per set to accomplish. You can vary the sequence, concentrate on legs or arms, abs or shoulders, where-ever you need the improvement. The strength that you gain will add to your sense of vitality, sense of self and sense of success in other athletic pursuits.

For those of you who develop hives at the mere thought of going to a health club, I suggest that you design a strength training sequence for your home. The same general principles apply. The only equipment that I advise is a set of variable weight dumbbells, a bar for chin-ups and an exercise mat. We can produce the same set of exercises at home, just as we did in the health club.

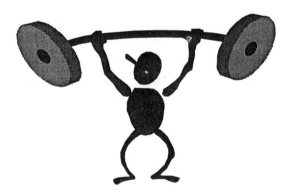

1) Lat pull downs – Do a chin-up instead. The same muscle groups are worked. If you can't do a chin-up, assist with your legs just a bit. Do what you can and build from there.

2) Chest press – Lying on the floor or on a bench, press dumbbells in both hands slowly upward. Squeeze and release slowly. Do a set of 8 – 10 reps.

3) Leg extensions – Seated in a chair, hook your toes under a sofa and try to lift the sofa up. Unless you are particularly strong, you will not be able to do it, but you will be working your quadriceps muscles in the attempt. Do a set of 8 – 10 reps.

4) Leg curls – Lying prone on your exercise mat, extend your leg at your hip. Attempt to raise your heel as high as you can. Do a set of 8 – 10 reps. The hamstring and gluteal muscles are worked with this exercise.

5) Deltoid raises – With relatively light weights in hand, lift the weights laterally and up in an arc, to the point where your arms are parallel with the ground. Squeeze and release slowly. Repeat and do a set of 8 – 10 reps.

6) Leg adductors – Using a partner, have your partner resist your squeezing your knees together. Your partner should provide enough resistance to make the exercise difficult but not impossible. Do a set of 8 – 10 reps.

7) Leg abductors – Again using a partner, have your partner apply resistance to your moving your knees apart. Again, do a set of 8 – 10 reps.

8) Pectoralis flexors – Lying supine, with weights in hand, arms fully extended to your side, lift in an arcing motion, bringing the weights above your chest. This exercise differs in form from the chest press in that the press is a forward pushing motion, while this is an arcing motion. Do 8-10 reps.

9) Biceps curls – Seated, with your elbow placed on your thigh, moderate weight in hand, move the weight from full extension of your arm to full flexion. Exercise one arm, then the other. Guess how many. Remember to squeeze, then release

10) Triceps extensions – Push-ups are ideal. Vary the resistance of your push-up by the placement of your feet. A push-up done with your knees on the ground offers less resistance than one with your feet on the ground. Placing your feet up on a chair offers more resistance yet. Do 8-10 reps.

11) Calf raises – Using the stairs, place your toes on the tread, then raise and lower your weight with your calves. Do I need to suggest a number?

12) Resisted toe raises – Again, hook your toes under the sofa while standing, then try to lift the sofa by raising your feet with your heel as the fulcrum.

13) Abdominals – Lying supine on your exercise mat, do crunches. With hands lightly behind your head, raise your head and shoulders off the floor and hold for five seconds. For greater resistance and difficulty, extend your arms over your head. Do twenty.

14) Back extensions – Lying prone on your exercise mat, lift your head and shoulders up 4 – 6 inches off of the mat. Hold for five seconds and release slowly. Do ten.

With a little practice you will be able to garner the same strength training stimulus from these home exercises as you would from doing similar exercises at a gym. An additional benefit of learning this set of exercises is that they may be done anywhere – home, hotel, or office.

Writing Your Own Aerobic Training Prescription

Determine your fitness category – Begin your program design by determining your fitness category: low, medium, or high. You can probably estimate your aerobic fitness level from how active you have been for the past six months: not very active (low), walking regularly (medium), good, vigorous exercise participation (high). You may also take the walk a mile as fast as you can test (Appendix).

Choose your aerobic exercise – With an understanding of aerobic metabolism, of the aerobic training effect and of the benefits of achieving an aerobic training effect; you may select and design an aerobic program suited to your preferences, schedule, and needs. You have almost limitless latitude of choice. Do you want to walk, jog, bike, jump rope, or do a step class? How long? How often?

Design your program based on FIT – Remember the principles of aerobic exercise: FIT - frequency, intensity and time (duration). Ideally, aerobic exercise should be performed four times per week, but three times is acceptable. The intensity should approximate 70-80% of VO2 max as determined by your heart rate (70-80% of your age-predicted maximum heart rate). The duration should be long enough to spend adequate calories for your fitness level (low fitness requires 100-200 calories; medium fitness requires 200-400 calories and high fitness requires 400-600 calories). Select an activity with an energy rate expense of at least 7.5 cal/min to ensure an aerobic training effect. Use the exercise planning charts to help plan your program. Let me demonstrate some different plans.

Examples of Exercise Programs

Initial Questions:
1) current level of fitness?
2) what you want to accomplish?
3) realistic time available?

Example 1

fitness - low, beginner
goal - increase strength, appearance, weight loss, general well-being
time - 5 hours per week (one hour per day for five days)

Program:
Stretching - 7 days per week, at home in the morning
Aerobic - 3 days per week, for weight loss and well-being
Strength - 2 days per week, for strength and appearance
Duration - 8 weeks, sign the contract

The aerobic portion of the program will use 100 – 200 calories per workout because the exerciser is a beginner in the low fitness category. Walking one to two miles will satisfy that calorie requirement, and walking is a great exercise for beginners. We already know how. Stationary bicycles are an excellent choice, too. A twenty-minute ride will spend 100 – 200 calories.

Strength training would be best accomplished at a gym where weights and machines are available. Sometimes the gym atmosphere can be intimidating, and your home may offer a non-threatening environment for the beginning exerciser. One set of the fourteen exercises outlines in the section on weight training is a fine start. Within one or two weeks, increase to two sets and perhaps three sets by the third or fourth week. There's no rush.

Keep records and review every two weeks (weekly if you are truly obsessive). Reward yourself for success.

Example 2

fitness - medium
goal - increase strength, tone, appearance, improve athletic performance
time - seven hours per week

Program:
    Stretching - 7 days per week
    Aerobic - 4 days per week
    Strength - 3 days per week
    Duration - 8 weeks, sign the contract

The aerobic portion of the program will use 200 – 400 calories per workout because the exerciser places in the medium fitness category. Riding a stationary bicycle for thirty minutes, walking rapidly for thirty minutes, or working on a rowing machine for twenty-five to thirty minutes will satisfy the caloric requirement. A ten-calorie per minute intensity is a reasonable output of energy, affording good aerobic training stimulus.

Again, I feel that a gym atmosphere is the best for weight training. Everything you need is available and the social environment is stimulating. For recluses, stay at home, but you will need the minimum home equipment. Start the program with two sets of the fourteen exercises and progress to three soon. Vary the exercises or add some others. Add weight when you are able to do ten repetitions. On occasion do more than three sets.

Keep records. Review your progress. Reward yourself. *Get a Life!*

Sample Form for Exercise Prescription and Recording

Fitness level _____

Goals _____

Time available _____

Basic formulas: Strength: 3 sets, 2-10 reps, every other day

Stretching: every day

Aerobic: every other day

Weekly Schedule: Sun   Mon   Tue   Wed   Thu   Fri   Sat

Stretching ____|____|____|____|____|____|____

Strength ____|____|____|____|____|____|____

Aerobic ____|____|____|____|____|____|____

Aerobic Training

Activity _____

Rate of calorie use _____

Calories to be used _____

Strength Training

Exercise	Weight	Sets	Reps
Lat pull downs	_____	_____	_____
Chest press	_____	_____	_____
Leg extensions	_____	_____	_____
Leg curls	_____	_____	_____
Deltoid raises	_____	_____	_____
Leg abductors	_____	_____	_____
Leg adductors	_____	_____	_____
Pectoralis flexors	_____	_____	_____
Biceps curls	_____	_____	_____
Triceps extensions	_____	_____	_____
Calf raises	_____	_____	_____
Resisted toe raises	_____	_____	_____
Abdominals	_____	_____	_____
Back extensions	_____	_____	_____

Integrating Activities and Sports into Your Program

Any physical activity or sport proves a valuable inclusion or addition to an exercise program. Properly performed they offer aerobic or strength training effects. Practiced beneath the training thresholds, while offering no aerobic

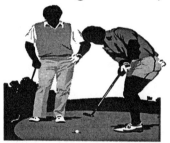

benefit, they still use calories. Activities are fun, offer variety, promote socialization, and build coordination. All activity becomes valuable and useful. Be aware of how your chosen sport or activity benefits you and your exercise program. What is its relative intensity? How many calories does it use? Knowledge affords you the opportunity for better choices.

Here is a list of sports and activities with the energy expense for each endeavor (energy requirements). Increase or decrease the energy requirement by 10% for each 15 pounds above or below 150 pounds.

Activity	Energy requirement (cal/min)
Sleeping	1.2
Sitting	1.3
Eating	1.5
Standing	1.5
Talking	1.8
Light activity	2.6
Showering	3.4
Sweeping floors	3.9
Ironing	4.2
Mopping floors	4.9
Gardening	5.6
Chopping wood	7.5 – *Minimum intensity for
Digging a hole	7.5 aerobic training
Walking up stairs	10.0

133

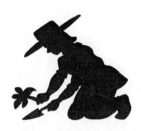

<u>Sports</u>

Golfing	4.0
Walking (3.5 MPH, 17 min/mile)	6.0
Swimming (leisurely)	6.0
Walking (4 MPH, 15 min/mile)	7.5 – ***Minimum intensity for**
Water skiing	8.0 **aerobic training**
Cycling (10 MPH)	8.5
Tennis	9.0
Mountain climbing	10.0
Racquetball	10.0
Cross country skiing (6 MPH)	12.0
Jumping rope	12.0
Wrestling	14.4
Running (7.5 MPH, 8 min. mile)	15.0
Running (marathon pace)	30.0

Quietly, for a professional lifetime, Gary W. carried mail by foot to the residents of Chatham. Upon his retirement at age sixty-five, he thought it would be a good idea to have a general physical because he suspected some heart disease in his family. He wanted a treadmill stress test to have the best chance at diagnosis or to offer greater reassurance of health.

I'm here to tell you that a stress test is physically demanding. When I was in my forties and in great shape, I could only get mid-way through stage seven. Gary calmly proceeded to mid stage nine, nearly completing a test that most professional athletes would struggle to finish.

The moral of the story – routine, lifelong exercise works. His stress test was as negative as it could be, not so much as a blip out of place. He continued to walk after his retirement as if he still worked.

Whom Should You Trust? How Do You Select an Advisor?

"Thrust ivrybody, but cut th' ca-ards."

❖

Finley Peter Dunne

Get a Life, America! can't teach you everything, although I wish it could. I can't be there to answer questions that may arise. I can't be present to motivate your exercising, but I hope that you know my joy if I had anything to do with your exercising. Periodically, you will need someone to whom you may turn for questions, encouragement or advice. Who is your smart monkey in the jungle?

My philosophy is and always has been: TRUST YOURSELF, FIRST! Of course, we cannot be expert in all aspects of our lives, but we can educate ourselves to a point of being able to judge others' levels of expertise. Progressively educate yourself about your health and exercise program. Read at your leisure. Subscribe to selected magazines like *Walking, Runner's World, Outside* or *Women's Sports and Fitness*. They are full of information. Question as you read, making sure the answers you find are consistent with your degree of knowledge and understanding.

Currently, no universally accepted certification for expertise about exercise, and no requirement in the fitness industry for such a certification exists. At some point certification will be the norm. Until then, it's buyer beware. We assume health club personnel, personal trainers, coaches, advisors, and TV "fitness pros" all have some background in exercise, but how do we judge the adequacy of that background?

The American College of Sports Medicine offers certification in many areas of exercise. If an individual has such a certification, that is to his and your advantage. Beyond that certification, ask the individual for a copy of his Curriculum Vitae, his formal training and experience. Read it. Write down your parameters before seeking advice, and then review after discussion with the individual to determine his "score" for you. How easy is it to talk with him and to work with him? Try to get a sense of his motivation, philosophy and direction. Be cautious of people with unbridled enthusiasm, an agenda or a product to sell. Evaluate many different people until you find one with whom you feel comfortable. Their background, philosophy and personality are equally important in your choosing them as an advisor. No one program, idea or person is entirely correct or can provide all of what you need.

135

In conclusion

We can change the face of our individual health, and we can change the face of our nation's health. Both efforts begin with us and begin with our choosing to develop more active lifestyles. Keep this philosophy in mind as you read the remainder of *Get a Life!*, thinking of prospective ideas to facilitate our evolution to better national health. I ask for your ideas in the last chapter. Help me help you to *Get a Life, America!*

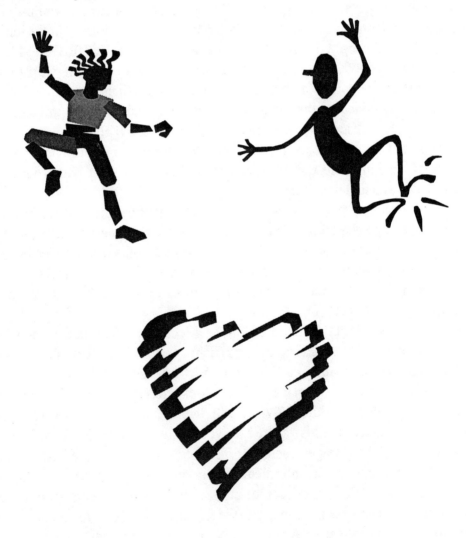

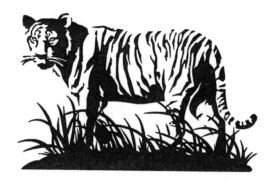

Chapter IV

"Through the Eye of the Tiger"

*"Fight for your highest attainable aim,
But do not put up resistance in vain."*

❖

Hans Selye, MD

This is a chapter about stress. Duh! Of course it is. You will learn what stress is. Ha! You will learn that stress is as difficult to define as it is to capture an ethereal butterfly delicately between your thumb and forefinger. We'll talk about the physiology of stress, how abnormal thought patterns make stress worse, how communication styles help or hinder your stress, the danger of peak performance, but mostly we'll focus on *Getting a Life!* as we find health, happiness and love in a stressful world.

Did you know that the stress of tax time raises accountants' blood pressure and cholesterol to dangerously high levels? Did you know that stress kills by the same biochemical mechanism as does cocaine? Did you know that you are blindly subject to the insidious effects of this stealthy killer on a day to day and hour to hour basis? Stress lurks as an omnipresent danger, yet we seem to ignore the lethal risks of stress because it has become integral in our modern day existence.

Like a hungry tiger, it's a vicious killer. So let's *Get a Life, America!* and ferret out some life saving information about this wily adversary.

I have never read a dissertation about stress introduced with an allegory other than the one about the caveman and the saber-toothed tiger, an allegory so well used as to be threadbare. You know the one – tiger surprises caveman who has an immediate alarm reaction – heart racing, pupils dilating, adrenaline surging, and caveman running to escape. Yes, the alarm reaction is a protective mechanism that worked well for the caveman, but in modern man the same extreme response to perceived threat has become maladaptive and even counterproductive. Let us begin, however, in the same prehistoric epoch and launch our study of stress through the eyes of the tiger.

Tigris Eatalotofus pads stealthily through the dense growth of a prehistoric forest. He is a marvelous specimen, five-hundred pounds of hungry killing machine. Just ahead in a modest clearing two cavemen pause for a brief rest, having spent their morning in a futile search for small game. *Tigris* enters the clearing, surprising the cavemen, and himself. Biologic emergency alarms sound in all three. *Tigris* salivates because he sees the potential for food. The cavemen, let's call them Lunch and Dinner, quake with fear. In unison all three feel the rush of adrenaline, the quickening of their pulses, and they spring to action. Dinner happens to be a bit quicker than Lunch and escapes. Lunch, quickly seized and killed, is lunch. *Tigris* eats his fill and drags the remainder of Lunch to his lair for his mate and cubs. Mindful that he had come upon two cavemen, *Tigris* returns to the clearing, catches the scent of Dinner and follows it to Dinner's cave. Unable to gain entrance to the cave because it perches high upon a cliff, *Tigris* marks the spot and returns to his lair. Knowing that food waits in that unreachable cave frustrates *Tigris,* and he returns daily for a month hoping to find a way into the cave. Dinner sits inside, paralyzed with fear in anticipation of the return of the tiger. Gradually the frequency of *Tigris'* visits lessens, but Dinner's fear grows. He begins to feel fatigue, his diet suffers, he develops stomach pain and eventually an ulcer. His ulcer bleeds and he dies. Dinner, a prehistoric caveman, dies the death of a twentieth century businessman, hemorrhage from a stress-induced ulcer.

This simple allegory demonstrates many principles about stress. What would Hans Selye, MD, the "father of stress," have to say about this sequence of events? He would probably say that it is a silly story, but in its silliness provides entertainment, a stress reliever in itself. He would see the presence of the General Adaptation Syndrome (GAS) that he described in his early work on stress. The

GAS is a nonspecific response of the body in response to a wide variety of stimuli, the purpose of the response being adaptive in nature. The adaptive response in the cavemen was to attempt to protect themselves while the adaptive response in the tiger was to feed himself. Both responses attempt to ensure the survival of the species.

The physiologic response to the stressors in each of the participants was strikingly similar, demonstrating the pan-species consistency of the stress response. The non-specific bodily response is nearly identical in rats, tigers, and man; in prehistoric times or in the present day. All species are vulnerable to stress and react to it by a common pathway stress response.

The tiger had good stress while the cavemen had bad stress, yet their physiologic responses were the same. From the point of view of the stress producing activity it makes no difference whether the agent or situation we face is pleasant or unpleasant. It seems incongruous that such contrasting stimuli should produce a common response in different individuals. Yet, this is indeed the case, for it has been demonstrated that certain reactions of the body are common to all types of exposures.

Although Dr. Selye postulated the stress response to be universal, and it is to a large degree, recent research has added specificity to the individual response, especially in man. Through socialization, learning, experiences, and personality development, individuals learn to modulate their stress responses. It is through the individual modulation that specific target organ systems become involved in the response. In modern society we have learned to mute the magnitude of our stress responses and unconsciously redirect the stressor effect to target organs. Gastrointestinal disorders, strokes, heart attacks, headaches, and increased susceptibility to disease in general are the modern result of "learning" to channel stressors.

Not only do we "learn" to channel stress to target organ systems, we also "learn" to perceive stress. With the evolution of man's ability to think, he has developed the propensity to attach his own emotional finger print labels to events. Perceiving that the tiger would eventually, somehow, capture and eat him, created Dinner's paralytic fear. If Dinner had thought logically, he would have realized that the tiger could never enter his cave because it was too high. He was actually safe. In large part, man's cerebral evolution has led him to the emotional position where **stress is perception.**

The implication is inherent in Dinner's circumstance that the repetition, intensity, and duration of the perceived stressor were integral in his deteriorating health. The stress response evolved to protect the organism from immediate

139

danger, but the perpetuation of the stress response over time results in "dis-stress." The organism's ability to adapt and to cope is severely taxed, and its protective immune system becomes dangerously compromised. Who knows what other as yet undiscovered stress related effects lurk within the dark reaches of our physiology and psyche?

Such a simple story as I have just spun carries with it far-reaching principles and implications. So it is with stress. What seems apparent and simple actually masks a very complex and secretive issue.

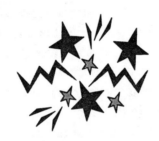

What is Stress?

Everybody knows what stress is, and nobody knows what stress is. The word stress, like success, failure, or happiness means different things to different people. With the exception of a handful of scientists who study stress, no one has attempted to define it clearly. Still, however, it has become part of our daily vocabulary. Stress is effort, pain, fear, humiliation of censure, physical injury, or unexpected success like winning a lottery. Each of these conditions can be singled out as being the "it," the critical essence of stress.

How can we expect to cope with the stress of life if we cannot even define what we are dealing with? The pressured executive, the threatened caveman, and a wife who helplessly watches as her husband dies of cancer are all subject to stress. Their problems differ, but the internal biochemical reactions they all experience are similar. The factors that demand adaptive changes in each of these individuals are called stressors. The reaction is the stress response.

Stress is not simply nervous tension. It is not the non-specific result of damage. It is not always evident. Often the effects of stress go unnoticed, or become evident only after long term exposure. Stress is not to be avoided necessarily, for complete freedom from stress is death. We can meet it efficiently and selectively. We can enjoy it and learn how to adjust and to adapt.

Although we see ourselves in individual lights, in reality, our existences are quite common. As humans, we have similar experiences, fears, frustrations and stressors. What are stressors common to us all? Here are just a few – change, loss of a loved one, feelings of helplessness, feelings of loss of control, illness, anger or frustration, too much stimulation or too little, and unpredictability.

Each of us is unique in our threshold of response according to temperament, early life experiences, personality, recent life changes and our social support from family, friends, or professionals. People differ markedly, too, in how they respond by different organ systems. We should always be alert for these widely divergent bodily expressions of stress – feelings of anxiety, chest pain, headaches, high blood pressure, rapid heart rate, weight loss, loss of appetite, loss of sexual desire, fatigue and depression, sleep difficulty, shortness of breath, and frequent colds. These stress related symptoms exact a huge personal toll, and also are associated with significant losses to our society.

Stress Exacts an Exorbitant Social Toll

According to the American Association of Family Practice, stress related symptoms prompt at least two-thirds of office visits to family doctors. Industry leaders have become alarmed by the cost of such symptoms manifested in employee absenteeism, company medical expenses, and decreased productivity. Based on national samples these costs have been estimated between $75 and $150 billion per year, more than $1,000 per year for each worker. Corporations are being asked to foot this rapidly escalating financial burden.

We know stress to be a major contributor, either directly or indirectly, to coronary heart disease, cancer, lung ailments, accidental injuries, cirrhosis, and suicide – six of the leading causes of death in the United States. Stress plays an aggravating role in such diverse conditions as multiple sclerosis, diabetes, and herpes. It has been quoted that "our mode of life itself, the way we live, is emerging as today's principal cause of illness."

The upheaval in society's most basic values adds greatly to the general level of anxiety. Even our pleasures are often fretful. The results of a New York University study about sources of stress revealed that the greatest source of stress to married men and women was the change in society's attitude towards sex, including sexual permissiveness and "the new social roles of the sexes." While stress may have once taken the form of an occasional calamity, it is now a "chronic relentless psychosocial situation." Stress is so omnipresent that we are evolving to a point of addiction to stress, addiction to our own adrenaline secretion. Stress, in addition to being itself, and the result of itself, is also the cause of itself.

If stress looms so nebulous and ethereal, a diaphanous veil shrouding clear vision of our lives, how do we measure it? In the 1940's and 1950's psychiatrist, Thomas Holmes, and psychologist, Richard Rahe, attempted to quantitate the effects of stress through the development of the now widely used Holmes-Rahe (aptly named) scale. Leading the scale with an assignment of 100 points is the death of a spouse, followed by a 73 point divorce and a 63 point prison sentence. Positive stress scored well, too, with marriage rating a 50, pregnancy a 40, and my favorite, Christmas, at 12. High scores on the scale carry predictive value of stress-related illness and accidents.

The Holmes-Rahe scale may not be as accurate as a well-Windexed crystal ball, but it provides a good and useful prognosticator of relative risk. Their scale also proves a good tool for initiating awareness about stress in our lives. Remember that stress occurs not only from major life events but also from the accumulation of everyday annoyances and hassles of our lives.

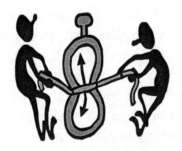

.... It is not the large things that
send a man to the
madhouse ..... no, it's the
        continuing series of
small tragedies
that send a man to the madhouse

        ....

not the death of his love
but a shoelace that snaps
with no time left.........

Stress poses a significant risk of disease and death. Stressors are often not isolated events but carry with them a ripple effect. Divorce is not an isolated event. It is accompanied by some social isolation, often drastic economic changes, and sometimes the complications of being a single parent. This combination of results becomes a chronic strain on the individual's life. Joblessness has a similar ripple effect. The greatest source of stress is not the actual loss of the job, but rather the waterfall series of associated changes.

The ripple effect extends beyond individuals, to society. The chronicity of stressful problems is expressed in rates of diseases. A sociologic study in the 1940's documented that for each 1% increase in the unemployment rate, there were 1.9% more deaths from heart disease and cirrhosis, 4.1% more suicides, and an upturn in the number of first-time admissions to state mental hospitals. The chronicity of stress eventually overwhelms our ego defensive coping capacity, and diseases become manifest.

The trials and tribulations of our lives, however, are less important than how one deals with them. How an individual adapts to and copes with a stressor is more important than the stressor itself. Certain populations are known for their good health and longevity. Mormons, nuns, symphony conductors, and women who are listed in *Who's Who* have been particularly notable in this respect. Something in the lives of these groups supports their collective longevity. Faith, pride in their work and accomplishments, and creativity may play a role in the attenuation of the effects of stress. Conversely, it is known that widows die at a rate 13 times higher than their married counterparts for every known cause of death. Psychologists postulate multiple reasons. Among the reasons are a sense of being out of control of their lives, not having a network of friends or family to provide "social support," and lacking such personality factors as flexibility and hopefulness.

Attitude and social support carry enormous prognostic influence over illnesses. A lack of closeness to parents and a negative attitude toward one's family have been strongly linked to cancer, mental illness and suicide. People with few close contacts die two to three times faster than those who regularly turn to close friends.

Isn't it odd to think of friends in terms of the chemical advantage they might offer to us? Our chemical reaction to our perceived stressors may have other effects, too. The stress mediated jolt of excitatory chemicals released into the bloodstream could be causing more fat to be released into the blood, thereby raising the risk of deposition of the fat in the blood vessel walls, the end result being hardening of the arteries. Caffeine, a popular drug of the stressed person, is a risk too. Two and one-half cups of coffee doubles the circulating level of epinephrine. **The combination of high demands and low control in our lives raises our risk of heart disease the same order of magnitude as smoking or having high cholesterol.**

I don't think that we have to make the case that stress is an ambiguous, often unconscious, life threatening entity any stronger. It simply is, and more.

Before we begin to study the physiology of stress let me offer a Stress Index Test to pique your interest. Score each item from 1 (almost always) to 5 (never) according to how much of the time each statement applies to you.

_____1. I eat at least one hot, balanced meal a day.
_____2. I get seven to eight hours of sleep at least four nights a week.
_____3. I give and receive affection regularly.
_____4. I have at least one relative within 50 miles on whom I can rely.
_____5. I exercise to the point of perspiration at least twice a week.
_____6. I smoke less than half a pack of cigarettes a day.
_____7. I take fewer than five alcoholic drinks a week.
_____8. I am the appropriate weight for my height.
_____9. I have an income adequate to meet basic expenses.
_____10. I get strength from my religious beliefs.
_____11. I regularly attend club or social activities.
_____12. I have a network of friends and acquaintances.
_____13. I have one or more friends to confide in about personal matters.
_____14. I am in good health (including eyesight, hearing, teeth).
_____15. I am able to speak openly about my feelings when angry or worried.
_____16. I have regular conversations with the people I live with about domestic
        problems, e.g. chores, money, and daily living issues.
_____17. I do something for fun at least once a week.
_____18. I am able to organize my time effectively.
_____19. I drink fewer than three cups of coffee (or tea or cola drinks) a day.
_____20. I take quiet time for myself during the day.

_____TOTAL

To compute your score, add up the figures and subtract 20. Any number over 30 indicates a vulnerability to stress. You are seriously vulnerable if your score is between 50 and 75, and extremely vulnerable if it is over 75.

Physiology of Stress

The physiology of stress represents the series of checks and balances that allow people to adapt to change. Charles Darwin initiated the seed of this concept with the notion of adaptiveness or fittedness of bodily mechanisms to the environment. Claude Bernard, in *Principles of Constancy*, introduced the concept of homeostasis, the idea that organisms strive to maintain an internal equilibrium. He stated, "It is a need of all organisms to keep the interior *milieu* steady and constant. The whole organism, amoeba or man, must govern and synchronize the range of physiologic fluctuations in its past to prevent disruption of its integrity. It is the internal regulation for preservation of the norm, a balance, homeostasis." Sigmund Freud concurred. "Human behavior," he commented, "is governed by pain and pleasure, and fine tuning of response is regulated by thermostats."

In the 1940's Walter Canon enunciated the body's response to emergency, the fight or flight principles, and of specific homeostasis – the tendency of each of the body's systems to operate so as to maintain stability, but while also being able to respond to demands. The modern view of the stress response is a series of positive and negative feedback mechanisms, mediated through complex interrelationships of hormones and enzymes.

The stress response is a relatively simple interrelationship of the brain, hypothalamus, pituitary gland, and adrenal glands. The relationship, governed by a feedback system among chemical mediators, is individualized in each organism. The unique manifestation of the organism's stress response depends upon his temperament and experience, and is modified by sophisticated cerebral pathways. These pathways involve the autonomic nervous system and the neuroendocrine system. The autonomic and neuroendocrine systems are further regulated by the brain's three major integrating systems; the reticular activating system (RAS), the limbic system, and the hypothalamus.

The RAS is the gatekeeper that determines whether a message about potential threat gets through to the brain cortex and becomes consciously perceived as such. If the RAS allows information about a potential threat to enter the brain, it also alerts the limbic system. The limbic system, in turn, tags the message with an emotional label and then mediates a series of outgoing messages. The hypothalamus, the third subcortical system that mediates individual responses to stress, is responsible for the somatic (bodily) expression of stress.

In primitive man, perceived danger triggered a well-coordinated, prepared response of the brain and body. The same response occurs in modern man to the same perceived threat. The heart rate increases, blood pressure rises, pupils dilate, epinephrine rises, blood is diverted to vital organs, glucose is mobilized from the liver and platelet levels rise. **The problem arises for modern man in that he has developed a frontal neocortex in his brain capable of thought and maladaptive over-anticipation, which can trigger the stress response without the actual presence of danger.**

This root of maladaptive behavior can have far-reaching and potentially disastrous consequences. Examples of maladaption to stress are:

1. Anxiety or depression that interferes with function.
2. Functional disorders such as gastrointestinal problems, fatigue, headaches, or insomnia.
3. Exacerbation of organic disease.
4. Irritability.
5. Regression or dependent behavior.
6. Thinking pattern dysfunctions.
7. Nightmares and traumatic flashbacks.
8. Antisocial, criminal, or deviant behavior.

The ability to adapt, to habituate, evolves as another individualization of the stress response. A first stressful experience like a job interview, sales efforts, or asking for a raise may be quite stressful. With repeated efforts, however, the magnitude of the stress response attenuates and the individual is considered to have adapted or habituated to the stressors. Normal people learn to "turn off" from repeated stressors, while neurotics continue to respond to repeated stressors as if each one was new. With the evolution of man's frontal neocortex and his ability to think, and to over anticipate, the physiology of stress may have joined forces with man's stressors and dangers.

Abnormal Thought Patterns Contribute to Our Stress

Man's development of the neo-cortex, his development of the ability to think, has been a double-edged sword. While it has enhanced his ability to develop, invent, conceptualize and think in abstract terms, it has also potentiated the stress response. Simply by his perception of stress, even in the absence of physical danger, he may precipitate a stress reaction. His ability to think and reason is not always true and accurate. Can you see yourself participating in any of the following examples of abnormal thought patterns?

All-or-Nothing Thinking – You engage in all-or-nothing thinking when you evaluate your performance or personal qualities in extremist, black-or-white categories. A prominent student who received a B on an exam concluded: "Now I am a total failure." All-or-nothing thinking is clearly illogical because things are not usually completely one way or another. No one is completely attractive or totally ugly. Similarly, people are neither absolutely brilliant nor hopelessly stupid. All-or-nothing thinking forms the basis for perfectionism. It causes you to fear any mistake or imperfection, because you will see yourself as a complete failure or feel inferior and worthless. You may become depressed if you don't achieve your absolute standards.

Overgeneralization – You arbitrarily conclude that a single negative event will happen over and over again. A shy young man mustered up his courage to ask a girl for a date. When she declined, he was destroyed. He thought, "I am never going to get a date. Girls are always turning me down." One event defined a future lifetime of failure.

Selective Negative Focus – You pick out the negative details in any situation and dwell on them exclusively. You conclude that the whole situation is negative. A severely depressed college student heard some graduate students making fun of her roommate. She became furious because of her thinking, "That's what human nature is like, cruel and insensitive." Of course she had forgotten the fact that in the previous few months, her classmates and professors had been exceedingly congenial to her roommate.

Disqualification of the Positive – This rises as one of the most amazing and magical of all of the thinking errors. When a depressed individual is confronted with information, which clearly refutes her negative self-image and pessimistic attitudes, she quickly and cleverly finds some way to discount the information.

A young woman who was hospitalized for chronic depression claimed that no one could possibly care for her because she was such a despicable person. Upon her discharge from the hospital, she was paid warm tributes and given high praise by the staff for her recovery. The young patient's reflex reaction was to parry the compliments by claiming that they only paid her those compliments out

147

of their professional sense of duty. She further discounted the praise of her family and friends by saying that they wouldn't be offering her compliments if they knew the "real her."

Arbitrary Inference – You jump to an arbitrary, negative conclusion that is not justified by the facts or the situation. Two types of arbitrary inference are mind reading and negative prediction.

- Mind Reading – You make the assumption that you know what other people are thinking. You assume that they look down on you. So convinced you are about your assumption that you forget to check out its validity. You may then respond to this imagined rejection by withdrawal or counterattack. These self-defeating behavior patterns may act as self-fulfilling prophecies, setting up a negative interaction when none originally existed.

- Negative Prediction – You imagine that something bad looms in the near future, and you take this prediction as fact, even though it may be quite unrealistic. During frequent anxiety attacks, a college student assured herself that she would either pass out or surely go crazy. She had no history of fainting, nor did she have even the remotest signs of impending insanity. Her predictions were highly unrealistic.

Magnification or Minimization – This distortion can be called the "binocular trick," because you either blow things up out of proportion or shrink them. You magnify your imperfections and minimize your good points, resulting in your feeling inadequate and inferior to other people.

Emotional Reasoning – You take your emotions as evidence for the way things really are. Your logic is: "I feel, therefore I am." Examples of emotional reasoning include: "I feel guilty. Therefore I must be a bad person." "I feel overwhelmed and hopeless. Therefore my problems must be impossible to solve." Such reasoning is erroneous because your feelings simply reflect your thoughts and beliefs, not what is the present reality.

Should Statements – You make the effort to motivate yourself to increased activity by saying, "I should do this or I must do that." Such statements cause you to feel guilty, pressured, and resentful. Paradoxically, you end up feeling apathetic and unmotivated.

Labeling and Mislabeling – Personal labeling involves creating negative identity for yourself, which is based on your errors and imperfections as if these revealed your true self. Labeling is an extreme form of overgeneralization. The philosophy behind this tendency is: "The measure of a man is the mistakes he makes." Mislabeling involves describing an event with words that are inaccurate and heavily loaded emotionally. The man on the diet who ate a rather large dish of ice cream was so consumed with self-disgust and revulsion that he spoke of himself as a pig. He became so upset that he ate the entire quart of ice cream.

Personalization – You relate a negative event to yourself when there is no basis for doing so. You arbitrarily conclude that the negative event is your fault, even if you were not responsible for the event and did not cause it.

Control Fallacies – You feel extremely controlled and you see yourself as a helpless victim of fate. Or, you feel you control everything and are responsible for the pain and happiness of everyone around you.

Fallacy of Fairness – You feel resentful because you think you know what is fair, but other people will not agree with you.

Fallacy of Change – You expect that other people will change to suit you if you just pressure or cajole them enough. You need to change people because your hopes for happiness seem to depend entirely on them.

Being Right – You are continually on trial to prove that your opinions and actions are correct. Being wrong is unthinkable and you will go to any length to demonstrate your rightness.

Heaven's Reward Fallacy – You expect all your sacrifice and self-denial to pay off, as if there were someone keeping score. You feel bitter and resentful when the reward doesn't come.

All the above are examples of distorted thinking that can predispose us to stress and potentiate our stressors. What are some signs of distorted thinking?

What can you do about it? Here are some clues to be vigilant for and a couple of suggestions for promoting awareness.

Be vigilant for:

- ➤ Painful emotions – nervousness, depression, chronic anger, disgust.
- ➤ Certain worries that you play over and over like a broken record.
- ➤ On-going conflicts with friends and family.

To promote your awareness:

- ➤ Notice what you say to yourself about the other person.
- ➤ Notice how you describe and justify your side of the conflict.
- ➤ Police yourself for faulty logic.

What can you do about it?

- ➤ Recognize it.
- ➤ Choose to change.
- ➤ Read on.

Spotting faulty thinking in yourself can help to prevent stress and assist in dealing with stress that may have crept into your life. Spotting faulty thinking is becoming aware of a behavior that is dysfunctional. When we become aware that something is amiss, we may address its need to be changed. Before we attempt to make those changes, we would best be armed with decent "tools" to make the change. "The right tool for the job makes the task a lot easier," my dad used to tell me.

Communication Styles Affect Stress Management

Communication style functions as a critical tool for the prevention or management of stress. How we communicate our needs or wishes may determine in large part whether or not our needs are met. If we do not achieve our goals, meet our needs, or have the opportunity to express our thoughts, we may become frustrated and stressed. Communication style is key to all three efforts. Communication, just as behavior, comes in three "flavors:" assertive, aggressive, and passive. Let's look at each of these styles of communication and see how each works, or doesn't work, in specific relation to stress management.

Passive communication is unclear, often taking the form of implication. Direct statements don't exist, because the person making the statements fears her request being rejected. Passive communication protects her against rejection because she can deny that she was actually making a specific request. The passive communicator is unsure, has a fragile ego, and is phenomenally needy and dependent. Passive communication includes "body language," posturing to communicate needs or wishes, and often includes the game of "read my mind." The passive communicator hopes or expects that her partner implicitly "knows" what she wants. When she doesn't get what she wants, she may become sullen, resentful, angry, dejected, or depressed. This is anything but clear communication. It is the epitome of defensive behavior and usually results in frustration, anger, and additional stress.

Aggressive communication is angry communication, most often ending in a counter-productive manner. Aggressive communicators run roughshod over their associates and mates, or at least they attempt to do so. Their method of communication is so onerous that it is seldom rewarded. If short-term gains are achieved by aggressive communication, it is most certainly at the cost of long term gains or relationships. People tend to avoid or ignore aggressive communication. Avoidance is the recipient's method of coping with a barrage of verbal aggression. The aggressive communicator is angry, frustrated, domineering, lonely, and manipulative. He doesn't have many friends, and has little understanding or empathy for others. This is relatively ignorant communication. He just doesn't know any better, and certainly is unaware of assertive communication.

Assertive communication is loving communication. Honest and vulnerable, assertive communication is an open, clear, thoughtful statement or question. It conveys the thought, question, request, or hope succinctly and without threat. When communicating assertively, we automatically consider the feelings of the person to whom we are speaking. We do not want to offend arbitrarily. Even if the subject of our discussion is mutually distasteful, but is better aired than not, we may proceed with necessary honesty. It is the communication that we all strive for. Assertive communication is almost universally well-received because care has gone into its preparation. We think before we talk when we offer assertive communication. Frequently, assertive communication is confused with aggressive communication, but they differ like night and day. Simply remember that aggressive is angry, and assertive is loving. Assertive communication requires confidence, thought, a reasonable sense of self, and the ability to love.

Assertive communication, once understood and practiced, becomes a tool that makes our task of stress management easier. Assertive communication can help us function quite nicely in our lives, allowing us to be productive, while protecting us from higher perceived levels of stress.

Peak Performance, Flameout and Burnout

Two rather obvious clues that one needs to address the stressors in their lives are flameout and burnout. Peak performance provides a subtle clue to these unnecessary states. Our perception and chosen reaction to life's "circumstances" locates our performance on the perceived stress vs. performance graph (Figure 1). Where do you sit?

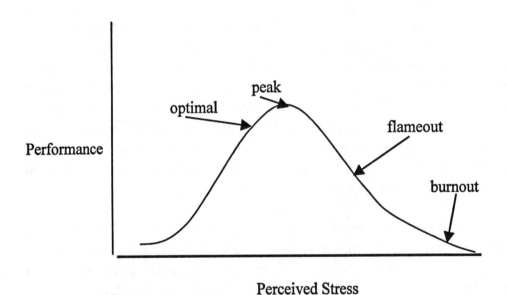

Figure 1

As perceived stress increases, our ability to function increases to a point, and then rapidly declines.

This graph illustrates the location of optimum performance, peak performance, flameout and burnout. Flameout is the earlier diminished function with continued stress, while burnout becomes an inability to function with excessive stress over time. Peak performance occupies a precarious position. Performance maximizes but sits too near the fire of flameout and burnout, thus one risks potential vulnerability to small increments of increased stress. I suggest that you consider aspiring to the optimal performance range, allowing yourself a buffer zone for unforeseen stressors.

What predisposes us to flameout? Psychological defense mechanisms that dull or diminish our self-observational acuity, coupled with certain personality characteristics increase our potential for flameout. Any or all of the following will predispose an individual to flameout, so look out for:

- Lofty goals
- High levels of motivation
- Over-commitment
- Over-dedication
- Over-scheduling
- Inflexibility
- Rigidity of role application
- An omnipotent God complex.

How does one know or suspect he may be flaming out? Run through this screening test. You can do it blindfolded, left-handed and backward. Score each item from 5 (almost always) to 1 (never) according to how much of the time each statement applies to you.

Flameout Screening Test:

_____ 1. I feel dull, but I don't know why.
_____ 2. I really don't care about things like I used to.
_____ 3. I feel like I should have advanced farther in my job than I have.
_____ 4. I am tired most of the day, even when I get up in the morning.
_____ 5. People irritate me.
_____ 6. Everything seems to be the same, I am bored.
_____ 7. I am between a rock and a hard place.
_____ 8. I can't seem to solve my problems.

_____ 9. I have no choices.

_____ 10. My confidence is gone.

_____ 11. Maybe I'll cheat and steal to get ahead.

_____ 12. I would feel more at home with a bunch of sheep.

_____ 13. I feel lonely most of the time.

_____ 14. I can't relax.

_____ 15. My boss has me doing too much work.

_____ 16. My job is no longer satisfying.

_____ 17. My marriage is horrible, but I can't do anything about it.

_____ 18. I want someone else to take care of me and my life.

_____ 19. I find myself drinking more alcohol and taking sleeping pills.

_____ 20. I have had a lot of colds lately, or been in the hospital.

_____ 21. I feel depressed.

_____   TOTAL

To compute your score, add up the figures and subtract 21. Any number over 30 indicates a vulnerability to flameout. You are seriously vulnerable if your score is between 50 and 75, and extremely vulnerable if it is over 75.

Flameout is bad enough, but burnout is much worse. It's much more devastating, more painful and more difficult from which to recover. Because the pathway from decent functioning to flameout and on to burnout is a progressive sequence, many of the clues to burnout are the same as those for flameout, only more severe. A near paralytic inability to function should be an obvious warning sign.

What predisposes an individual to burnout? Time does. The duration of the stress proves critical in the etiology of burnout. Sprinkle in a little ignorance and, _voila_, burnout. Burnout victims allow external factors to have a major influence in their lives. For example, bureaucratic factors, long hours, heavy work load, difficult and unreasonable clientele, adherence to a Protestant work ethic (if I just work a little harder and a little longer, then everything will be OK), all stand as external factors increasing the likelihood of burnout.

Internal factors begin to augment the external ones. Disillusionment, questioning of one's competence, loss of autonomy, no self-recognition or rewards for doing a good job, lack of collegiality among peers, a sense of entrapment and unrealistic expectations erode the essence of who we thought we were and .... snap, crackle, pop .... we have burned out.

It is curious that we can be so blind, so ignorant of warning signs along the way, that we eventually land in the pile of burned out people. I find it rather sad because burnout isn't necessary, and we can learn to live successfully in a stressful world.

> When I met Bill Howard he was retired, but not retiring. At seventy-two he was active physically, sharp mentally, and involved emotionally. Early in his career he was a businessman, imprisoned in a position of high stress. Realizing his health risk from the daily and relentless stressors of his high-pressure city job, he quit and became a counselor for troubled youth. Not only did he remove himself from the stressful environment that threatened to eat him alive, he chose to serve his fellow man through counseling. Altruistic and healthful in its own right, choosing to serve society bequeathed value to Bill, but reclaiming his perception of control of his life afforded Bill the greatest healthful benefit of his stress management.

How to Live Successfully in a Stressful World

Yes, we live in a stressful world. I promise you that we can thrive in spite of our stressors, that we can learn to live in concert with them, and that we can indeed *Get a Life!* Once we have discovered awareness, we have limitless choices available to us for stress management. As with all other elements of health and wellness presented in *Get a Life, America!,* no single stress management technique exists. In *Get a Life, America!* we have a cornucopia of choices.

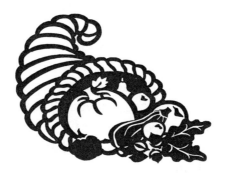

No two people's lives are identical, and even if they were, no two people will respond in the same manner to their life circumstances. Therefore, coping with stress is an individual expression of self. Of necessity, one must choose his or her own stress management techniques. The technique that works best for you is the one that you design and use for yourself.

Successful stress management begins with principles and progresses to specific techniques. The principles of stress management are:

1) **Awareness provides the basic foundation for stress management.**
2) **Stress is perception, not events.**
3) **Perception is subject to choice.**
4) **We all have freedom of (and responsibility for) choice, perception included.**
5) **Stress management is coping, bending and blending, not avoiding, denying, and ignoring.**

Offering multiple perspectives of stress management for your choice, I will begin with preventive efforts, progress to some philosophical offerings of the masters, and end with a listing of stress busting techniques garnered from just about everywhere.

Preventive Efforts Against Stress

We begin by examining a prospective approach to the management of stress in our lives. As we do, let us also consider that we might possibly use stress to our advantage. Stress can be a legitimate motivator. We do not want to eliminate stress from our lives, but it would be nice if we had more control.

Always remind yourself that you have choices – "Beyond that wonderful, glorious five second rage, everything is choice", quotes Dr. Kubler-Ross. I never knew that. I thought that if you were mad, you were mad. If you were sad, you stayed sad until the feeling gradually went away. To think that we might have control and choice about how we feel was not even a distant idea to me. I just didn't consider the possibility until I happened upon the quote by Dr. Kubler-Ross. It's powerful and elegant in its simplicity. We are allowed the luxury of our emotions, but they do not imprison us.

Dr. Kubler-Ross, author of the book *On Death and Dying*, remarks that "very few people have done what they truly want to do." They haven't because no one told them that they could. Knowing that we have choices, in each and every aspect of our lives is liberating, empowering and stress relieving. Frustration, anxiety and depression about what we think we "should and must" do in our lives dissipate when we realize that "shoulds and musts" are merely products of our perception. "Shoulds and musts," as opposed to positive choices, result from our perception that we are not in control of our lives and our futures. Understanding, accepting and believing that we are free to choose, eliminates the bondage of "shoulds and musts."

Making choices is positive, assertive, and self-supportive behavior. How many times have we heard ourselves utter, "I had no choice. I had to do it." Facing financial catastrophe, filled with despair, a small business owner opts for filing for bankruptcy. "I had to do it." Could he have borrowed, negotiated scheduled payments, searched for a better job or worked a part-time job? Those demonstrate but a few options, different from his very polar choice. How about suicide, a more popular "no choice" behavior from the depression era of the 1930's. Was that their only option? I think not. We must mindfully search for and turn over a few rocks. Choices wait patiently for our discovery.

Sometimes, amidst the din and chaos of our lives, I must admit it is difficult to be mindful that we do have choices. What can we do then? An interesting and useful technique to remind ourselves about choices is to establish a personal signal, a designated reminder. A ring, a particular necklace, a scarf or a photo, anything we designate has the power to remind us of our freedom to choose. We may choose from a full menu in life. We may select emotions, friends, jobs, mates, thoughts, styles, attitudes, and even our personality. We may choose to remain as we are or choose to change, but whatever we choose, we must make the choice consciously.

Shorten your downtime – Shortening your downtime is a corollary to Dr. Kubler-Ross' opening quote. We are not obliged to wallow in a quagmire of negative emotions. We may choose how long to allow that emotion to live with us. How many of us have allowed a negative experience to ruminate through our thought processes for days? It creates terrible discomfort and decreases our productivity and our happiness. We don't have to do the unhappy dance marathon.

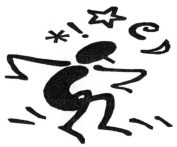

The phrase, "shortening your downtime," means that we may recognize the negative aspect of an event, acknowledge it, and feel it. We may choose our level of emotion to apply to the experience. Then we may choose how long to allow the presence of the emotion. Don't waste a perfectly good day fuming over a petty argument with your spouse or anyone else. It probably isn't worth spending that much time being upset. Learn to recognize your emotions, allot a time value to them, determine if any remedial action is necessary, then get on with the enjoyment of your life.

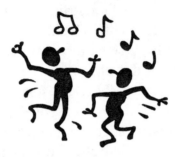

Remind yourself, "How do you eat an elephant?" – You eat an elephant one bite at a time. What do you do when you face a task so imposing and resistant that accomplishing it seems impossible? Many of us procrastinate or avoid the task entirely, because we view its enormity as overwhelming. Where does that view take us? Nowhere. We cannot allow ourselves to travel through our lives avoiding some potentially wonderful gains because we did not know how to address large issues and projects.

What do we fear when we face the elephant? We fear the enormity, the unfamiliar, the possibility of failure, and more, the potential of succeeding. Should we fear? Will we experience physical pain? Will it kill us? No, no, and no!

How would we answer if faced with a small problem, one that might be a part of the larger whole? More than likely we would see no difficulty in solving the small problem, solving it expeditiously. The advantage of the concept of "eating the elephant one bite at a time" perceptually dissects a large problem into a series of smaller ones. We distract our focus from the larger, imposing whole and place it on smaller, more familiar units. The diversion of our focus allows us to operate in a more comfortable realm.

The component parts of a whole are more manageable, less imposing, and less fearsome. In the process of breaking down the whole to its parts, we learn more about the whole. Taking something apart and then reassembling it educates us, just as reassembling a puzzle teaches a child.

We support our sense of control by creating and handling manageable, less threatening parts of the whole. With a series of baby steps, eating the elephant one bite at a time, we offer ourselves success in the long run.

Interpersonal relationships can be an elephant, very complex, fearsome and imposing. Relationships evolve over time, step by step. Consider the perceptual plight of a single mother longing for permanent companionship, who cries, "I want a relationship now, and I don't want to wait." Unfortunately, for her, relationships don't just happen. Relationships grow. What can she do? Eat the elephant. Bite one – join a social group. Bite two – call a friend who might be able to introduce her to someone. Bite three – take the initiative and ask someone she likes for a date. Bite four – do some fun things together. Bite five – keep at it and eventually a relationship is born and growing.

How about starting a business? That is an elephant! Is it too big to even consider? No, get out your fork and knife. Bite one – ask for advice. Bite two – create a business plan. Bite three – read your business plan. Does it make sense? Bite four – start small. In the process of starting small and accomplishing the small tasks, we learn the flow of the business, which we may then apply to an expanding effort.

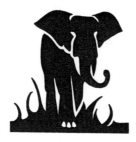

So, remember to eat the elephant one bite at a time. It's more manageable and less imposing. It teaches us a process, and teaches us about the elephant. In the long run, it teaches us that we are in control.

Thinking distortions add to stress – We understand thinking distortions, and that those illogical thinking patterns cloud our perception of the reality of our circumstances.

Practice assertive communication – We know the three flavors of communication, and that we want to practice only one of those flavors – assertive communication.

Learn to live with stress – Stress management is largely coping and adaptation. It's not eliminating stress and it's not making absolute behavior changes. It's modification of the stressors and of our responses. We seek a satisfactory locale somewhere between two extremes on a continuum, an area of our selected comfort.

Stress is perception – We know, but let me repeat that stress is perception, not an event. Two people experiencing the same event will react differently, depending upon their genetic make-up, their background and their experience. Perception is our choice. "Beyond that wonderful five second rage, everything is choice." With our ability to think and to reason, we can decide how we perceive events in our lives. We can consciously attach whatever emotional labels we wish to the events in our lives.

When we individuals can accept our ability and responsibility to consciously choose our perceptions of events, we will have granted ourselves greater control of our lives. **Perception is our choice and it allows us control.**

Do not isolate yourself – Socialization is a key principle in stress management and modification. We are social animals, not intended to be isolated, physically or emotionally. We need the physical proximity of friends and family, and we need their emotional support.

People unfortunate enough to suffer a terminal illness often become isolated. Their friends don't know what to do and say at such a difficult time. Friends, well-meaning but confused, tend to stay away. When asked what they would most desire, the terminally ill universally answer, "Company." One cancer victim said that he felt so lonely and isolated that he simply wanted a warm body near him. It didn't have to talk or touch him. He just wanted it to be there. We need people in health and in sickness, and I contend that the presence of people in our lives prevents illness.

Exercise and nutrition are key – I have presented chapters on exercise and on nutrition. They are not isolated entities in our lives but are integral parts of health and wellness, of *Getting a Life!* Exercise, especially aerobic, but also strength-training, is a documented stress reliever. Exercise can function as one of the catalytic behaviors that potentiates other desired behaviors. Similarly, nutrition affects our ability to handle stress. Nutrition affects how we feel, how we perform, and contributes to our reserve capacity. Carrying excess weight depresses and stresses us. Caffeine intake augments our anxiety. In essence we are what we eat, or at least we are affected by what we eat.

Guided visual imagery – This is just plain fun, your free travel ticket to anywhere you want to go. Quick and easy, guided visual imagery is a conscious, purposeful daydream.

When my daughters were younger, I would put them to bed at night with a guided visual imagery send-off. As they lay relaxed on their backs in bed, I would ask that their world become my voice. We began by focusing on various parts of their bodies, making a leg very heavy, or an arm very light. They felt the weight of their heads sinking into the pillow. Then it was time to fly. With bodies becoming lighter than air, they saw themselves rising through the roof of the house, floating skyward, and weaving a pathway through the clouds. Floating ever so lightly, so gently, they might meet an eagle soaring with them. They make eye contact with the big bird, nothing more. The world is their view from on high. Nothing threatens, for their existence in that moment is ethereal warmth and safety. Periodically, I calmly remind them that their world is my voice, only my voice. We travel lightly, safely and happily together. No boundaries, no distances, and no time, we are simply existing and sensing in those moments. Then it is time to come back to earth, to the weight of their bodies, to the comfort of their beds. The landing was always soft and gentle, and they went to sleep so easily after those imagery trips.

I think that you get the idea. You may send yourself on a trip anywhere you wish. Ask a friend to guide you. From deep inside of your soul to the farthest reaches of space, no limits restrict your guided visual imagery travel.

Meditation, the best preventive effort against stress – Many forms of meditation are practiced throughout the world, including transcendental meditation, yoga, Zen, Subud, Scientology, self-hypnosis and the relaxation response. Mindfulness meditation, in my opinion, is the most easily practiced on a daily basis. The details of mindfulness meditation are presented shortly, immediately after Dr. Eliot's comments about stress.

Be Your Own CEO – You are not intended to be alone in this world, although at times the world may feel quite lonely. To counter the sense of being alone, I suggest using the power of numbers and of team. You are the captain of your ship, the manager of your athletic team, the CEO of your corporation. It is you who are responsible for selecting, contracting with, placing into position and instructing your team members. It is imperative that all of us develop two personal teams, one for daily living, and another for crisis management. I do not mean simply to have a perception of who these players in your life may be. Select them and write your line up on a 3 x 5 card, one side of your card for your daily team and the other for your crisis team.

Let's consider first our daily team, our **"first team."** What is its function? At the very least, our first team allows us to avoid loneliness, but it provides much more. Our first team gives us emotional support, provides us family and friends with whom we may talk, and allows us readily available mirrors for seeing ourselves. Our carefully selected first team offers us a key ingredient to *Getting a Life!* – fun.

Who is on our first team? Our primary partner, husband, wife or significant other leads off. Children are right in there, too. Write their names down, don't just list "children." Who is significant in your life in your work environment? Do you have a pet special enough to be listed? Who among your friends deserves to be designated on your first team? Do you volunteer your time or services to the community? If so, are there meaningful people there who belong on your list? Are you a member of an organization? Write each of your first team member's names down, then review the list in one week. Make any additions or deletions.

It would be lovely to go through life without any crises, but there aren't enough rose colored glasses to go around. When a crisis occurs we need to know immediately where to turn for help. Crises are not the time to scramble and search for people to help us. We must already know who they are. It is time to "Circle the Wagons," just like in the old West. Each wagon has one of your **"crisis team"** members driving it and each driver serves for your protection. Whom do you select? Here are some example categories to which you might add your own.

1) Mentor
2) Lawyer
3) Medical source
4) Accountant
5) Key family member
6) Insurance agent
7) Special friend

One other important part of your CEO management plan remains, to select your **"personal oasis,"** a spot where you may go to renew, to think, to meditate.

It could be your office, a particular room in your home, your favorite coffee shop, a nearby country setting, your rooftop, or your church. My former partner in medical practice would occasionally leave our office and go to the town fish pier where he could sit in back of Willard Nickerson's Fish Market, alone and thinking, or alone and not thinking. It was his oasis. We all need one. Choose yours and write it down.

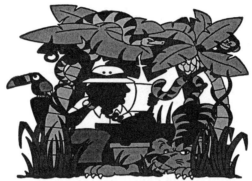

The idea of having your own teams, first ones, crisis ones and your oasis gives comfort and reassurance. The perception of being alone in life is depressing, and of being alone in a crisis, is quite fearful. Connecting to a spot on this mother earth, your oasis, affords some sense of security in a very chaotic world.

As part of the responsibilities inherent in your CEO management position, you must be mindful of and open-minded to other stress management philosophies and techniques. Let's now look at some different presentations of coping with stress.

Dr. Robert S. Eliot's Thoughts About Stress Management

I will always remain amused by Dr. Eliot's description of his having a stress related heart attack – "There I was, in the hospital, looking up from the wrong side of the sheets." It helps to be a doctor to appreciate the irony in his statement. None of us ever thinks that he will end up on the wrong side of the sheets. We think that we have some divine entitlement to health, our own "Get-Out-of-Jail-Free" card. Often it takes a heart attack to wake us from our denial. It did for Dr. Eliot. He learned from his experience and has shared some of his thoughts in his book, *Is It Worth Dying For?*

Dr. Eliot pioneered research about the effects of stress on cardiovascular disease and identified the "hot reactor." The "hot reactor" reacts in a severe cardiovascular manner to minor or moderate stress. Blood pressure elevates, vascular resistance increases and heart rate climbs. These individuals have a high risk of cardiovascular disease. Approximately 18% of our total population are "hot reactors" and 33% of our "professional community" are also. Of even greater concern is the fact that "hot reactors" who have an "anger-in" personality stand an alarmingly high risk of sudden death.

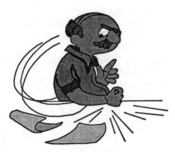

Dr. Eliot has aptly concluded that stress poses grave danger to our cardiovascular system and has developed his own philosophy and techniques for coping with stress. Here are some of Dr. Eliot's ideas:

Don't sweat the small stuff, it's all small stuff – Once we have departed this world, was there really any difference in magnitude to the various aspects of our lives. Did our worrying about anything make a difference?

Practice the five T's of stress management – We must learn to take the **time** that we need for ourselves in our lives. It is OK to take time for ourselves. Taking time to nurture ourselves is not selfish. It's our responsibility to ourselves and to those near and dear to us.

Choosing to and learning to **trust** is critical. We are not intended to be alone in this world. We need people. Trusting other people, as we would trust ourselves, provides necessary emotional support during stressful times.

Teasing is playful fun and frolic. We must learn to be light-hearted and to have fun. It's quite difficult to feel stressed when you are frolicking with a friend.

Always **talk**. A vehicle for self-discovery, talking forces thinking and organization of thought. It facilitates awareness. It allows us to share our troubles, and to give some of those troubles away in the process.

Touch is magic. Try it. You can almost feel stress physically leaving your body. Give hugs and request hugs. Touch someone's hand or shoulder. Give a foot massage. Accept a foot massage.

Deal with anger as the Japanese do – First, smile. Second, smile and bow. Third, shrug your shoulders and indicate that you "don't understand."

Play – Learn how and do it. Play a game. Play with your children. Play with your dog.

Keep your own 3 X 5 card with your successes listed on it –

- List your ten best qualities on the front side.
- List your five happiest moments and
- List your five greatest accomplishments on the other side.
- If you ever have negative brain messages, read what you have placed on the card.

I visited Dr. Eliot's facility when it was located in Denver. After debating whether I should visit as a clinical observer or go as a patient of his facility, I chose the latter. Yes, I was identified as a hot reactor, but I had suspicions before I went. His facility taught me many functional lessons for the management of my own stressors.

Coping With Stress, a Mindfulness Approach

About a year before I attended Dr. Eliot's cardiovascular stress management facility, I stumbled upon a unique experience at the University of Massachusetts Medical School. I happened upon an ad in a medical "throw-away" magazine, which read: "Stress reduction for physicians. It will involve an entire weekend. Wear loose clothing and bring a pillow." Intrigued, I went.

Jon Kabat-Zinn, Ph.D., conducted a weekend retreat in meditation for physicians. Having no previous experience with meditation, I was a bit (a lot) skeptical and apprehensive. Jon disarmed me totally that weekend and introduced me to one of the most wondrous disciplines available to man, mindfulness meditation.

I would like to share my joy with you. It is easy to learn, easy to understand, and easy to practice. Sit as still as you can in a comfortable position with a straight back, head erect and listen to Jon Kabat-Zinn talk.

"Being aware of your breathing, of the 'in breath' and of the 'out breath;' being aware of any sensations in particular regions of the body; being aware of the body as a whole; hearing silence and sounds; observing thoughts and feelings as they move in and out of the mind, moment by moment, not getting involved in the content, but observing them as thoughts, as feelings; when you notice that the mind has drifted into fantasy, etc., gently bring it back to alert attention in the present moment."

Jon teaches that meditation begins with the **non-judgmental observation of life** from moment to moment. When you find that the mind is being judgmental, pushing away things it doesn't like, and holding on to things it likes, simply observe that this is occurring. Meditation is an effortless and choiceless awareness of the totality of life's expressions within you and around you in any and every moment. It is a state of being, not an activity. Meditation is not something to do; it is allowing yourself to just be. Be sure you understand that this is not a tuning out process. It is being fully present with a larger perspective grounded in the sense of being.

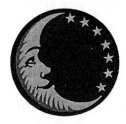

He recommends that it is helpful to sit quietly in this way one or two times a day for fifteen to thirty minutes. Do it at regular times, every day. By doing it every day, whether you feel like it or not, you allow a sense of strength and balance to develop in your life which goes beyond moods, emotional turmoil, busyness, and beyond the particular experiences, pleasant and painful, in your life. This quality of mind or sense of being is naturally independent of being still or moving. It is awareness in each moment, the simple remembering of your completeness as a human being. If you notice yourself resisting or avoiding a daily period of silent awareness, bring your attention to the resistance itself and observe it. By sitting in this way daily you will establish a more relaxed and balanced tone for your day's activities and encounters.

An extension of the effort of mindful meditation is relaxation, a practice to be done as many times a day as you can. You will develop the skill to scan your body with precise and concentrated attention. When you notice tension in specific regions, use breath to dispel the tension. Dispel the tension on the "out breath."

Allow ease and relaxation to express on the "in breath." You may do this at any time of day, under any circumstances. It only takes an awareness of the body, and a few diaphragmatic breaths. Try to breathe diaphragmatically (allow your abdomen to expand as you inhale) as much of the time as possible during the day. Again, this should not require effort, simply awareness.

Remember that the deepest relaxation is a sense of being comfortable with your own being, in your own skin. It goes beyond external circumstances and internal mental states, which may at times cause feelings of tension and unpleasantness, and at other times feelings of relaxation and pleasure. By directing your energy into the detached observation of these fluctuations of circumstances and mood, you are developing this deeper level of relaxation, which is really an expression of wisdom.

Mindful walking is another extension of the meditation process. Again, do it as often as possible. It is helpful to observe yourself as you are walking, then slow down a little and remind yourself, "here I am, complete in this moment." Notice the way you carry your body, the feeling in your feet, legs, chest and head as you walk. Do what you are doing mindfully. Be open to the sights and sounds around you. This can be done anywhere. Try it while shopping, walking down the street, going up or down stairs, or while standing and waiting for something or someone. Of course, this can be combined with an awareness of breathing and the diaphragmatic breath.

Mindful eating is just like mindfulness or mindful walking. It is awareness of our existence. You might want to pay attention to the quality and the quantity of the food you put into your body, and what functions eating performs at any moment. Do you eat to nourish your body and to keep it finely tuned? Do you eat to satisfy cravings for taste sensations, to feel more full, more complete, more secure? Are you aware of the source of the food you are eating? Does much of it come out of factories? Have the substances you eat been processed? If so, how much? What has been removed? Are chemicals really harmless in food? Do you pay attention on this level?

Try eating with greater awareness, and somewhat slower than usual. As an experiment, you might try intentionally eating one meal a week in silence with your family, just to experience the eating itself. Also, you might consider not reading or watching TV during meals. This will help you become more sensitive to how you eat. Not watching TV is a catalytic non-behavior. By not doing something, we can still potentiate other aspects of our lives. Share your experience with others and bring your increased awareness about eating to them.

It may help to ask yourself every day, "What is my body like right now? How is my health right now? Do I know? Do I need an expert to know? Am I allowing some aspect of my body or mind to be in an unhealthy condition through neglect, inattention, or inactivity? Is greater wellness a goal of mine? What am I doing today to realize the goal?" Ask the questions and commit the answers to paper. Practice mindfulness and awareness. "A problem once recognized is half solved."

Stress management has no one most important facet, but without awareness we are doomed to failure from the beginning. No one plan encompasses all of stress management, but all plans are based on awareness. Stress management has no end point, but awareness and the consciousness of choice make it possible for us to live in harmony with a stressful world.

Regular sittings to practice mindfulness meditation are essential to benefit from this wondrous discipline. Dr. Kabat-Zinn used an oriental chime to signal the end of a sitting during our weekend retreat. The sound of the chime transcended the aural sense and became an all-encompassing feeling of warmth and love. The benefits of meditation are not solely limited to the meditation period. You may take the principles of mindfulness with you throughout your day. With practice, you will begin to live a mindful life. As you practice, consider implementing Jon Kabat-Zinn's principles.

Breathing and other internal clues – Be mindful of internal cues informing you that a particular situation is stressful. Remember the possibility of a measured, mindful response rather than a knee-jerk reaction. Be mindful of the breath at these times in particular. How you are breathing can be a very sensitive barometer of stress. Shallow breathing is stressful breathing.

You are complete – Try to remember as often during the day as possible that you are a complete, infinite being who loses nothing by allowing your fullest sensitivity and love to express themselves.

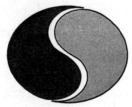

Be alert for judgmental feelings – Notice judgmental feelings of liking or disliking; wanting or rejecting. When they are present be aware of how they get expressed in your activities and behavior, i.e., your tone of voice and the choices you make. Be aware of the consequences of these activities and behavior. For example, if you immediately form a strong negative impression of someone, does this prevent you from really knowing and seeing the whole person clearly? When someone flatters you, does this result in your doing things you really do not want to do? Be aware of the presence and strength of the "Wanting Mind" during the day. Notice your feelings of incompleteness. Are they accurate?

Seek intuitive knowing – Be aware of the realm behind activity and thought where awareness is strong and clear, grounded in peace and stillness. Be aware of the realm where there is a sense of intuitive knowing. It is available if you seek it.

Connect with your emotions – Be aware of how much our moods and reactions to events influence how we feel physically. Be in touch with how you carry yourself, how you look, how and how much you eat, drink and talk. Use the breathing to tune in to the body. This is not the same as being self-conscious. Do you understand the difference? Take some time and reflect upon the difference. Being in touch with yourself is loving yourself, respecting yourself.

Be aware when you are feeling:	You may choose:
Fearful, angry, jealous	enthusiastic, peaceful
Envious, lazy, low-energy	open, infinite energy
Agitated, bored, anxious	calm, secure
Worried, insecure, greedy	satisfied, caring
Hateful, vengeful, aggressive	fearless, joyful

Notice how strong and overwhelming the emotions on the left are when they come up. Notice how much blindness and inaccuracy they usually entail. Then notice the quality of the emotions on the right when they happen. Are they as strong? How can the emotions on the right side be supported, strengthened, nourished? Is there also blindness and inaccuracy in these realms? Emotions can be dreadfully inaccurate. Ask yourself why you may allow the inaccuracies.

Do not live in the past or the future – Notice how much the mind dwells in memories of the past or anticipation of the future. How much of all thinking revolves around "I," "me," "mine." Notice how much of the day is spent

169

calculating ways to strengthen this aspect of your being. Is it necessary? Do you suffer for it? Be aware of the "Judging Mind."

Be where you are, in the present – Practice using awareness of the breath to help ground you in the present moment. Ground yourself in the right now. Nothing else matters, not the past, and not the future. The past is past and no one has promised you a tomorrow. You only have today.

Be alert for depression and anxiety – Notice the thoughts that are associated with moods of depression and anxiety. Are these thoughts accurate? What thoughts might you think to support your self-esteem and sense of well being? Are these thoughts more accurate?

Maintain a peaceful mind – Imagine that you could die at any moment. You could, as we all could. How would you want your mind to be at that moment? Can you think of practical steps to allow this goal to be realized in every day life? How about right now? Today! Such a simple question carries with it rather far reaching implications.

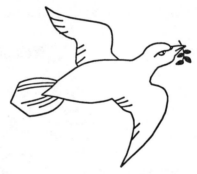

Allow yourself the normal ebb and flow – Remember that the learning process is irregular and consists of steps. Ups and downs are expected. We may become discouraged and feel like quitting, but we must not. We may have slipped back to the original condition at times, but these regressions will become rarer and rarer. It should be anticipated that new difficulties will be encountered for such is the way of life. Would we want it otherwise? Our consciousness may have previously rejected or suppressed what we now discover. That rejection may have been because of fear or pain, but as our self-confidence grows, the probability mushrooms that we will greet new opportunities in our lives.

Be in concert with the forces of Nature – Blend with the natural flow of life and Nature. Swim with the stream, not against it. Run with the wind. Congregate, don't isolate. Embrace all of your emotions, not exclusively love.

Being in concert with the forces of Nature blends nicely with the philosophy of Dr. Hans Selye. The "father of stress," Dr. Selye has many lessons to teach us.

Hans Selye's Prescription for Enjoying a Full Life

Dr. Selye practiced what he preached. He lived by his principles that he developed throughout his professional life. They served him well. He exercised, ate well and was a loving, assertive communicator. Could we live our lives as Dr. Selye learned to live his? Could we.....?

Release frustration – "Even if you systematically want to hoard love, don't waste your time trying to befriend a mad dog."

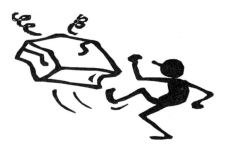

Recognize a hierarchy – "Admit that there is no perfection, but in each category of achievement something is tops. Be satisfied to strive for that."

Embrace simplicity – "Do not underestimate the delight of real simplicity in your lifestyle. Avoidance of all affectations and unnecessary complications earns as much goodwill and love as pompous artificiality earns dislike."

Prioritize – "Whatever situation you meet in life, consider first whether it is really worth fighting for. Do not forget what Nature has taught us about the importance of carefully adjusting syntoxic and catatoxic attitudes to any problems of a cell, man, or even a society."

Enjoy the pleasantries of life – "Try to keep your mind constantly on the pleasant aspects of life and on actions which can improve your situation. Try to forget everything that is irrevocably ugly or painful." This is perhaps the most efficient way of minimizing stress by what he has called voluntary mental diversion. As a wise German proverb says, "Imitate the sundial's way; Count only the pleasant days."

Take stock of your successes – "Nothing paralyzes your efficiency more than frustration. Nothing helps it more than success. Even after the greatest defeats the depressing thought of being a failure is best combated by taking stock of all your past achievements which no one can deny you. Such conscious stocktaking is most effective in reestablishing the self-confidence necessary for future success. There is something even in the most modest career that we are proud to recall. You would be surprised to see how much this can help when everything seems hopeless."

Don't procrastinate – "When faced with a task that is very painful yet indispensable to achieve your aim, don't procrastinate. Cut right into an abscess to eliminate the pain, instead of prolonging it by gently rubbing the surface."

Performance determines value – "Realize that men are not created equal, though they should, of course, have a birthright to equal opportunities. After birth, in a free society, their performance should determine their progress. There will always be leaders and followers, but the leaders are worth keeping only as long as they can serve the followers by acquiring their love, respect and gratitude."

Adopt a natural code of conduct – "Finally, do not forget that there is no ready-made success formula which would suit everybody. The only thing we have in common is our subordination to those fundamental biological laws, which govern all living beings, including man. Hence, a natural code of behavior based on nonspecific mechanisms of adaptation comes closest to what can be offered as a general guideline for conduct."

Dr. Selye's philosophy of life and how he lived his life was based on three simple principles:

1. Find your own stress level – "Work as hard as you feel is natural for you and pursue the aim of your own preference, without being sheepishly guided by what society expects of you."

2. Altruistic egotism – "Admit that all living creatures are built so that they must look out for themselves first. You can do that without developing inferiority or guilt complexes even if you do things for your own good, as long as they assure you the esteem, good will, and love of others. Incidentally, this is the only capital that cannot be devalued or taken away from you."

3. Earn thy neighbor's love – "The time honored wisdom of the biblical command, 'Love thy neighbor as thyself,' can still be used in our scientifically oriented society. We admit that it is impossible to love on command. However, just as the ancient Eastern and Hebrew versions of this expression of 'The Golden Rule' had to be translated into languages understandable by contemporary people, so the essence of this prescription can be rephrased from loving on command into a code of behavior that can give you worthwhile motivation for all your activities throughout life, namely: 'Earn thy neighbor's love.'"

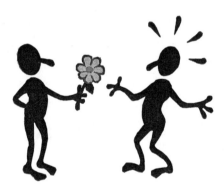

Dr. Selye formulated his personal philosophy of conduct in terms of the simple jingle:

"Fight for your highest attainable aim,
But do not put up resistance in vain."

We would be wise to adopt some if not all of Dr. Selye's philosophy. Perhaps we could use it as a foundation for developing our own philosophy for surviving in this crazy, stressful world.

This World is so Crazy, How Can I Possibly Survive the Stress?

Stress management is pragmatic, utilitarian, functional. We do what works for us. We do what we know. We mimic what we have witnessed in our parents and in our peers. It is for that reason we are at risk of the "generational compulsion to repeat." Our behaviors, thoughts, prejudices, coping skills, and even language will mirror those of our parents and their parents, and theirs. If their behaviors were good, then we are lucky. If they were dysfunctional, then we have some work to do. The odds are against our being the fortunate recipients of functional family dynamics because psychological studies estimate that ninety-percent of families are dysfunctional in their dynamics. Most of us start out behind the eight ball.

Don't despair, for help is within your reach. Because we are capable of thought, reasoning and understanding, we can change the tide of the "generational compulsion to repeat," offering better behavior dynamics to our children and theirs. Here is a list of techniques that you may choose to employ in your life to cope with and adapt to your stressors.

1. Distract yourself – We all harbor a set of bad mood thoughts that surface when we are feeling down. We can benefit from techniques that stop or divert us from focusing on those negative reflections. Norman Cousins watched Marx Brothers films to recover from what his doctors described as a terminal illness. A sporting event, a funny book, or good movie can serve as a pleasant distraction. The *Far Side* series by Gary Larson or Ellen DeGeneres' recent book, *My Point, and I Do Have One*, are laugh-out-loud funny. Ellen's book, in particular, helped me with laughter to the point of tears during some very frustration periods of writing this book. Writing a book was included in her "list of things that sound like a good idea at first, but really aren't." I defy you to feel stressed or depressed when you are in the midst of a hearty belly laugh.

2. Change your environment – Depression is more frequent in cities and alcoholism is more frequent in rural settings. No matter where you live or what your stressors are, a brief change of locale may help. If you dwell in the city, go for a walk in the park, a ride in the country, or a picnic by the lake, river or sea. If you reside in the country, plan a dinner or a theater outing in the city. Say "hello" to a stranger. Go to an art museum or walk along urban streets with a note pad and camera. Look, listen, and record.

3. Reach out and touch someone – Yes, physically touch someone. It is powerful medicine for you and the person that you touch. A Purdue University study demonstrated that physical contact, no matter how casual or from whom, almost immediately makes a person feel better. Physical contact lowers blood pressure and heart rate. So when you are feeling stressed, depressed, or generally down, give a hug, ask for one, or get a relaxing massage.

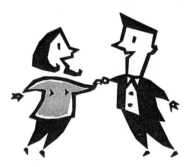

4. Learn to procrastinate and do it well – Finding a way to reduce seemingly insurmountable tasks and responsibilities is putting off until tomorrow (or never) what you feel you "should" do today. This creates time for you to do things important for you. It may be as simple as taking personal time to relax, think, reflect, exercise, see friends, cuddle with your mate, or one of my favorite fantasies, do nothing at all. Incidentally, my suggestion of procrastination counters the philosophy of Dr. Selye. Choose what works for you.

5. Get to the root of the problem – Sometimes a blue mood seems to arise spontaneously. Concentration on the clues to one's blues may be appropriate. Body signals like chest pain, abdominal pain, diarrhea, and headaches are clues to internalization of body stresses. Be aware of maladaptive thoughts like, "They caused this" and "I should be perfect." Think logically. Rather than focusing on potential failures, focus on successes in the past and apply those facilities to the present dilemma.

6. Float your blues away – It's a special treat, submerging your body in the protective dark womb of an isolation tank. The solutions in the tank are so strong with salt that your body bobs on the surface like a cork. Some researchers claim that endorphins are released during soaking periods in these tanks. Whether producing a pleasurable placebo effect or not, these relaxation tanks have gained common acceptance as useful and legitimate modes of stress therapy. Even if you can't find the time for a hyper-osmolar soak in a tank, a comfortable respite in a scented bath may offer similar stress relief.

7. Choose your colors with care – Without question colors affect our moods. Red is known to stimulate our nervous system. People feel warmer in a red room than in a blue one. Yellow stimulates anxiety centers in the brain, so avoid yellows when tense. Pastels, blues and pinks are soothing. Complimentary color combinations promote comfort, while discordant color combinations precipitate anxiety.

8. Meditate – As I have described meditation done regularly offers some of the best results in stress management efforts. Plain and simple, it works. Not at all difficult, anyone can meditate, lotus position not required. Reread the section on meditation to reinforce your familiarity with this fascinating modality.

9. Relax and observe – Make time to take time. People watch, paying attention to whatever happens around you, locally, world-wide, moment by moment, without hanging on to it, without judging it. Practice mindfulness and awareness. The goal is to be aware and to experience without attaching emotive labels to the event we witness. This is powerful stuff. Try to be aware and experience your environment anew, as if for the first time, with awe and wonder. Walk down a street and take in everything; trees, colors, light, people. Experience your world as if you were a tourist in your own life.

10. Tune in – Soothing music is wonderful as a relaxation aid. Keep a collection of well-selected tapes or CD's at the ready, in your car or at home. Take frequent "music baths" by lying down in front of your speakers and allowing the music to flow over you. Or revert – go back to a happier more carefree time in your life and play the music of that era. Do you remember the popular music when you first fell in love?

11. Improve your diet – Review what you have been eaten lately. Have you migrated to more fats and simple sugars? Simple sugar consumption leads to mood swings, sugar highs, and hypoglycemic lows. Increasing your intake of complex carbohydrates and protein can attenuate the amplitude of your mood swings. Remember protein can come from vegetable sources, low-fat cheeses, soups with the emphasis on legumes, and rice. Use meat only as a garnish.

12. Put on a happy face – Try smiling, even if you don't feel like it. It is surprising how many of the body functions will follow the lead of your smiling face. Smiling is catalytic. Smile and say hello to a stranger. It will probably be returned in kind.

13. Take a hike – One of my main themes is exercise. I favor exercise as a regular part of our lives and schedules. Regular exercise serves to prevent anxiety and depression, but on occasion those rascals poke their heads up. Exercise, whether a brisk walk, a game of tennis, roller-blading, or strength training has a dependable and predictable mood lifting effect. The effect is quick and true. If you don't feel better after a physical effort, maybe it is time to join the "Prozac Parade." Exercise and kick start the circulation of those wonderful endorphines.

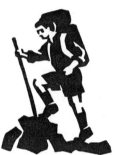

14. Try a little sunshine – Many people are victims of SAD (seasonal affective disorder). Once thought to be an "imaginary excuse" for depression or that it was "all in one's mind," SAD has been documented as a significant chemical syndrome, linked to a lack of light and relieved by exposure to sunlight or artificial sunlight. During the short daylight hours of winter, if you feel down and sad, try going for a walk at lunchtime in the sunlight. When you can't get out, try sitting in front of a full spectrum light source such as Vitalight.

I have experienced SAD and it took me eight years to diagnose it. Living on Cape Cod, with fog, frequent clouds and drizzling rain, I finally recognized the insidiously depressive nature of the environment. Winter turned everything to gray, the landscape, the ocean, the sky, the people and their attitudes. Yes, I sought more light, but I finally moved to Arizona. Thank goodness!

15. Don't worry, be happy – This little phrase embodies at least two of my principles, attitude and choice. If our attitudes are positive we will achieve positive results. What if our attitudes are poor? If they are, it was our choice.

Remember Dr. Elizabeth Kubler-Ross' offering, "Beyond that wonderful five second rage, everything is choice." Gradually, gently, with practice and support we may learn and accept that choice is available to us. So, choose a positive attitude. Choose happiness and freedom from worry. Choice is always, always, always available to us.

There is more. Not only must we be aware that choice is available, we must also accept that choice is our responsibility.

16. Let go of your fantasies and enjoy the moment – We all have fantasies, those snapshots of what we feel our lives should be. They are usually unrealistic and unattainable, covered with "shoulds and musts." If your fantasies are unrealistic, simply let them go.

Often we are not consciously aware of our fantasies, but we furiously and futilely struggle to achieve them. We become so involved in attaining the fantasy goal that we are oblivious to the trip. Nothing may be wrong with your fantasies and goals, but for goodness sake don't miss the trip there.

George, an up and coming corporate type, who was "destined to become CEO," became so consumed with that goal that he missed his children's youth and his wife's love and affection. He lost his health through inattention, had a heart attack at age 55 and is now a cardiac cripple on disability. Jane, a working mom with three kids, lived with the vision in her mind of a tidy house, obedient children, a successful husband and her own success at work. Rather busy, she reasoned that she could spend "quality time" with her children and "quality time" with her husband. "Quality time" with her children was reading stories and doing puzzles for sixty minutes by the clock every day. "Quality time" with her husband evolved to a ten-minute sexual endeavor on a weekly basis, just before falling bone-tired to sleep. Gradually, as she became more successful in her work, the "quality time" with her husband declined. In her declining years she rued the days past, the days that she did not take the time to enjoy and fully appreciate the true gifts and moments of her life. The solution was available at any point in her (or our) life. Let go of the fantasy and enjoy the moment.

17. Be where you are – One of the major causes of irritability is an inability to focus on the present. Irritable people brood over the past and fret about the future. It's impossible to tend to our own or anyone else's needs if we are preoccupied with the past or future. The message is simple. Pay attention to the now of our lives in body and mind. It can be quite enjoyable and rewarding. This is especially true and applicable with children, for they require periods of our full and dedicated attention, the nows of their and our lives. Give those nows to them by your own choice.

18. Seize the moment – We don't have to plan big trips, big events, or significant gatherings to make our lives meaningful. Spontaneous little moments possess the greatest power for fond memories and present fun. Recall as a child your favorite times and memories. I'll bet they weren't a trip to Disneyland or the family week vacation at the beach. Rather, I suspect the fondest memories are of time spent with your parents, doing little or nothing, or of time enjoyed playing with your siblings. Those are the truly good times of our lives. Take them and remember them.

19. Accept your own authority – When it comes to children, accept your own authority. Uncertainty causes stress in parents and in children. With young children, parents have the responsibility to make the rules and to enforce them. Accepting that role reduces the anxiety about the myriad of choices that a parent must make. It is her role and her responsibility. Accept it.

20. Play – Play with your children. Play with your mate. Play with your dog. Roll in the leaves with your children, romp on the beach with your mate, play "tuggies" with your dog. I challenge you to keep a straight face, not laugh, and not thoroughly enjoy yourself.

21. Take control of your time – Don't over schedule. Be selective about what time you commit. Always save ample time for yourself and your family. We can give little else so precious as our time. Give it generously to yourself and to your loved ones. Sure, schedules get busy, but periodic, prospective review and modification can correct errant allocations of time.

23. End of day stress busters – Here is a series of quickie efforts to relieve the stress of a busy day, assuming you allowed the day to get to you. Remember with good coping skills, we are less likely to be stress victims. Sing, laugh, daydream, pep talk yourself, put your worries away (write them on a piece of paper, then throw it in the trash), snack, focus on your loved ones.

24. Be aware of overload and stress points – Consciously search for patterns in your daily life that trigger a stressful reaction. Be proactive not reactive. Don't wait for the bodily expressions of stress to become obvious. Be alert for those body signs of stress should they occur and admit, acknowledge and accept stress signals when they are present. Pay attention, examine them. In the mindful attentiveness that we give them, the magnitude of the stressors will naturally diminish.

25. Learn to say no – Perhaps one of the most difficult words to get past our lips is "no." We are not conditioned by our families or by society to say, "no." Who ever would ask something of us expecting "no" as an answer? All requests and demands in our lives carry with them an implicit expectation of a "yes" response. Saying "no" makes us vulnerable to rejection, and who likes rejection? However, developing the ability to say "no" carries with it a great sense of individual power and sense of self. We do not necessarily need the approval that comes with "yes." If we can be comfortable in saying "no" we are probably reasonably secure with ourselves.

You can become an artful deliverer of a "no" response with what I call "no, but." "No, but" recognizes the validity of the request made of you, that you have given the request careful thought and consideration, even to the point of offering a modification of the request.

For example, you are under tremendous pressure to complete a project at the office, working late every night, and your daughter will be playing softball one of those evenings. She really wants her father at the game. "Dad, this is the finals. Everybody will be there." You fear that you will have to say "no." The question remains, to whom will you say "no?" Thinking quickly, you conceive a barter plan. "**No**, Mr. Chesley (your boss), I can't work Wednesday night because my daughter is playing softball and I want to be there for her. **But,** I have put my assistant to work on the project and I will be in two hours early in the morning to assure its completion."

"No, but" is assertive communication.

This little tale illustrates another important principle of living – **family is first**. Once a family event has passed and you have missed it, recapturing the moment is impossible. It's gone – history. If you are working diligently and Mr. Chesley cannot respect your dedication to family, it may be time to consider a job switch, or at least an honest, assertive discussion with Mr. Chesley. I recall H. Ross Perot affirming his view that family is the primary responsibility of a young man. "You can always continue to pursue your career when your family is grown," he commented.

26. Learn and use organizational skills – Simplify whatever and wherever you can. Delegate if possible and try to create a supportive atmosphere, at home or at work. Asking associates and family members to be part of your team compliments them. Generally, they will feel good and accept the compliment that you have intended for them. Technique is key. People perceive and receive asking for assistance quite differently than demanding or commanding.

27. For every complaint, offer two solutions – Don't be a whiner and a complainer. Don't expect other people to solve your own problems. Ultimately, you will solve all of your own problems by yourself. You may need help, and that is where friends and family come in. Reflect on the problem at hand. Look at it this way and that way. Write it down. Write down possible solutions. Then ask a friend or family member to listen to you, to your assessment of your problem and to your potential solutions. Ask for their input and if they might have additional insights. Use all of your available resources, but formulate two positive solutions for each complaint you may have. Offering solutions establishes your position as part of the "management team" of any organization, especially your organization.

28. Ask your mate for help – It is quite legitimate, you know. This is one of the responsibilities of being a marriage partner, helping the other person. It would be wonderful if our mates were intuitive enough to sense when and how we need help, but that is living in the fantasy world of playing "read my mind." It doesn't work. Mind readers are a rare commodity. Consider for a moment the risk of being married to a mind reader. Scary! It's OK to ask for help. It's good to ask.

29. Take 15 minutes twice a day to shut out the world – Relax completely. "Smoke a long cigar." One of my venerable medical mentors, when facing the imminent death of a terminal patient, and was pressured by anxious nurses to "do something, doctor," sat back and said it was time to "smoke a long cigar." Amidst the din of the chaos, if we can learn to sit back and relax, life (and death) will take care of themselves. Smoke the cigar (this is only a figure of speech, for I vehemently oppose smoking).

30. Reduce your intake of caffeine and alcohol – These and other exogenous drugs combat our bodies' efforts at homeostasis. They augment the emotional and physiological swings that we normally experience. This amplification of normal physical and emotional variations eventually causes discomfort, stress, and anxiety.

31. Cultivate a sense of humor and fun – Try not to take life too seriously. Set a goal of saying at least one funny thing per day.

Let's not forget Red Skelton's approach to worry. When he rose to face his day, he might have six things to worry about. Of the six, five never occurred. Of the sixth, he commented, "Why worry, none of us gets out of life alive, anyway?" What profound messages in comedy!

32. Develop self tolerance and discomfort tolerance – Life is not easy, smooth, or always pleasurable. Neither are we. We will experience pain, difficult times, and failures. Some we cannot change. We must learn to accept those.

33. Don't magnify your failures – Failures are failures. Don't dwell on them and increase their magnitude. Let them go.

34. Give yourself credit for past accomplishments – Much like the news media, we tend to give emotional headlines to our failures, relegating our positive accomplishments to the tiny print in the third column on the back page. Accomplishments are front page, headline news.

35. Consider negative outcomes, in order to prepare for constructive responses – Don't be blind-sided by a surprising outcome, especially a negative one. Anticipate all of the possibilities. Surprises cause stress.

36. Don't expect future failures based on past unsuccessful experiences – This is one of the thought distortions, negative predictions.

37. Minimize expectations of yourself and others – Not to suggest that you should not have high ideals, I would suggest that periodically you cut yourself and others around you some slack.

38. Consider the following factors that may enhance your ability to handle stress:

- Eat a low-fat, high-carbohydrate, high-fiber diet.
- Get 7 – 8 hours of sleep every night.
- Give and receive affection regularly.
- Have at least one friend or relative within 50 miles on whom you can rely.
- Do not smoke or use drugs or medications.
- Be the appropriate weight for your height.
- Appropriately adjust expenses to meet revenue.
- Have one or more friends to confide in about personal matters.
- Be in good health.
- Be able to modify unrealistic thinking when angry or worried.
- Do not be alone.
- Have regular conversations with the people you live with about domestic issues (chores, money, and daily living issues).
- Do something for fun at least once a week.

39. Look at yourself and your environment more positively – Beat stress before it beats you. How you perceive yourself and your environment is your choice.

40. Keep a journal – It's a powerful tool to stimulate awareness and provides an audience when you don't have one at hand. It forces you to organize your thoughts while committing them to paper.

41. Biofeedback – This obviously requires sophisticated technical equipment and a professional to administer it, but it can be of great use in reinforcing the learning of new behaviors. I found my own biofeedback laboratory in the cockpit of my airplane.

One of my passions is flying. To fly is relatively easy. To fly well requires a phenomenal marriage of knowledge and skill. During my instrument training, as my workload in the cockpit increased, my stress level increased. Unaware of my stress until I looked at the altimeter, I noticed that the unconscious muscular tension in my body had translated to an altitude error of 400 feet above my intended flight level. The altimeter became my biofeedback tool to remind me to physically relax while paying attention to the tasks at hand.

42. Take progressive "news breaks" – Have you ever paid attention to how you feel after watching the evening news. It's all so upsetting. I find myself feeling tense and irritable. The solution – don't watch it.

43. Use an intermediary – If you know that a confrontation is eminent, that it will add to your stress level, and that you don't need the additional stress, ask a neutral party to represent you. The confrontation will occur and you won't be there. You will be represented, and you will pay far less emotional currency in the process.

44. Get rid of lists – Lists, although valuable, if kept compulsively can add to stress. Eliminate them. Better yet, make a list item that says, "Do nothing."

45. Buy flowers – Flowers aren't exclusively for women or for special occasions. Flowers will brighten any day or any room.

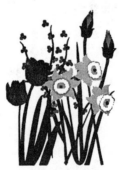

46. Have a massage – How yummy! How luxurious! How wantonly extravagant? No, how critically necessary! Massages are relaxing and have been proven to have therapeutic benefit.

47. Realize that a stressful event has already happened – It's done. It's past history. We have no ability to change what has already occurred. Choose to get on with your life.

48. Simplify – Life's more fun this way.

49. Acknowledge the negative, but focus on the positive – It's your choice.

50. If you are not going to be mad later, why be mad now?

51. Play the six months to live game – Imagine that you only have six months to live. What must you do before you die? What do you want to do before you die? What do other people want you to do? Concentrate your activities on what **you want to do.**

52. Identify your stressors, then choose to eliminate them – You may begin with the smallest stressor first, or you may begin with the greatest stressor first. You choose.

53. Use the Hermit Crab Concept – For those of you who live on the flat lands, a hermit crab is a resourceful crustacean who uses the discarded shells of other sea dwelling animals as his temporary house. He utilizes what is already available.

Why reinvent the wheel each time we seek a solution to a problem? Let's use what is already in place and build upon it. It's a very simple idea that has been available to us for all time. Occasionally, we forget.

The next time you face a problem, remember the hermit crab. Ask yourself what has already been done to solve the problem. Could you use any present knowledge or structure to assist you in the solution?

54. Use The Tuition Concept of Learning – We all do dumb things. We all make mistakes. Some are small and some are large. Some are free and some cost money. Allow yourself the education of making initial mistakes.

The cost of the mistake is the tuition paid to the School of Experiential Learning. In our society, "higher education" costs dearly. If we repeat the mistake, then we enter a remedial class called Stupidity 101. We may accept paying tuition for the initial learning, but to pay it again is sheer folly.

55. Circle the Wagons – Circling the wagons is a crisis management technique. When all hell has broken loose in your life, the roof falls in, the earth trembles beneath your feet, the Indians attack your wagon train; all I want you to remember is the phrase "Circle the Wagons." Do you recall the Saturday morning westerns on television during the late 1950's? The Indians were always attacking the wagon train. The wagon train leader would then yell, "Circle the wagons! Circle the wagons!"

Circling is a natural, often defensive, mechanism. Porcupines and hedgehogs roll up in a ball when threatened. Zebras usher their young and infirm members into the center of a circling herd to protect them from predators. Whales swim in circles to condense other fish into a smaller area, then swim up through the middle of the concentration of fish to eat them.

When we remember to "Circle the Wagons," we are assuming a defensive posture and protecting ourselves from injury. We've already learned that a member of our "crisis team" drives each wagon, and that we should use the necessary members of our "crisis team" for our defense. Simultaneously, we are stimulating awareness that our homeostasis has been dangerously disturbed. While we reflexly protect ourselves from injury, we may begin to formulate a plan to reestablish our balance.

I love stress. It is my choice. That short statement may sound paradoxical, but when we are aware and alert, participating fully in our lives, we are most alive. By acknowledging our stressors, learning to live with them, managing them successfully, we experience the joy of living. Living with our emotions, loving our families and friends, lamenting our losses, are all part of a fuller existence. It's all a matter of our choosing to participate in our lives, rather than opting to observe. As we learn to make these choices, we *Get a Life, America!*

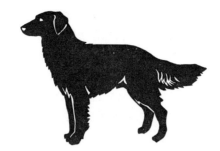

Chapter V

"Denial is Not Just a River in Egypt"

"I'm afraid the black dog has really got me. Churchill's image of despair suits me better than "the black hole." A black hole just swallows you up. Would that it were that easy, to sink down into darkness, as if sleeping. But this dog, this dog! It crouches in the corner of the room, waits for me to make a move. Or lies at the foot of the bed, like a shadow, until I try to get up."

Growls, and will not let me up.

I go nowhere alone; he's at my side. He stands between me and any other, while I'm looking good, staying calm, smiling to disarm his ferocity.

Little things overwhelm me: I can't find the mate to my sock. I break the yolk of the egg. The doorbell rings while I'm on the phone. I can't cope with the little things while he's there.

I have a lunch date.

I cannot see how to get dressed for it.

The dog stands in the way.

I can't figure out where to put the baby down so he's safe ....."

❖

from the Prologue of *On the Edge of Darkness* by Kathy Cronkite (yes, Walter's kid)

A chapter about depression? Yes. In this chapter we'll reveal a well-kept secret – that depression affects one in five of us, yet we steadfastly deny its existence. Depression, still viewed as a personal weakness by many, denied by most, ruins lives and kills. We'll look at bringing this sinister visitor out from the darkness into the light of day. We'll learn that much like the night stalking vampire, depression shrinks from the light of day, the dawning of awareness and acknowledgment of its presence. We'll learn how to recognize it, and we'll learn how to prevent it and to combat it. If nothing else, this chapter will free you from the shackles of shame for your depression.

Michael Jordan appeared in a skit on *Saturday Night Live,* one about positive affirmations with Stuart Smalley. Stuart questioned Michael about any apprehensions he might have on the basketball court. "Are there nights when you feel sub par?" queried Stuart. "No," calmly responded Michael. "Are there nights when you feel inadequate about your skills or scoring," he pressed on. Again, "No." "Well, are there times when you worry that other players will get the best of you?" Stuart searched with growing frustration. "Not really." Stuart snapped his head to Michael and chided, "Michael, denial is not just a river in Egypt, you know."

In a book focusing on prevention, health, and wellness, it may seem paradoxical to include a chapter on depression. Having presented a theme, assuming health as the norm, then building upon that foundation to maintain a higher level of health and function, I offer insights and information about depression. Why? Of insidious nature, the omnipresence of this debilitating condition, as well as our steadfast denial of its existence, demands exposure.

I met Mary late one evening in the ICU of Cape Cod Hospital. She couldn't talk. She was unconscious, a tube in her trachea, ventilated by a respirator. Her parents provided me with background about Mary. Five years prior, at eighteen, she was unhappy. Now twenty-three, isolated and depressed ,yet to no one's knowledge, suicidal, she tried to take her life by an overdose.

She had taken a massive quantity of pills, enough to kill a horse. Only through the providence of early discovery, she was rushed to the hospital, treated and supported. By all rights she should have died, but she lived.

I don't know why, but her post hospital psychotherapy served as a catalyst to turn her life around. She found a good relationship, got a job writing for a prominent travel magazine, and last I knew, was living a healthy productive life.

Mary's is a common story. Unfortunately, many depressed people attempt suicide. Most people close to the patient never suspect the depths of depression, and certainly never expect suicide.

It's our steadfast blindness to depression and denial to its existence that makes depression so dangerous. Mary's story is uncommon in its happy outcome. Boy, did she *Get a Life!* You can, too.

Old as Dirt

Depression, a relatively recent medical diagnostic category, is old as dirt. For centuries the condition was called melancholia, from the ancient Greeks' humoral theory of the temperaments. Melancholia was thought to reflect an excess of black bile. Modern clinicians sometimes use the term melancholia to define the most severe cases of primary endogenous depression. Depression, a much broader term than melancholia, now occupies a position of common usage in our modern society.

Many studies conclude that between 4% and 14% of patient visits to primary care physicians are prompted from some form of depression. One study in particular demonstrated the overall prevalence of clinically depressive symptoms in primary care visits to be 21%, while only 1.2% of the patients cited depression as a reason for the medical visit. Reasonable estimates indicate that depression in some form may be as high as 20% in a setting of primary care providers. Can these estimates be extrapolated to the general population with similar percentages?

Outside certain socioeconomic milieus, namely upper middle class urbanites who provide the New York City psychiatrists with a fine living and loads of funny stories for their cocktail circuits, depression and other psychiatric disorders remain strongly stigmatized, especially among older individuals. Because of the stigmata attached to depression, it is possible, even probable, that the prevalence of the condition may be significantly underreported. Consequently, our national statistics on depression may be erroneously low.

We are loathe to admit to medical professionals, let alone to ourselves, that we might be depressed. We view depression as some sort of emotional weakness, an inability to function normally in society. Moreover, we fear that society will deem us weak. Valid concerns about discrimination in employment (if you are an airline pilot and acknowledge depression, the FAA will yank your "medical" and you are out of a job!), security clearances, insurability and reduced rates of third party payments for treatment are among the reasons for non-reporting of depressive symptoms. I am a member of the post World War II baby boom generation and live among the first part of a succession of generations who have discovered and acknowledged that depression is a part of many of our lives.

Depressive disorders are highly prevalent and associated with significant mortality and morbidity, exacting a huge toll in human suffering and economic terms. Sixty-percent of suicides are attributable to major depressive disorders, and up to 15% of people with depression severe enough to be hospitalized will eventually commit suicide. Men are at particular risk, but as women integrate into corporate environs, they compete with the men for risk. Suicide ranks as the third leading cause of death in the 15 to 35 year-old population subgroup. Depression is a costly, chronic disorder with a high probability of recurrence.

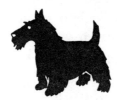

It Costs a Bundle!

The social costs of depression include charges for hospitalization, institutionalization, visits to doctors, visits to non-doctor counselors, drug treatments, as well as the indirect costs of lost productivity. The total cost of mood disorders on a nationwide scale has been estimated at $16 billion annually. Other studies like that of Greenberg in the 1990 article in the Journal of Clinical Psychiatry estimate the costs to be much greater, on the order of $43.7 billion annually. We can debate the specific numbers but cannot debate the fact that depression and mood disorders cost money.

OK, so a lot of people out there have it, and it is a big dollar item, but what is it? Depression refers to a range of disorders of mood, spanning a spectrum from a mild case of the blues, to being discouraged about a loss by your favorite professional sports team, to the most severe uncontrollable, blackest of feelings that seem to come from nowhere. The bleak, utter despair, the dark abyss that demands death, or the insidious uncontrollable bipolar undulations of manic depressive illness are expressions of emotions beyond our ability to cope, depression at its worst. The Black Dog!

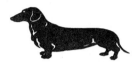

Often our ego defense mechanisms of denial and internalization contribute to our depression, augment it, and obscure our early recognition of the process. Here is a list some of the major categories of symptoms that should tip us off to the presence of depression. Do you see yourself here? Do you see friends here?

1) Depressed mood, or irritable mood in children and adolescents. Irritable mood in adults who act in a juvenile manner, most of the day, every day as indicated by self-observation or by the observation of others.
2) Markedly diminished interest or pleasure in activities that were formerly pleasurable.
3) Significant weight loss or gain when not purposely dieting, or change in appetite on a prolonged daily basis.
4) Change in sexual desires or habits.
5) Change in sleep patterns.
6) Fatigue or loss of energy. Fatigue in an otherwise healthy, robust appearing individual is a leading symptom of depression. Fatigue and the attendant medical evaluation is a very expensive part of the Gross National Depression Medical Product (my term for money spent on depression).
7) Feelings of worthlessness or inappropriate guilt.
8) Diminished ability to think, concentrate or make decisions. Increasing tendency to make mistakes or errors.
9) Agitation, excitability, tremors or shaking.
10) Recurrent thoughts of death, not just a fear of dying. Recurrent suicidal ideations without a specific plan, or a suicide attempt.

Depression is very common. Be alert for it. Look in your emotional mirror with the above list in hand. Do any of the symptoms fit? Are you at risk? Do you know someone who has any of these symptoms? Let me give you a little more information about the types of depression and then we shall explore ways to eliminate or cope with depression. Unrecognized and untreated, depression is debilitating.

Classification of Depression

Various classifications of depression, all useful in their own right, have historically filled the psychiatric literature. Classification allows us to understand a vast array of clinical presentations and to better manage our specific problem. If we suffer from depression, our ability to function, to be productive, and to enjoy our lives is markedly diminished. If only for the reason of being better able to enjoy our lives, I highly recommend our self-scouting for depression. Do you fall into any of these groups?

Melancholic depression is more common among older individuals and is primarily characterized by a prolonged loss of enjoyment of life and an inability to experience pleasure.

Psychotic depression involves delusions and/or hallucinations. It tends to have genetic predisposition and, therefore, runs in families.

Catatonic depression describes a condition in which the individual may be stuporous or extremely withdrawn.

Atypical depression affects mostly younger persons and is differentiated by two hallmarks. The individual may display a vegetative personality (over-eating, over-sleeping, weight gain) or he may display extreme anxiety (difficulty sleeping, phobias, and generalized hyperactivity of organ systems).

Seasonal affective disorder (SAD) has become widely recognized and diagnosed. Characterized by repetitive annual depression usually related to decreased available light days, it's most common in the winter months and in gray, cloudy, rainy climates, and it's very responsive to light therapy (or moving to Arizona).

Post-partum depression affects 10% to 15% of women within three to six months of delivery. It can be catastrophic. The most severe case that I can recall was a young mother who purposely walked in front of a train, leaving her infant son and his father to survive alone.

Depressive disorder not otherwise specified (DDNOS) is what we in medicine call a "waste basket" diagnosis. Not meant to be demeaning, the term describes those diagnoses that do not fit into other categories and need a place to be filed. This large, very important category, encompasses many people who have no idea that depression affects their lives. These persons may not have symptoms severe enough to achieve the status of the other, more easily definable classifications, but still suffer from diminished performance and enjoyment of life. I suspect that a vast portion of our population could be placed in this category. In one study of the general population, fully 11% satisfied the criteria for DDNOS.

Bipolar disorder is the new terminology for what was formerly called manic depressive disorder. These disorders are marked by swings between profound depression and periods of uncontrollable mania (psychic and emotional hyperactivity so severe as to appear psychotic). In reality, the manic episodes of these unfortunate victims are replete with absolute panic and fear.

Panic and fear, common to all depression, often precede catastrophe. Feeling boxed into a corner, depressed persons all too frequently attempt suicide.

I received a call from the hospital late one night, it's always late at night, telling me that one of my patients was there with an overdose. Twenty-four dreary miles later, I arrived at the Emergency Room to see my patient. This was a man whom I saw regularly in my office and around town. When I looked at him on the stretcher, I didn't recognize him. So, I went back to check the chart. It was a match, right chart, right patient. The best that I can offer here is that people don't look too good when they try to kill themselves.

Do yourselves, your family, and your doctor a favor and don't attempt to kill yourself. There are better choices. In this case, we made the better choice after a near catastrophic wake-up call of his suicide attempt. Our better choice with this particular gentleman was to arrange to see him in the office every Friday morning for an hour of talking. He brought two donuts and I provided coffee. Well, I provided something else, too, something glaringly absent from his life, friendship and love. He did die about two years later at age eighty-four of natural causes, and happier I might say.

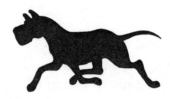

How Do You Recognize Your Depression?

Armed with the above knowledge about depression, how do you determine if you suffer from depression? Ask. Ask yourself, ask your friends, ask your family. If you have any inkling that something in your life just doesn't feel right, ask. "Am I behaving differently? Do I irritate you?"

A simple screening technique was offered to me at a medical meeting a few years ago. The professor said, "You all know those patients and people who simply irritate you, who seem to get under your skin without half trying, those that for some unidentifiable reason, you rue the thought of seeing. All you want to do is to get them out of the office quicker than they came in. There is a high probability that those persons are depressed. The behavior that is so irritating to you, that you want to avoid, is a manifestation of their depression. If you can bring yourself to see these people in that light, then you may be in a better position to help them." I pass this insight along to you to use in any social interaction. Depression is common and so is irritating behavior. Could there be a tie that binds the two?

Let's look at this lesson from a different perspective. If you find that people are avoiding you, it's possible that you may be guilty of similar abrasive behavior. It's possible that you may be depressed. In your subconscious attempts to cope with your depression you may be altering your personality. "Yes," you counter, "but there are also some people in this world who are just plain jerks!" Right you are, and we can't fix that, can we?

If you are concerned about your own potential for depression, many commercial screening tests for depression are available, but usually only available though a professional therapist. In a turf protection move, those therapists will tell you that it is only they who can interpret the test results (and charge you a lot of money). You certainly can screen for depression on your own. The graphic nature of the results, a specific number score, can serve as a catalyst to your seeking help, self or professional. Once recognized, most depression can be handled by yourself. Professional help in dealing with depression can be excellent, but make it your positive choice. Take the following 20 question screening test for depression and see how you score.

Depression Questionnaire

Directions: for each of the following twenty questions, phrases or statements indicate a numerical score between one and ten with one representing the least positive situation and ten representing the most positive. Don't spend a lot of time on any one by being too analytical. Read and answer quickly.

1. Oh, how I love to get up in the morning ...
   1____2____3____4____5____6____7____8____9____10____
   Too tired, don't want to   Can't wait, let's go

2. Hi Ho it's off to work I go ...
   1____2____3____4____5____6____7____8____9____10____
   Yuk   Whoopie

3. I am late, I am late for a very important date ...
   1____2____3____4____5____6____7____8____9____10____
   Oh, no!   No big deal

4. Frankly, Scarlet, I don't give a damn ...
   1____2____3____4____5____6____7____8____9____10____
   I don't care either   I give a damn

5. Uh, Mrs. Robinson, you've got your bra off ...
   1____2____3____4____5____6____7____8____9____10____
   uh, oh   oh, boy!

6. A little bit of sugar helps the medicine go down ...
   1____2____3____4____5____6____7____8____9____10____
   I hate medicine   Thanks for the help

7. Oklahoma! Oklahoma!
   1____2____3____4____5____6____7____8____9____10____
   Too loud, be quiet   Sing it again

8. My Country 'tis of Thee, Sweet land of Liberty ...
   1____2____3____4____5____6____7____8____9____10____
   Go away, don't bother me   I'll stand while you sing

9. I've got a bluebird on my shoulder ...
   1____2____3____4____5____6____7____8____9____10____
   And it just crapped   How pretty

10. Fly high ... you are the wind beneath my wings ... fly high ...
    1____2____3____4____5____6____7____8____9____10____
    I am too tired to fly   I appreciate you so much

11. I must be overly sensitive because my feelings seem to get hurt a lot ...
    1____2____3____4____5____6____7____8____9____10____
    It really hurts   I can take it

12. Happy, Happy, Joy, Joy ...
    1____2____3____4____5____6____7____8____9____10____
    The bluebird is still crapping   Let's dance

13. It seems that bad things are constantly happening to me, only to me ...
    1____2____3____4____5____6____7____8____9____10____
    Nobody else   Tomorrow's a better day

14. When I look in the mirror, I like what I see .....
    1____2____3____4____5____6____7____8____9____10____
    No   Yes

15. When I see myself naked in the mirror, I ...
    1____2____3____4____5____6____7____8____9____10____
    Want to throw up   Am glad that I exercise

16. I treat myself well and expect others to treat me well, too ...

1____2____3____4____5____6____7____8____9____10____
No, they mistreat me   Of course

17. I love to fall in love ...

1____2____3____4____5____6____7____8____9____10____
Too scary   Can't wait

18. If a stranger said, "Hello," would you respond in kind?

1____2____3____4____5____6____7____8____9____10____
Hang my head and walk on by   Good morning to you

19. I like flowers. I like colors. I like bright blue skies ...

1____2____3____4____5____6____7____8____9____10____
I want to go back to bed   Show me more

20. I'm late for work. The boss is on a tear. The dog just pooped on the rug.

1____2____3____4____5____6____7____8____9____10____
That's it, I can't take any more!   Poor doggie, couldn't get out, sorry

Now add up your total score and divide by twenty. This gives you a numerical placement along the continuum scale from significantly depressed (1) to blissful lunacy (10). You may generally view the importance of your score as follows:

1.0 to 2.9 – You are significantly depressed. Consider professional help, soon.

3.0 to 4.9 – You are displaying depressive thinking, interpretation and attitude.

5.0 to 6.9 – Obviously the middle ground, but these questions and statements are generally upbeat in themselves, and even neutral responses may tip off a depressive viewpoint.

7.0 to 8.9 – This is where I would like you to be, reasonably positive, but not wearing rose-colored glasses.

9.0 to 10 – Time to take your Lithium (the drug that treats the mania associated bipolar disorders). You're wearing blinders, not rose-colored glasses.

How to Prevent and Combat Depression

Depression is not an obligatory component of our daily existence. Beyond modest limits it is abnormal, detrimental and just plain no fun. And, it is within our realm of control to manage and to virtually eliminate it from our lives. We do have this choice. While I may risk nauseating repetition about the sequence of behavior change, please allow me to review it quickly here, for it applies directly to coping with depression.

1. **Capacity** – One must possess the capacity to recognize and initiate the process of coping with or preventing depression.

2. **Awareness** – "Once recognized a problem is half solved," quoted George Washington. Without awareness of our problems, we are issued a life sentence of being imprisoned by them.

3. **External motivation** – As with behaviors, something in our world must be suffering due to our depression; a relationship, work or our health.

4. **Internal motivation** – We must acknowledge and accept the depression as our own and be internally motivated to change.

5. **Execution** – Make a plan and do something about it.

The biggest problem in managing depression is our blindness to the fact that depression hangs its hat in our closet. The insidious nature of depression, then, nurtures and prolongs its own existence. Assuming your capacity to change, however you become aware of depressive tendencies in yourself is unimportant. Awareness and acceptance are the initial goals.

If you spot it by looking in the mirror, a friend tells you that you have changed, you notice physical changes (e.g. energy decrease, palpitations, loss of appetite), or you have taken my screening inventory, at least you have begun to look. You may benefit from reviewing the section on awareness in the chapter on behavior modification for other techniques to promote awareness. Once you are aware and believe that depression may be a problem for you, what can you do about your discovery? How can you deal with it?

No single solution to depression awaits us. The solution lies in the incremental summation of multiple efforts. The summary process eventuates in the amelioration of the depressive mood disturbance. Add up a whole bunch of little fixes and you have a big fix. Remember, too, the concept of **synergy**. Some of the preventive and therapeutic techniques that you employ will potentiate others. The result will be a whole, greater than the sum of the parts. Be mindful of the concept of **catalytic behaviors.** Performing certain behaviors will facilitate the incorporation of other behaviors into your coping armamentarium. Select as many as you wish from the following list of anti-depressive behaviors.

Talk – It may be cheap, but its value is priceless and limitless. It is the best. Talking leads my list of therapeutic interventions for depression and stress management. It works. It aids in self-discovery. It is the basis for psychologic therapy. Talking to a good listener, one who is compassionate, not prone to interruption or "solving" your problems, one who may be able to ask appropriate questions to guide you or to explore areas you may not have considered important, is the best therapeutic and preventive emotional effort I know. Sure, I have just described the ideal psychotherapist. But unless you are severely depressed and suicidal, the "therapist" doesn't have to have letters (Ph.D., M.S., M.D., L.I.S.W.) behind his name to be effective for you. A good friend may be your best listener.

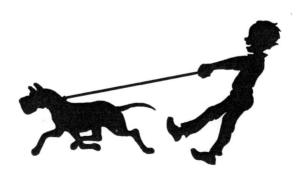

Listen

When I ask you to listen and you start giving advice,
      you have not done what I asked

When I ask you to listen to me and you begin to tell me why

I should feel that way, you are trampling on my feelings.

When I ask you to listen to me and you feel you have to do
      something to solve my problems, you have failed me,
      strange
      as that may seem.

Perhaps that is why prayer works for some people,

Because

God is mute and He doesn't offer advice or try to fix things,

He just listens and trusts you to work it out yourself.

So please just listen and hear me. And if you want to talk
      wait a few minutes for your turn and I promise I'll listen
      to you.

The meaningful answers that we find in our lives are the answers that we uncover of our own accord. A friend may offer the identical solution, but answers assume greater "validity" if we discover them on our own. Is there a reason for how I feel? Did something happen in my life, in my relationships? If so, can I change it? How can I change it? What if I can change my circumstances, then what might I expect? Talk, explore, take some time, reflect, then talk and explore some more.

Good marriages or partnerships are founded upon and grounded in a base of good communication. Talking, exploration, and listening are regular and routine. Potential problems and negative emotional reactions to them may be averted by good, regular, honest, assertive communication. Good communication seems self evident to emotional health, but less than 10% of relationships practice good, assertive communication.

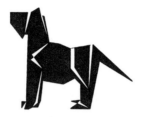

Exercise – Step over the black dog! Regular aerobic exercise has been proven to relieve and prevent depression. The generation and release into the circulation of endorphins produces a mood elevating effect that lasts for much longer than the immediate exercise period. The associated benefits of increased muscle tone and performance ability add to the neurotransmitter effect of the endorphins. Better mood, better performance, more strength, and greater endurance all support the emergence of an improved attitude, demeanor, and self-image.

Although strength training may not result in endorphin release, the increased muscle strength, tone and efficiency allow us to perform the usual daily activities with less attendant fatigue. You will stand straighter, walk more briskly and feel better about yourself. Refer to chapter III on exercise to review the hows of establishing and maintaining an exercise program. Are you already exercising? Vary your program. It can add thyme to your life.

Improve Your Nutrition – Review your diet. Have you regressed to old or bad eating habits? Are simple sugars and fats (snacks) becoming staples in your diet? Is caffeine (coffee, sodas, chocolate) consumption becoming increasingly common? Snacks and caffeine constitute a common depression diet. That diet, nutritionally catastrophic, promotes your feeling physically wretched. The rapid rises of blood sugar with obligatory, precipitous "sugar lows" occurring shortly after snack consumption produce internal biochemical chaos. Compound that chaos with a blast of caffeine, then wait for the caffeine withdrawal in the evening when you aren't drinking coffee. It's a roller coaster ride. These paradoxical physiologic reactions produce an uncomfortable and unacceptable biochemical undulation, which exacerbates depression.

Eating significant quantities of fat is a problem, too. Fat intake has been proven to decrease physical performance when compared to complex carbohydrate intake. Decreased physical abilities contribute to depression. All of the nutritional factors mentioned are at least additive, if not potentiating, in their effect on depression.

Let's take control. We can attenuate the amplitude of the sugar highs and lows, the caffeine highs and lows, by eating a diet high in complex carbohydrates. The complexity of the molecular structure of complex carbohydrates dictates a longer period of time for their metabolism to glucose, thus avoiding rapid fluctuations in blood sugar. Limit caffeine intake and decrease fat intake. Evidence, albeit anecdotal and circumstantial, that high protein diets aid in treating depression has been has been frequently offered. One psychiatrist that I interviewed a number of years ago felt that he achieved a 15% improvement in depressive symptoms in his patients if they adopted a high protein diet. **Note:** anyone who opts for a high protein diet must remember to drink high volumes of water for kidney protection.

Depression is often consequent to our perception of being out of control of our lives. By "eating right" we gain the additional psychologic reward that comes from our perception of being in control of our lives.

Choose a Preventive Philosophy – Aver that you are in control and wish to have good physical and mental health. View your emotional health in a preventive fashion. Do not view your life with a retrospectoscope, finding and fixing things that went wrong. Think ahead and plan ahead.

Do preventive maintenance. Plan vacations ahead, regularly, when you don't "need" them. Don't wait until you are so emotionally inundated and crippled that you have to "take some time off." Have you ever felt that you were emotionally under water, breathing through a straw? Vacations are for (should be for) prevention, not for repair. It's simply a matter of choice. It's a matter of simple choice.

"Beyond that wonderful, glorious five second rage, everything is choice." – Don't ever forget this quote from Dr. Kubler-Ross. Such a simple statement may save your life.

Write – Keep a journal of your thoughts, ideas, happinesses, unhappinesses, hopes and aspirations, fears and fetishes. Write letters to friends and to family members. Write letters to yourself. This is powerful. It's amazing what you might tell yourself. Write a poem and frame it on your wall. Write a fantasy. Do it again. Discovery and expression greet you in your writing.

I sat down to work on this book one morning in my office, which incidentally is located at my local airport (one of my favorite places, and my positive choice to be here). Not feeling terribly motivated to work on the book, I began typing a short fantasy story. Three hours later I didn't have a lick of work done on this book, but I had such fun and was allowed a very interesting look at myself.

Socialize – Don't isolate yourself. Throw a party. Invite your friends to your house. Having a party affords you not only an environment with people, but also the benefit of doing something nice for other people. Giving of yourself is very rewarding. Go to the theater with a friend. Live theater teems with excitement, a very positive social environment. Call someone that you like and ask them out on a date. If you are married, ask your mate for a date.

My friend suffered a terrible tragedy. She returned home to find her brother hanging by his neck from the balcony of her living room, an obvious suicide attempt. With the aid of the paramedics he was "saved" physically, but now suffers from significant brain damage. She became his caretaker, and lives with the present burden and responsibility of her brother's care, and with the indelible memory of the event. Every day she "sees" him there, hanging by his neck from her balcony. What to do? She threw a party. Her friends, her friends' friends, the more the better, everyone was invited. Great party! Good time! Now at least she can remember the party in her house, the festivities, the laughter, not the tragedy.

One of my favorite people, Harry Blank, an older gentleman when I knew him, selflessly shared so much of his wisdom with me. We were together at the ICU when his wife died there one afternoon. I have been present at so many deaths, and I am never sure what to do, what to say, what to expect. Well, Harry turned to me with half of a smile and asked if he could take me to lunch at the Hyannis Yacht Club. I asked myself, "What? Lunch? Don't you know that your wife just died?" Of course he did, but he explained to me that he and his wife loved to sail, loved the water, and loved people. Where better would she want him to be? Later that year Harry booked a six-month cruise around the world. He chose not to withdraw from life. He kept himself busy with people and activities.

Don't isolate yourself – "A warm body in a room is better than being alone." Depression can be akin to terminal illness because it is so abjectly lonely. You need people. I related the story of the terminally ill person, whom, when offered a private room in a hospital quoted, "I fear being alone. I want to be in a room with someone, if only a warm body, for it's far better than being alone." If you are depressed, do not, do not, do not, be alone!

Take a newsbreak – Go for a day, a week, two weeks without reading newspapers or watching television news (or television at all). What information have you received from news sources that was meaningful to your life? Other than "being informed," news only serves to create and promote anxiety. All of the news that sells is bad news. Wars, murders, crashes (economic, aviation and auto) and natural disasters are all "news." Have you ever gone on a two-week camping trip to find upon your return that you had not thought about news happenings for the entire time? Were you at a loss for not having received news for that time? It is doubtful. Were you more relaxed? Probably you were.

Avoid depressants – If you are taking any medications, review them in the *Physician's Desk Reference* (available at most libraries) to identify any pharmacologic depressant effect of the drug. Look it up yourself, and don't depend on your doctor or pharmacist to warn you. Address that possibility quickly. Avoid alcohol because you will probably be a morose drunk, and that does no one any good. Avoid "nay sayers" and anyone who has a negative effect on you. This is not the time to try to repair difficult relationships. Seek supportive, understanding, forward thinking persons. You need to be stroked with the direction of your fur, not against it. Have you ever tried petting an animal against the direction of their fur?

Ask for help – Speak up! Ask! You are highly unlikely to get what you don't ask for. Few of your friends are intuitive enough or insightful enough to recognize what you need and when you need it. We universally fear asking for help, lest someone reject our pleas. Sure, it is possible that our request may not be granted. However, not receiving what we requested is simply not getting what we asked for. It is not personal rejection. Personal rejection is what we interpret, what we truly fear. The worst that can happen in asking someone for help is simply not getting the help. What then? Ask someone else.

Delegate – If you are overloaded with tasks and responsibilities, then delegate (this is part of being your own CEO). Prioritize. Some of your "obligations" can wait. Some really don't need attention at all.

Eat the elephant – Do you remember how? Eat the elephant one bite at a time. Refer to Chapter IV on stress management for an expanded treatment of eating the elephant.

Play the six months to live game – Picture yourself with just six months to live. What do you truly **have** to do? Better yet, what do you truly **want** to do? You choose.

Use a middle man – If you are facing a potentially unpleasant, adversarial confrontation, use the middle man approach. Ask someone to be your spokesperson, someone who has no vested emotional interest in the confrontation. It's a great defusing mechanism for both highly charged adversarial combatants.

Seek newness – Look for something enjoyable and new to add to your life. Being cautious not to overload your circuits, consider learning to play a musical instrument, learning a language, enjoying new music, or traveling to a place that you have never been before. Find a new friend. Join an organization or volunteer at a hospital or food kitchen. Newness generates enthusiasm.

Seek beauty – I love this one. On a daily basis look for and allow beauty to enter and to be part of your life. Seek and appreciate beauty. Be mindful of the beauty in your surroundings. Did you ever stand in awe of the natural beauty of a tree? Have you watched the clouds constantly forming and dissipating as you lie supine on freshly mowed grass. Allow the smell of the grass to fill your senses. Bring flowers into your home. Plant them. Add more colors around you. Seek music, art and people beautiful to you.

I am fascinated with birds of prey and take special notice if I see one soaring. It is a very special beauty to me. If I am privileged on any day to see an eagle, I have what I call an "eagle day." I hold that if I have been blessed to view this unique beauty of Nature, I will carry that vision with me the entire day. That day becomes good and complete, regardless of the day's events. It is a matter of belief and perspective, but it works for me. Find what is beautiful to you and hold it next to your heart.

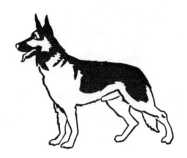

Fall in love on a daily basis – Allow yourself to love, someone or something. Seek and hold love in your life. Be it a family member, partner or clerk at the coffee shop, a host of lovable people cue up to be in your life. Invite them in. Look for and embrace love every day of your life. Do not be afraid to accept love offered in return.

Follow the lead of Leonardo Da Vinci – "Every now and then, go away, take a little relaxation, because when you come back to your work, your judgment will be surer. To remain constantly at work will cause you to lose power of judgment. Go some distance away, because then the work appears smaller and more of it can be taken in at a glance, and a lack of harmony or proportion is more readily seen."

Maintain a direction facing forward – At the close of each day, sit and review your day. Make an evening "I did" list rather than the customary morning "to do" list. Be able to list at least one, and preferably more, positive accomplishments for that day. For example, you exercised, walked the dog, called a friend, cleaned the house, planned a vacation. Give yourself credit for accomplishments. If you have a "do nothing day" then choose to do nothing. The choice of doing nothing becomes the positive effort for that day. Don't be a passive cork in the water, directed by external currents and winds. Your perception that you have choices and control your life empowers you.

Pick more daisies – Isn't it magic how poets express a myriad of thoughts and emotions in a few lines?

Daisies

If I had my life to live over, I would pick more daisies.
I'd try to make more mistakes, I would be sillier than
I had been this trip. I would relax, I would limber up,
I would take more trips, travel lighter. I would be crazier.
I would be less hygienic. I would take more chances.
I would climb more mountains, swim more rivers and watch
more sunsets.
I would eat more ice cream and less beans. I would have
more actual troubles and fewer imaginary ones.
You see, I am one of those people who live practically,
and sensibly and sanely, hour after hour, day after day.
Oh, I have my mad moments. And if I had it to do over again,
I'd have more of them. In fact, I'd try to have nothing else;
Just moments, one after another, instead of living so many
minutes ahead.
I have been one of those people who never go anywhere
without a thermometer, a hot water bottle, a gargle, a raincoat
and a road map. If I had my life to live over,
I would start barefooted earlier in the spring and stay that way
later in the fall. I'd play hookey more. I would ride more
merry-go-rounds and swing more. I would do more water and
sun and fun things. I'd turn more somersaults, and roll in the
grass, and go barefoot all over. If I had my life to live over,
I'd spend more time at fun places. I'd try to be more in touch
with God and those I love. I'd pray aloud more and not care
what people think or expect of me. I'd give more of me and
take more of you. I'd just be more and more ....
Yes, I'd pick more daisies next time.

Nadine Stair

Seek a good therapist – If, in spite of attempts to improve your depression, you find yourself sinking ever deeper into the dark abysses of depression, and certainly, if suicide passes across your vision screen, get professional help. Don't wait! As you know, I remain philosophically opposed to unnecessary drug treatment, but I rage against suicide resulting from depression. Suicide simply is not necessary.

While I feel that antidepressant drugs are over-prescribed and over-used in general, I recognize their role and effectiveness in major depressive reactions. Unfortunately the popularization of drugs like Prozac by the lay press, the widespread availability of these drugs and the reluctance and laziness of practitioners to seek the root causes of depression, has led to "quick hands" in prescribing drugs for depression. I simply wish that the drugs were used with greater thought and care.

Search for a good and compassionate therapist, one with whom you feel you can work. If you are not satisfied with the first one, seek a second opinion. Which reminds me ... Rodney Dangerfield wasn't happy with his diagnosis of gastritis and said he wanted a second opinion. His doctor said, "OK, you are ugly, too."

Laugh – This last little anecdote reminds us all to laugh. You can't cry when you are smiling. But you can *Get a Life!* when you're laughing and smiling.

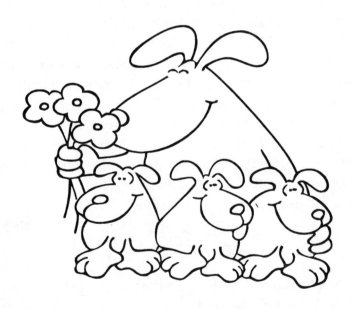

A Matter of Fat

"Cholesterol"

❖

by: Charles Albert Appel
Lt. Col. USAF, WW II

Arthritis, bursitis and seventy-two years;
Those aches and those pains, they gave me no fears.
But now I am panicked, my back to the wall,
Horror of horrors, I have Cholesterol.

Cholesterol was unknown when I was a lad;
Today all I know is that it's something bad.
Seriously, I knew it wasn't something small,
When I was told: I had Cholesterol.

Something I don't know scares the hell out of me,
And cholesterol falls into that cat-e-gory.
Up to that time, I had no worries at all,
Until I was told: I had Cholesterol.

Dairy products are out, no more eggs for me,
And marbled red meats are taboo, you see.
My diet must change, menus and all,
Since I was told: I had Cholesterol.

Asparagus, broccoli, but no Hollandaise;
Tomato is fine, but no mayonnaise.
The gloom that descended is draped like a pall,
Since I was told: I had Cholesterol.

It isn't contagious, or that's what they say,
But somehow I notice my friends fade away.
None of them write and few of them call,
Since I was told: I had Cholesterol.

As healthy as a horse and strong as an ox,
Yet recently I've become sly as a fox.
For seventy-two years, life's been a ball,
Until I was told: I had Cholesterol.

In this very critical chapter, we'll focus on the simple chemistry of lipids (fats), what the component parts of cholesterol are, and how exercise affects lipids. We'll offer irrefutable epidemiological evidence supporting the value of lowering cholesterol levels. We'll understand that a low cholesterol diet may not be a cholesterol lowering diet. We'll examine genetics, and look at cholesterol in women, children, and seniors. We'll end with an affirmation to *Get a Life!* by showing you **how** to lower your cholesterol.

In the 1980's cholesterol and fats were big news stories. We haven't heard much lately. Why? Are cholesterol and fat still important? Absolutely they are! We've unfortunately been lulled to sleep on these issues. In fact, according to Harvey Hecht, MD, of the Arizona Heart Institute, a guest on my *Get a Life!* radio show in Phoenix "More heart attacks may be related to cholesterol abnormalities than we once thought. And, the relatively tight NCEP (National Cholesterol Education Program) guidelines may not be strict enough, especially when it comes to LDL."

Dr. Hecht's comments underscore a renewed emphasis on controlling our cholesterol. Yes, it's a tedious job, but in spite of seemingly meager added years to our lives, I offer that the reward is well worth the effort.

Why Bother Cutting Fats to Live a Mere Eleven Days Longer?

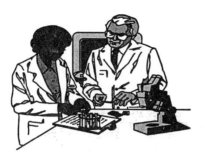

Researchers in Montreal found that reducing saturated fat intake to 10% of calories consumed could add from eleven days to 4 1/2 months to the average life-span of a man free of heart disease. A woman's potential life-span similarly increased, although less, from 3 1/2 days to 2 months.

In contrast, the same study found that cessation of smoking could add from 2 1/2 to 4 1/2 years to the life of the average male smoker and from 2 1/2 to 3 1/2 years to the life of the average female smoker. We could deduce that the disparity in results could encourage a smoker to stop, but at the cost of one's turning a deaf ear to dietary modification. Studies like these reinforce the lax attitude of physicians towards dietary counseling. It seems we gain so little.

There is, however, a lot more to life than living longer. It might not be so awful to die of a heart attack at age 80, but to have one at 35 and live the remainder of your years as a "cardiac cripple" is thoroughly repugnant. Quality of life and quality of health are the gifts we receive from making dietary changes.

I propose a study that computes the life-span gain from more stringent saturated fat intake, like 5% to 7% of total calories. I predict that we would see a more significant increase in life-span. A 10% saturated fat intake, only a modest restriction, represents a marked reduction from the American norm of 20% saturated fat intake. To my knowledge long duration studies of what I would term significant restrictions of total fat and saturated fat intake have not been accomplished, because potential study subjects become increasingly rare as available fat in their diets decreases. People, unwilling to live without their steak, milk, butter, eggs, creamed sauces and high-fat salad dressings, drop like flies from such stringent studies. Much lip service is paid to cutting fat from diets, but precious little performance follows.

Gains from performance tantalize public health officials. While benefits to the individual, on average, are meager, the expected population benefits from reducing fat and saturated fat intake may be quite substantial. Despite seemingly small individual gains in life expectancies, universal adoption of a modest low-fat diet in Canada could save 373,000 to 505,000 person-years of life for men over the lifetime of the current population. Considering the economic benefit alone, and estimating $30 thousand productivity per man-year, the economic savings to Canada would be between $11 billion and $15 billion. That produces an economic impact of up to $15 billion, not even considering women. In the United States the incidence of fat-related cardiovascular disease (CVD) costs between $50 and $100 billion annually in medical treatment and lost wages.

Consider, too, that the studies only compute average life extension in the overall population. What if you identify yourself as a high-risk individual, eating high on the hog, loving the couch, hating your job. Wouldn't it make sense to expect much greater than "average" results if you modified your diet, especially if you make significant changes to the 5-7% saturated fat level? Remember, "average" is for statistics. None of us is "average" if we have information and control.

Definition of Hyperlipidemia (High Blood Fat or Cholesterol)

OK, given that we have control, what are we controlling? Traditional medicine has defined hyperlipidemia as an increase over a designated blood lipid concentration of cholesterol or triglycerides or both. Traditionally, persons have been diagnosed as having high cholesterol or hyperlipidemia (hyper = high; lipid = fat; emia = in the blood) if their blood levels of cholesterol or triglycerides exceeded the 95th percentile for their population group. We classified people as having "normal" lipids if they fell anywhere below the 95th percentile level. This definition is based on a statistical comparison of lipid levels in our population, a population that leads the world in deaths from heart and vascular disease. In the United States I assume that having "normal" lipids meant that one would have a "normal" heart attack.

Let's give ourselves credit, however, for we have nearly made the "normal" cholesterol designation an antique. Now we refer to **desirable** lipid levels, and differentiate them from the statistical norms. Desirable levels have a much greater significance in their relationship to the incidence of heart disease than did the broad normal range. Current desirable total cholesterol is below 200 mg/dl. Heart disease is virtually non-existent in persons with levels below 150 mg/dl.

I am not terribly ancient, but can recall in my early days of medical practice telling people that their cholesterol of 240 mg/dl was "normal." That was the current medical opinion in the early 1970's. Should I have known better? Probably so, but I was just a young medical pup, barely paper-trained, trying to spit back at the public the best medical dogma that had been given to me.

I liken this mind-set to that of smokers' who smoked for years until the Surgeon General's report of 1969 told them that it was bad for their health. The universal response of the smoking community was, "Gee, I didn't think that smoking was bad until the Top Doc said so." Are we so ignorant and blind that we cannot see when something is hazardous to our health? Must we be told everything? Sadly, it seems so.

A more recent Top Doc, C. Everett Koop, MD, quoted, "Knowledge is the best prescription." Let's heed his advice as we learn how our bodies handle fats and cholesterol.

Lipid (fat) Transport

Although lipids are vital components of many of our body tissues, they are insoluble in water. The body's fluids are water-based, and in order to achieve transport to tissues, lipids must be carried by attaching themselves to molecules that can move through the aqueous (water) medium. These transporting agents are the lipoproteins, complex aggregations of lipid and protein. Basically, by attaching fat to protein, the fat can be transported in a water medium. Lipid transport in the bloodstream is designed to transport water insoluble fats to cells for energy use, storage or synthesis, or to the liver for conversion and excretion.

As defined by their density (weight per volume) on ultracentrifugation, five major lipoprotein families can be identified:

1. the chylomicron, and the following lipoproteins
2. VLDL (very low density lipoprotein)
3. IDL (intermediate density lipoprotein)
4. **LDL** (low density lipoprotein) **("bad cholesterol")**
5. **HDL** (high density lipoprotein) **("good cholesterol")**

Of this list, two are most important, **HDL** and **LDL**. HDL is a heavy, dense small molecule when compared to LDL, which is a larger, lighter, less dense molecule. Although each of the five lipoprotein families takes part in the transport process of cholesterol, LDL plays a key role. It provides cholesterol to sites that have an LDL receptor, both in the liver, but especially in the vascular intima (the lining of the arteries) where deposition of cholesterol leads to atherosclerosis (hardening of the arteries) and eventually to narrowing of the arterial lumen. HDL plays a counter-balancing role to LDL by removing the deposited cholesterol from these tissues and returning it to the liver for storage or metabolism.

HDL is synthesized by the liver and in its early form is incomplete, lacking certain surface markers and additional cholesterol. As HDL "matures" in the circulation, it takes on additional cholesterol from various tissues, including cholesterol from the vascular intima. HDL may transfer the cholesterol that it scavenges during the maturation process back to LDL molecules, or return the cholesterol to the liver for excretion. The removal of the cholesterol from the tissues, and its ability to deliver that cholesterol to the liver for excretion describes HDL's reverse transport of cholesterol. One can consider HDL a cholesterol vacuum cleaner.

The greater portion of cholesterol removing lipoprotein one possesses, the less the probability of developing progressive atherosclerosis. Reversal of the process that was born of excess LDL may be accomplished in part by increasing the artery-cleaning agent, HDL, above former equilibrium levels that initiated and caused the diseased status of the arteries.

Despite its image as a villain, cholesterol has several important functions in body chemistry. It is an essential component of nerve cells, cell membranes, and hormone synthesis. The villainous nature of cholesterol is born of the excesses of blood cholesterol and the random deposits in the delicate lining tissues of our small arteries. High LDL can be potentially damaging to the small and medium sized arteries of the vascular tree. It is crucial that levels of potentially damaging cholesterol be kept low to prevent the deposition of cholesterol into the arterial walls.

Our diets supply twenty to forty percent of cholesterol, the major portion being produced internally. The liver, and to a lesser extent the intestines and other tissues, synthesize about one gram per day. Only about one half gram of cholesterol is provided by the average diet. For simplicity we may say that cholesterol is 1/3 diet and 2/3 liver produced.

If primarily the liver synthesizes HDL, and LDL is in large part a result of dietary intake, what is the significance of that fact? Traditional medical teaching answers that genetics determines HDL levels in individuals. What you have is what you got. According to most doctors, we have little control of our HDL levels, but we may lower LDL with diet and drugs.

My answer is quite different. In my practice, I have documented elevation of HDL levels from the mid-forties to the mid-eighties with three months of regular aerobic exercise. Supported by additional documentation in clinical research, the simple good news is that **aerobic exercise raises HDL levels significantly.**

Exercise and Lipids

The research supports my opinion and experience. Numerous scientific studies have attempted to define the relationship among exercise, lipids and cardiovascular disease (CVD). The results are not definitive in terms of establishing a causal mechanism between exercise and risk of CVD, but an inverse relationship does exist. Other study results are thoroughly exciting and very positive in confirming a positive relationship between aerobic exercise and improved blood cholesterol levels.

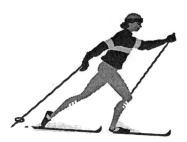

Researchers have found a relationship between HDL and physical activity, the greater the aerobic activity product (intensity x duration), the greater the beneficial effect on HDL. No positive relationship exists between strength training and one's cholesterol profile, but a positive relationship for an activity threshold of 1,000 calories per week has been reported. Other cholesterol fractions are affected, too. LDL is lowered with the same level of aerobic exercise. Total cholesterol remains constant and is unaffected by exercise specifically. Usually, however, weight decreases with exercise, and a corresponding lowering of total cholesterol is recorded. Even if total cholesterol were to remain constant, a rise in HDL results in a lowering of the total cholesterol/HDL ratio.

How long does it take to produce a lipid response to exercise? One study of walkers participating in a 500 km, ten day, walk documented an increase of HDL from 62 mg/dl to 70 mg/dl during that time. Most studies have focused on longer periods of time, and the consensus seems to be that for meaningful changes in lipid profiles, the equivalent of jogging ten miles per week for several months is necessary. At first glance that seems like a lot of exercise, but it is only a 1,200 cal per week effort, the equivalent of walking two miles a day for six days. Walking twelve miles in a week is not an overwhelming task. That level of exercise can be easily maintained with modest lifestyle modification.

Workouts of 300 or more calories offer the advantage of increasing high density lipoprotein (HDL) and increasing fat metabolism. Paffenbarger found that exercise intensity must exceed 7.5 cal/min (450 cal/hr) to reduce heart disease risk, with progressive protection at higher levels of intensity.

Although exercise does affect HDL, diet and weight (loss) are the primary influences and determinants of LDL levels. What does that mean to us? Again, the simple lesson is that dietary reduction of cholesterol and fat, especially saturated fat, will reduce LDL levels and total cholesterol. We do find a small reduction in HDL with dietary modification to lower fats, but this is more than offset by a greater percentage reduction in the LDL. One can also compensate for the minimal decrease in HDL from diet by performing routine aerobic exercise. Our primary goal should be changing the balance of the LDL – HDL – total cholesterol milieu to favor health rather than disease. We achieve this goal through diet and exercise.

Cholesterol Profiles, What do They Mean?

From a fasting blood sample (12 hour fast) reasonably accurate direct determination of total cholesterol, HDL, and triglycerides is available. Inherent errors in cholesterol testing of perhaps 5 – 10% do exist, so I have always recommended recording cholesterol measurements over time and watching for trends.

What are desirable levels of the specific lipids that we measure? Total cholesterol should be under 200 mg/dl, preferably under 180 mg/dl. HDL levels should be at least 50 mg/dl, and I would prefer to see 60 mg/dl. LDL levels should not exceed 130 mg/dl, 100 mg/dl being preferable. Triglycerides should be under

200 mg/dl. Recall that total cholesterol levels of less than 150 mg/dl are rarely, if ever, associated with cardiovascular disease.

While the individual parameters are important and carry vascular disease risk implications, other computed parameters give more precise risk data. Ratios, which express the balance of HDL, LDL and total cholesterol, afford the best prognostic information.

The most common cholesterol measurement ratio used in medical practice is the total cholesterol/HDL ratio. Less common but still frequently employed is the LDL/HDL ratio. Cholesterol/HDL expresses what part of the total cholesterol is composed of the good, scavenger cholesterol, HDL. Obviously, the more HDL the better, and thus lower numbers are more favorable. Desirable ratios are currently 4.0 or less for cholesterol/HDL; 5.5 or greater is cause for concern.

The LDL/HDL ratio expresses how much more LDL is present than HDL. Desirable ratios of LDL/HDL are currently 2.5 or less; 3.5 or greater being cause for concern.

These ratios are an effective method for expressing the balance of "good" and "bad" cholesterol at any one time. We desire to have the equilibrium of HDL and LDL favor the HDL side. As an exercise, let's compute some ratios and observe the relative risks.

My total cholesterol (TC) is 190 mg/dl and my HDL is 50 mg/dl. What is my TC/HDL ratio? Divide TC by HDL to obtain the result.

TC of 190 mg/dl / HDL of 50 mg/dl = 3.8

My ratio is desirable, i.e., under 4.0, and as such, my risk of CVD based on cholesterol profiles is relatively low.

My daughter's TC is 140 mg/dl and her HDL is 60 mg/dl. What is her TC/HDL ratio? Use the same procedure.

TC of 140 mg/dl / HDL of 60 mg/dl = 2.3

Her ratio is very desirable, and she will not likely develop CVD until she is 100 years old, if then.

It seems that interest in health related issues runs in cycles of popularity. Ten years ago cholesterol constantly led the headlines in the medical and lay presses. Interest in cholesterol seems to have waned in favor of other media darlings like antioxidants and phytochemicals. Cholesterol remains critical as ever. Look at this epidemiologic evidence.

Epidemiologic Studies Support Cholesterol Lowering Efforts

Although it has long been known that a positive continuous correlation exists between circulating cholesterol levels and the incidence of cardiovascular disease (CVD), it was necessary to demonstrate that reducing serum cholesterol would correlate with decreasing the risk of CVD. A number of key studies have accomplished that charge.

The Coronary Primary Prevention Trial (CPPT) was carried out by 12 lipid research clinics in North America. Cholesterol levels were lowered by a combination of diet and drug treatment. This trial demonstrated a direct relationship between the degree of cholesterol lowering and the decrease in risk of CVD. In sum, CPPT demonstrated that **for every 1% decrease in cholesterol levels, a 2% decrease in CVD risk was achieved.**

The Oslo Study Group produced quite similar results. This study group was treated with diet only, no drugs. Average cholesterol decreased by 13% while CVD decreased by 47%. Some of the participants were smokers and the investigators estimated that smoking cessation during the trial was responsible of 1/3 of the 47% improvement in CVD risk, while 2/3, or 36% was due to lowering of serum cholesterol. This study produced results even better than those of CPPT.

The Helsinki Heart Study was a five year study of men given the cholesterol-lowering drug, gemfibrozil. Over the study period total and LDL cholesterol decreased by 8%, triglycerides decreased by 43% while HDL increased by 10%. Based on the 1:2 formula of CPPT one would have expected a 16% decrease in CVD. Surprisingly, the study produced a 34% decrease in CVD. This seeming larger than expected decrease was attributed to the changing of the LDL/HDL relationship to a much more favorable one.

The National Heart Lung and Blood Institute Type II Coronary Intervention Trial studied patients with known CVD and high cholesterol. With diet and drug therapy they achieved a 20% cholesterol reduction. Angiographic studies were done prior to the reduction and after achieving the reduction. Compared to the control group, the study group showed a **significant slowing of the progression of CVD.**

The Cholesterol Lowering Atherosclerosis Study (CLAS) studied people with known CVD and who had bypass surgery. Through maximal drug therapy to lower cholesterol the following results were achieved: a 26% reduction of total cholesterol, a 43% reduction in LDL, a 22% reduction in triglycerides, and a 37% elevation of HDL. Pre and post angiographic studies were done. Of the entire study group 16% actually **had regression of the narrowing of their coronary arteries** (compared to 2.4% of the control group).

The National Cholesterol Education Program's Adult Treatment Panel I of 1988 and NCEP ATP II of 1994 both identified LDL as the primary target of cholesterol lowering therapy. The 1994 study contained features that distinguished it from its predecessor. It focused on the relative relationship of degree of risk for CVD and cholesterol level, using risk data as a guide for intensity of cholesterol lowering efforts. It paid more attention to HDL as a risk factor and **established HDL of less than 35 mg/dl as an independent major cardiac risk factor.**

ATP II increased emphasis on exercise and fat (weight) loss as essential components of dietary therapy for cholesterol. They summarized that **for primary prevention, dietary treatment should by the predominant mode of cholesterol management.**

My favorite study, though, is the angiographic study of Dr. Dean Ornish. He demonstrated, through serial angiograms, the **reversal and regression of established CVD in patients who achieved significant cholesterol reduction.** In his study, however, the greatest degree of regression was accomplished in those individuals who decreased their serum cholesterol, who exercised regularly, and **who were able to change their world view** from victim to empowered, from competitive to accepting, from confrontational to loving.

Generally, epidemiologic studies bore me to tears. These studies are by contrast to most, vibrant, exciting and potentially life saving. Another piece of potentially life saving information that I wish to share to you is the difference between a low cholesterol diet and a cholesterol lowering diet.

A Low Cholesterol Diet May Not Be a Cholesterol Lowering Diet

It has been known for some time that dietary cholesterol is a relatively minor determinant of circulating cholesterol levels. Saturated fat is the major determinant in Western diets. Saturated fats stimulate the liver's production of cholesterol. Of even greater concern is that saturated fat down-regulates the number of LDL receptors in the body resulting in a compensatory rise in serum LDL. That's down right scary.

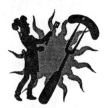

Most foods that contain saturated fat are of animal origin and contain cholesterol, too. Some plant foods like palm kernel oil, coconut oil, and palm oil (the tropical oils) contain large amounts of saturated fat, but no cholesterol. Because of their high saturated fat content, these foods will raise circulating LDL levels in spite of the fact that they contain no cholesterol.

Comparatively, certain foods contain large amounts of cholesterol but relatively insignificant amounts of saturated fat. Eggs are an example. Cutting back on eggs without decreasing saturated fat intake is unlikely to produce significant reductions in blood cholesterol. Taking the eggs out of the traditional farmer's breakfast of eggs, sausage, toast, and butter will have little beneficial effect of lowering cholesterol unless the sausage and butter are eliminated too.

The consumer still believes that dietary cholesterol is a potent factor in raising blood cholesterol levels. As we know, this belief is erroneous, but the educated eater assiduously avoids dietary cholesterol. Why? Good evidence suggests that dietary cholesterol intake is independently associated with the risk of coronary disease. The implication being that dietary cholesterol may have some other atherogenic effect, one not reflected in traditional cholesterol measurements.

Dietary cholesterol has been correlated with the appearance of a smaller, denser form of LDL that is thought to be even more atherogenic than normal cholesterol.

In the late 1980's researchers demonstrated that some individuals were particularly sensitive to dietary cholesterol, while others were not. Undoubtedly, some genetic predisposition to dietary cholesterol sensitivity and to the development of CVD exists. We have no means to identify those persons yet, so it seems prudent to limit cholesterol intake. What limit should we put on intake? NCEP (National Cholesterol Education Program) suggests limiting intake to 300 mg per day. The average American consumes 400 mg to 500 mg or more per day. I recommend an average maximum intake of 200 mg per day of cholesterol (One McDonald's Egg McMuffin breakfast sandwich has 230 mg of cholesterol!).

What about all of the advertising we see in the grocery stores that proclaim, "low cholesterol" or "no cholesterol?" If we read the food content labels of these products we are likely to find "hidden" saturated fats in those products. We know that saturated fats are far more deleterious than cholesterol in our diets. But, like lemmings running to the sea, we buy and eat those products because the big, bold letters on the packages bellows, "no cholesterol," while the small print on the food label whispers the truth.

Our lives depend on our understanding the difference between low cholesterol diets and diets that lower cholesterol. Low cholesterol diets are low in cholesterol, but are not necessarily low in saturated fats. **Cholesterol lowering diets are those which include limitations on both saturated fats and cholesterol.**

Genetic Predisposition Plays a Major Role in Lipid Profiles

Individual responses to cholesterol and saturated fat intake vary and make global conclusions about dietary intake difficult. Many of the conclusions about dietary impact on disease risk assume a more or less uniform response of individuals to various dietary factors. That just isn't the real world. As yet unidentified hereditary factors govern an individual's response to dietary intake of lipids.

Men and women differ in their responses to saturated fat intake. Lowering saturated fats results in a greater LDL decrease in men than in women. Low saturated fat diets in women particularly lead to greater lowering of HDL than in men. It is not clear yet whether this represents an increased danger to women, but the potential remains.

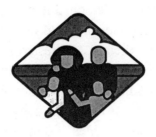

Age is a factor, too. Studies over a ten year period tend to track an increase in LDL, even though study subjects were on a total and saturated fat restricted diet.

Preliminary evidence supports the previously mentioned observation that certain individuals are particularly sensitive to dietary fat and cholesterol. Although these persons may have reasonable cholesterol indices, an increase in dietary fat puts them at greater risk of developing CVD than their normal counterparts who may eat similarly and have similar circulating cholesterol indices. So much remains to be learned.

Most of our lives, like football, are played between the twenty yard lines. Occasionally, we may approach the extremes, score a touchdown or relinquish one, live briefly at one or the other end of our life's spectrum. It's the extremes that we tend to notice, that we celebrate, that we chronicle. So it is with the seemingly mundane cholesterol, we chronicle the extremes, the unusual. Let us remind ourselves that most of us have normal genetic patterns, a great deal of control of our lipids, and consequently, significant control of our risk for CVD.

One in one million Americans, however, inherits two copies of a gene that causes familial hypercholesterolemia. This disorder hampers the ability of the normal lipid transport mechanism. Cholesterol levels may reach 1000 mg/dl or more. Artery blockages begin to develop by age two, and, sadly, in the absence of aggressive medical treatment these unfortunate recipients of a bad gene die in their teens.

By contrast, the "Methuselah" gene, which is even rarer than the one giving rise to familial hypercholesterolemia, affords the lucky recipient longevity. This gene prompts the body to make HDL at a rate three times normal, with HDL levels commonly reaching 200 mg/dl. Recipients of the "Methuselah" gene routinely live to 100 or more.

The Story of Valerio Dagnoli – Mutations of cholesterol genes occur, and one very fortuitous mutation was discovered in 1975 quite by accident. The little Italian village of Limone remained isolated between a range of steep, rocky mountains and the deep waters of Lake Gorda until 1931, when tunnels were blasted through the mountain allowing the villagers to make regular contact with the larger world. Hitherto, they had lived for hundreds of years in geographic isolation, with genetic inbreeding and crossbreeding. In 1780 Cristoforo Pomeroli and Rosa Giovanelli gave birth to a son with a genetic mutation that affected his cholesterol level significantly. This gene slowly infiltrated the bloodlines of the population of the small town and yet remained undetected for nearly 200 years.

Longevity was a hallmark of Valerio Dagnoli's family. Dagnoli, a 43 year-old railroad worker in Milan, sought relief for an irritable colon, but in the process of medical evaluation was found to have confusing and alarming cholesterol test results. His triglycerides were 600 mg/dl, total cholesterol was 300 mg/dl and HDL was a mere 12 mg/dl. His cholesterol/HDL ratio was 25. By all rights, he was dead and didn't have the presence to lay down.

Naturally, a study of his ancestry ensued, and the mutant gene controlling cholesterol was discovered. The study traced it to the 1780 birth of Cristoforo and Rosa's son. Fortunately, the Limone population was isolated for so long because such a tracing of genetic transmission would be impossible in modern, transient populations. The researchers in this study convinced everyone in the town of Limone to give a blood sample for the effort. Analysis of Dagnoli's HDL showed that genetic error had modified one of the surface proteins. While his HDL was made at a normal rate, it was quickly broken down, accounting for the low measured levels. Fortunately for the carriers of the gene and for Dagnoli, the HDL was super-efficient at its job, rapidly removing cholesterol from areas of deposition by the LDL.

Dagnoli and the rest of the recipients of the fortuitous genetic mutation were indeed blessed. But as an Italian lipid specialist studied the villagers in 1981, it was discovered that even those villagers who were not the beneficiaries of the mutant gene were rather long livers.

"Their longevity is partly due to the fact that they eat the ideal Mediterranean diet," concludes H. Bryan Bruner at the National Institutes of health, who also studied the Limone villagers. The Mediterranean diet is heavy in fish, grains, fresh fruit, and vegetables. Olive oil is the main source of fat (unsaturated) and wine is commonplace. These menu items are thought to contribute to lower rated of heart disease throughout southern Europe (Italy, Spain, Greece, and France).

The villagers also exercise whether they want to or not. It is part of their existence. Days in Limone are busy with villagers tending olive and lemon groves, hunting in the hills and manually making wine. The geography of the town consists of steep hills rising from the lake. Cars are restricted and most travel about town is by foot. It's an active life, much like living your life on a stair climber. Even villagers without the golden gene rarely get CVD and live routinely into their nineties.

What's the message from the Limone villagers? It is inescapable. Parents not only pass down genes to their children, but pass down habits, too. Habits often prove the more valuable of the two. Genetics and habits are undeniably important determinants of our health, but shouldn't we consider the contributions of age and sex on our cholesterol profiles, too?

Cholesterol in Women and Children

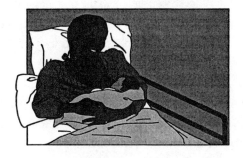

Prior to puberty, lipid profiles prove similar in boys and girls. At puberty, however, male HDL levels fall significantly owing to increased testosterone levels. By contrast, although exogenous estrogens can increase HDL in post-menopausal women, the rise in female estrogen levels at puberty is not associated with increased HDL.

Lipid changes in pregnancy are quite astounding with HDL rising and peaking by the 28th week of gestation, but with only a 15% total increase at delivery. LDL dips initially in pregnancy but averages 150% higher than prepregnancy levels at birth and remains elevated for at least eight weeks after delivery. Triglyceride levels may triple by delivery and if they reach alarmingly high levels, may predispose the new mother to pancreatitis. Despite the seemingly adverse effects of pregnancy on lipid metabolism, only a woman who has experienced at least six pregnancies appears to be at increased risk for CVD events. The transient nature of pregnancy induced hyperlipidemia probably discourages the development of CVD.

Menopause is the "coup de grace" in lipid metabolism for women. Lipid levels change with the altering hormonal milieu. As estrogen levels decline, HDL decreases modestly, but LDL levels rise significantly. The balance of HDL and LDL is negatively altered by a factor greater than the sum of the decrease in HDL and increase in LDL. **The increased risk of CVD for a woman is so great after menopause that the NCEP (National Cholesterol Education Program) has defined post-menopause as a significant risk factor for CVD.**

Estrogen replacement therapy (ERT) after menopause has a favorable effect on lipid profiles with decreasing LDL and increasing HDL levels. Triglycerides may rise but seemingly pose no CVD risk. Large studies of ERT and CVD found that ERT therapy lowers the risk of subsequent cardiac events by 35%. In women with preexisting cardiac risk factors (smoking, hypertension, sedentary lifestyle, diabetes, family history of heart disease) ERT may provide even greater benefit. NCEP now recommends ERT for post-menopausal women with elevated LDL who do not respond to lifestyle modifications.

Lifestyle modification is what I preach and what I teach. It is what I believe. I recommend the restriction of fat and calorie intake, increasing exercise, managing body composition, etc. By now you know the drill. In many clinical studies, however, women seemed to gain less than their male counterparts from the specific lifestyle changes. But, and this is a big but, in Dr. Dean Ornish's angiography trial, women experienced greater reversal of existing CVD with lifestyle modification than did men. I know why. Women can change more easily than men and can adopt and espouse love and peace in their lives.

As Dr. Dean so aptly teaches, lifestyle changes in the absence of an attitude change are unlikely to produce significant reversal of CVD. Only when one is able to change his attitudes, his world view, to a more accepting, harmonious, indeed loving perspective, can they begin to reverse their CVD.

While we are on the subject of changing attitudes, what is our attitude about our senior population? What is our thinking about cholesterol in our seniors?

Cholesterol and the Elderly, Does it Matter?

In the United States, contrasting China and Japan, we practice a callous disregard for our elders. We do not respect and revere our senior citizens, nor do we view them as a source of wisdom or advice. Rather, we push them aside, ignore them, and place them in long term care facilities until they die. How very unfortunate is our attitude. But it is this same disdain of the elderly, the nihilism that greets attempts to treat the cholesterol of people over 65, that dictates our attitudes and policies towards the elderly. We in medicine hold steadfastly to axioms dictating neglect of many legitimate concerns of the elderly, even though good clinical evidence suggests the opposite.

Here are two examples: 1) Scientific evidence has proven that the elderly benefit from exercise. Do we in medicine encourage exercise in the elderly, in nursing homes? Not really, we just ignore that aspect of their care. 2) The elderly have the same risk from lipid profile imbalances as younger people do. Do we address that risk? No, quite the contrary. The accepted medical axiom in practice is that measuring and lowering lipid levels in the elderly doesn't matter because they are going to die shortly anyway. In the scientific literature, those esoteric, not meant for lay ears publications, the message to doctors is couched in the terms, "cholesterol measurement and management is left to the discretion of the individual practitioner."

Similar studies have found that only one in four doctors monitors, treats or advises dietary modification for lipid management in the population at large. That 25% effort is concentrated on the younger population, those with a "future." To expect that doctors would spend their "valuable" time counseling the elderly about dietary modifications is akin to expecting a wolf to become vegetarian.

We know that certain physiologic changes occur with aging. Metabolism slows progressively. Steady caloric intake over the years coupled with a decreased physical activity level, produces an "inevitable" weight gain with aging. With respect to lipids, total cholesterol elevates, LDL elevates, and HDL decreases, creating a progressively greater risk of CVD as we age.

This background and information begs the question, "Do we simply sit passively, allowing these changes to occur and do nothing about the consequences? Or to take arms?" My answer as you might have guessed is to be an active, informed manager of your life at all ages. Obviously, don't wait until you are old to begin to monitor and manage your lipids. Make it a life long effort. I urge you that it is never too late to begin. The message is clear from me and from the scientific data. **It is important and essential to manage lipid profiles in the elderly. The same benefits accrue no matter what age.**

Someday each of us will sit at the upper end of our age time line, in old age. I trust that you agree with me that controlling our lipid profiles is a desirable endeavor now, before we arrive in our senior years. *Tempus fugit*, so we had better quickly find out how to manage our lipids.

How Do We Control Cholesterol?

How do we lower our cholesterol and produce a more favorable balance of HDL and LDL? Here is a simple approach of what to do and how to do it:

1) **Choose to take responsibility for fat and cholesterol intake**
2) **Eat smart**
3) **Get lean**
4) **Don't smoke**
5) **Drink only moderately**
6) **Monitor your own cholesterol**

Steve, a 35-year-old accountant, overweight, stressed, sedentary, with high blood pressure, and a pessimistic life view came to my office a few years ago. He said he just didn't feel well. To make a long story short, he was thirty pounds over-weight, had 175/105 blood pressure, with a total cholesterol of 240, HDL of 35, and LDL of 180. What to do? Start medications? Hardly, he was bright and motivated by how poorly he felt. So, we made one change and one change only, exercise.

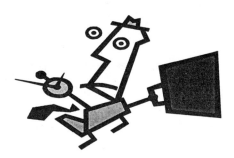

I knew the catalytic potential of exercise, but didn't share that with Steve. I wanted to let it work naturally on him. And, it did. Over the next four months Steve lost twenty-five pounds, became normotensive (blood pressure normal), lowered his total cholesterol to 180, raised his HDL to 60, and lowered his LDL to 100. He was so happy and enthusiastic I kidded him that we might have to start him on Lithium (the drug for bipolar disorders). A freight train steaming toward disaster, by taking control of his life, Steve demonstrated and lived the principles and practices of *Get a Life, America!*

Steve was successful. You can be, too. Here's an organized and integrated approach to cholesterol control.

Choose to take responsibility – Your choice to take responsibility for and control of what you eat is certainly the single most important factor in managing your lipid profile and managing the relative risk your profile poses to your health. It is free for the taking. How do you choose? You simply choose of your own free will. Choice and individual responsibility are two of the main themes of this book. If you don't accept that premise, then the book is as best a decent, casual story.

Eat smart – Keep total average fat intake below 20% of caloric intake, with saturated fats comprising no more than one third of the total fat intake. Saturated fats, those concentrated in meats and dairy products, the fats that are the single most important force in raising cholesterol, the villains that raise LDL, should be limited to a maximum of 7% of total calorie intake. Limit dietary cholesterol to less than 200 mg per day. Remember that saturated fat and cholesterol are listed on the food labels. Read the labels. Monitor your blood cholesterol initially, and if it remains above desired levels, adjust your fat and cholesterol intake downward. It may mean adopting a near vegetarian diet. Think of meat as a garnish. Vegetarians and people who stick to a very low-fat diet rarely have heart disease. Consider routinely eating oat bran. Most studies report a cholesterol lowering effect of 4 – 6% reductions in total cholesterol, with some enthusiastic studies reporting up to a 20% reduction.

Get lean – Lose body fat and change the ratio of fat to lean body mass. Target fat loss, not just weight loss. As fate might have it, low HDL is associated more with fat around the waist (body fat) than fat on the plate. So, lose the fat. Exercise is critical. Exercise helps to use calories, build muscle tissue, and use fat as a source of energy. Regular exercise helps to maintain a favorable balance of body fat and lean body mass. Be careful to avoid the "I am exercising, therefore, I can eat more" fallacy. Excess calories taken in are always stored as fat. Exercise also raises HDL whether through the modification of the body composition or through some as yet unknown mechanism. With the combination of changing body composition, weight loss and exercise, increases of HDL of greater than 40% are attainable.

Don't smoke – Among the legion of reasons against the habit is the fact that smoking significantly lowers HDL. It is too darn hard to raise your HDL to even consider sending your protective partner, HDL, up in a puff of smoke.

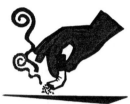

Drink only moderately – If you choose to drink, do it only moderately, a maximum of two drinks per day. Alcohol does raise HDL, and studies document that individuals who have two drinks per day have less heart disease than non-drinkers. Drinking greater quantities of alcohol increases the risk of cancer, accidents and stroke. The implication is obvious. Don't drink a lot.

Monitor your own cholesterol – We are not likely to do things where resistance faces us steadfastly. Traditional "modern" medicine maintains a tenacious strangle hold on control of medical testing under the guise that it takes a doctor to interpret the results of the tests. News flash! It doesn't!

All we medical types want to do is to maintain control of our patient population and get our economic slice of the pie. My point is that cholesterol testing should be readily available and affordable. Pharmacies and supermarkets could serve as convenient blood drawing stations. Samples could be taken daily to laboratories and results would be mailed to the person the same day. A full lipid profile should cost no more than $20 – $25. Currently, and depending on geographic location, it costs a minimum $50 visit to the MD and then $75 or more from the lab. I feel that this is prohibitive and wrong!

For now, make a deal with a medical lab to draw your blood sample. They should charge no more than $10 for drawing your blood. Tell them to send it to a reputable laboratory, and tell them that you want to pay the same rate as a large insurance company pays for the blood analysis, no more. With a little persistence, you will be able to negotiate an equitable deal.

Lipid profile information should be shared among family members, and a cholesterol family tree may be created. This is a quick, simple graphic way to scan your genetic horizons.

Routine testing should begin somewhere between 15 – 20 years of age, and should begin earlier in obese, sedentary or familially predisposed persons. Perform the testing annually for the first three years to establish trends, then every three to five years to keep yourself honest and informed. Nothing is wrong with doing it more often if you wish. Cholesterol indices are good and sometimes catalytic information. If you gain weight (and why did you?) you may educate yourself by observing what your lipid profile reflects. If you discover an abnormal lipid profile that does not respond to exercise and diet, more frequent monitoring may be advisable. It may be possible that you could be the unlucky rare recipient of a bad gene. If that is a possibility, then it may be time to consult a lipid specialist.

Just as we cannot sense or feel what our blood pressure registers, so too can we not sense our lipid levels. However, the intuitive person has a lot of indirect information available to her about what her lipid picture may be. What is your family history? Did members of your family die young of heart attacks, strokes, or did they live well into their nineties? What is your lifestyle? Are you sedentary or active, a worrier or calm? What is your diet like? Do you eat a lot of fatty foods, or do you consume vegetables and grains? How about body composition? Are you lean or fat? Are you an "apple" or a "pear?" What is your "gut to butt ratio?" Do you have fatty deposits around your eyes? This can be a sign of high cholesterol. All of these questions relate to our lipid status and are worthy indirect indicators of what our profiles might be.

Is this all worth the effort? Absolutely, definitively, no doubt about it, it is worthwhile. **"With diet and exercise,"** to quote **Dr. William Castelli of the renowned Framingham Heart Study, "most men and women in this country who are headed for a heart attack could avoid it."** Dr. Castelli, one of the good guys in medicine, has helped many of his study participants *Get a Life!*

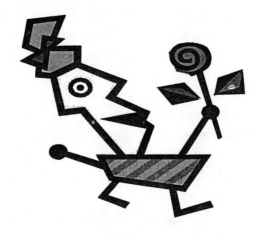

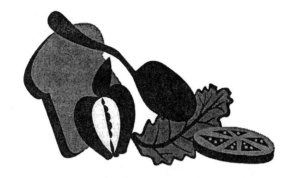

Chapter VII

Eating to Live,
Not Living to Eat

"Inside every fat man a thin one is wildly signaling to be let out."

❖

Cyril Vernon Connolly
The Unquiet Grave

In this chapter we will recognize, affirm, cast no doubt upon, the fact that the calorie (a unit of energy) is the common denominator to body weight and composition, and that obesity is a manifestation of energy imbalance. We'll simplify the energy balance equation. We'll look at nutritional considerations in weight management, warn against yo-yo dieting, examine some theories about obesity, stress the benefits of weight loss, and explain how to measure your body fat. Of course, we'll show you **how** to take control of your weight and body composition.

I pride myself on being fit, controlling my weight, and living a good life. I didn't always do that as I shared with you a few times. I confessed about the stressful period of my life when I remodeled cars in my parking lot. Well, I got rather large then, too. My weight ballooned from a normal of 205 to 250.

Every time I looked at myself in the mirror, I wanted to wretch. So I went on a severe diet. How dumb! Yes, I lost weight, all the way down to 185. Then I got pneumonia because my defenses were depleted from a rapid body change, one that was so demanding of the normal defenses that they succumbed and left me vulnerable to illnesses. Let's all say it together, "That was really dumb, Lennie!" That's no way to *Get a Life!* What follows is.

Calories, Fat and Us Americans

So profound is the relationship between disease and obesity that if the entire United States population were at optimal body weight, it has been estimated that coronary vascular disease could be reduced by 25% and congestive heart failure and strokes by 35%. In other disease processes a 15% decline in mortality is predicted as well as an additional 3 years of life expectancy. All of this would result from simple, better long-term weight management.

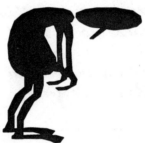

Our national data about obesity emerged from the second United States National Health and Nutrition Survey (NHANES II). A study conducted by the National Center for Health Studies between 1976 and 1980, NHANES II was a statistical cross sectioning of the United States adult population that found 24% of men and 27% of women to be overweight. Subsequent studies document a progressive increase in the trend towards obesity.

We err in our efforts to reverse the rush to obesity in the United States. Recent data suggests that the percentage of our population currently overweight approaches 33%. An alarming trend towards increasing obesity in our children has evidenced, while morbid obesity (weighing 140% of ideal body weight or more) affects 12.5 million people. Forty million Americans are obese and a similar number weigh more than they should.

Many factors contribute to this growing phenomenon, but the most significant are physical inactivity and increased consumption of fat. The percentage of fat in the American diet has risen from 30% in 1940 to 45% in 1980 and unfortunately remains about 45% in the mid-1990's in spite of a massive national education campaign about the deleterious effects of fat.

A weight greater than 20% above ideal body weight as defined by standardized weight tables based on disease risk (Metropolitan's actuarial data) poses a significant and increasing health risk. These risks include insulin resistance, non-insulin dependent diabetes mellitus, hypertension, hyperlipidemia, cardiovascular diseases, pulmonary disease, endocrine abnormalities, gallbladder disease, certain malignancies, orthopedic problems and obstetrical and surgical complications. Adolescent obesity remains a risk factor independent of adult obesity, and is associated with increased morbidity and mortality.

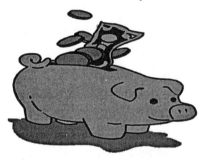

Obesity affects factors other than health. It costs money. The total estimated cost for obesity related diseases grew to $39.3 billion in 1986, representing 5.5% of the total health care costs for that year. In addition, our society spends more than an equal amount annually to combat obesity, about $40 billion (and growing). The sad news surfaces about the $40 billion expenditure in weight loss attempts, 95% or more of the lost weight is regained within one year. Frequently, more weight was regained than lost initially. About 65 million Americans are on a "diet" at any one time, with 40% of women and 25% of men trying to lose weight.

Factors involved in the onset and development of obesity include age, gender, heredity and environment. Statistically, each age group has an acceptable range of weights that correlates with lowest disease risks. These weights are termed "ideal weights" by the actuaries. Even if a person maintains a constant weight during his lifetime, his ratio of fat to lean mass usually increases due to progressive inactivity. The only legitimate physiologic reason for this change in ratio occurs when resting metabolic rates drop toward the later decades of life.

Men and women differ in their weight gain patterns, women gaining weight faster as they age, and particularly after pregnancies. Men are particularly vulnerable during their third and fourth decades of life, the providing years when career and family consume them, the years before their first heart attack.

The fact that excess fat is related to disease is not news. We have known that for a long time. Why, then, do we continue to allow ourselves to eat excess fat and become excess fat?

One reason is most certainly habit, a blind, unthinking carry-over from the generations of the 1930's and 1940's. Food was scarce during the Great Depression and World War II. Rebounding in the 1950's, the post-war decade of plenty, we had food and ate to make up for our perceived deprivation of the 30's and 40's. Meat and potatoes, butter and sauces, milkshakes and ice cream, vegetables never saw the light of day from underneath the hollandaise sauce. Boy, did we like chicken, breaded and deep-fried. Bite into that chicken leg, and fat dripped down your chin. Were we that dumb? Were we that ignorant?

I don't think so. I think we simply chose on an unconscious level to ignore what we knew was bad for us. How many people still smoke? Don't tell me we don't know smoking is bad. We are a population so adolescent that we persist in dangerous behaviors until our time expires.

The typical American diet is at least 40 to 45% fat, low in fiber, high in simple sugar, low in vitamins and high in caffeine. Little wonder that our disease rates are so alarmingly high and that we suffer from malaise, mood swings, insufficient energy, and a general insensibility. Ask yourself when was the last time that you really felt well, and moreover, felt well after eating.

The Weight – Energy Relationship

We can feel well after eating and we can feel well in our lives overall. Dietary mixes of foods, through complex chemical reactions, directly affect how we feel and how we perform. Camouflaged in the complexity, a common denominator exists among all foods.

All foods provide calories. A calorie is a measure or unit of energy, the amount of energy required to raise one kilogram of water one degree centigrade. How can too many calories make us gain weight? Can too much energy cause us to gain weight?

The answer is absolutely yes, because our bodies store excess energy. We must realize that all food has available energy, the amount of which is expressed in calories. When the food is broken down, the process called metabolism produces energy for work to be performed by our bodies. If excess food is present in the body and is not used for work, it is either excreted through the intestine (incomplete absorption) or stored for future energy needs.

How is it stored? It is stored many places and ways. Some is available as glucose in the blood stream, some as glycogen in the liver and muscle, and the remainder is stored as fat throughout the body. Amino acids are not stored, but the muscle mass itself (accounting for as much as 50% of body mass) is a large energy reserve for periods of caloric deprivation.

Our bodies extract energy from stored sources in our bodies as well as from the foods we eat. Different foods have different energy potential. Carbohydrate provides 4 calories per gram; protein provides 4 calories per gram, fat provides 9 calories per gram, while alcohol provides 7 calories per gram. Obviously, fat has twice the available energy as do protein and carbohydrate, which makes it a wonderfully efficient fuel source. We know, too, of the dangerous downside to this marvelous fuel. Excess circulating fat accelerates the clogging of our arteries, the atherogenic process. Too much stored fat results in obesity and all of the consequent risks of that condition.

Obesity is a manifestation of energy imbalance. Individuals gain weight because they eat too much or perform too little activity for the amount they have eaten. More commonly they do both, over eat and become a common slug. We shall focus on both sides of the energy balance equation, caloric intake and energy expenditure, to best understand the broad scope of the weight-energy relationship.

The **energy balance equation**, pictorially illustrated below, is a simple expression of the fact that excess intake of calories will result in stored energy (fat) and excess expenditure of energy will lead to utilization of the stores of potential energy (loss of fat stores). Increased food intake is often erroneously viewed as the chief cause of weight gain, but reduced energy expenditures are a significant contributor to the problem, especially as we enter our older adult years.

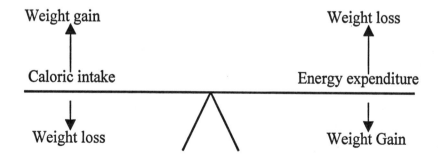

Child, adult or senior, total energy use is the sum of three parameters. These components of energy expenditure are:

1) resting metabolic rate (RMR),
2) thermic effect of food (TEF)
3) thermic effect of physical activity (TEPA)

RMR expresses the energy required for respiration, cardiac activity, general cell function and balancing of all the body's systems. It accounts for 60% to 75% of total daily energy expenditure, depending upon the activity level of the person.

Thermic effect of food refers to the energy used to process food, including digestion, absorption, transportation, metabolism, oxidation and storage of food eaten. TEF accounts for 5% to 10% of daily energy expenditure, regardless of "dietary mix." Although interesting, the fact that it takes more energy to store excess carbohydrate as fat than to store excess fat as fat, has little bearing on the 5% to 10% figure.

Comprising 15% to 30% of daily energy costs, the **thermic effect of physical activity,** the energy used in moving our bodies, is the second largest and

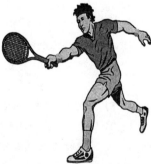

most easily manipulated component of the energy expense items. How much control do we have over the energy expenditure process in our bodies?

We have significant control, but let's understand a few things about RMR before we exert our control. We use the index of RMR to indicate the sum of total resting energy expense.

Normally, RMR is 1.2 cal/min for a person weighing 150 pounds (for each 15 pounds above or below 150, add or subtract 10%). RMR is directly correlated to fat-free body mass, the sum of lean body mass (muscle) and skeletal mass (bone). RMR in men is higher because they have greater fat-free body mass. Similarly, the decline in RMR with age results from the loss of lean body mass.

With advanced aging, the rate of energy usage drops, too. Certainly, we understand the significant hereditary component to RMR, because our body types and shapes are in large part genetically pre-cast. Other factors, not under our control, can influence metabolic rate from its steady state. Hormones, like thyroid hormone and testosterone, are examples. Hypothyroidism, a chronically low level of thyroid hormone, results in a slowing of the metabolic rate, slower usage of fuels, and eventually, weight gain. Testosterone, a male hormone, influences the building process of muscle mass. So, where is our control of RMR?

Through strength training, effecting increased lean body mass (muscle size) and increased bone density, we increase the amount of energy consuming tissues in our bodies. As lean tissue mass increases, the rate of energy use per unit of mass increases a bit, too. Aerobic exercise, when added to strength training gives an additional boost to the rate of energy usage by the muscles, an effect that lasts longer than the aerobic exercise period. This increase of RMR, referred to as the tail-off effect (or after-burn) of aerobic exercise, may be sustained for a longer period if the intensity of the aerobic exercise exceeds a minimum threshold of exercise intensity (70% of an individual's maximum heart rate). We actually burn calories faster than normal for a few hours after aerobic exercise.

If we increase our muscle mass and our bone mass, and perform aerobic exercise, we may achieve up to a 10% increase in RMR. This may not sound like a lot, but let's remember the principle of the summation of the parts.

Can we gain favor elsewhere? Although it is taught that we have no control of TEF (thermic effect of food), we actually do have some control. The relative timing of eating and of exercising is important. Exercising soon after eating increases TEF. How much? We don't know exactly, but we will take anything that is to our advantage. Interestingly, eating immediately before exercising creates a higher post exercise metabolic rate than the sum of the rate changes from eating and from exercising, individually. Not eating, and especially starvation slows the metabolic rate.

Physical activity energy expenditure, the sum total of all of our physical activity in a day, not just what we did at the gym, is entirely under our control. By choosing a more physical lifestyle, walking when we might have driven, climbing stairs rather than taking the elevator, playing games with our children and grandchildren (and great-grandchildren, for you are going to be healthier longer) we will increase our energy uses. Regular aerobic exercise spends calories but also gives us the aerobic training effect. Our simple choice of a physically active lifestyle will place our thermic effect of physical activity in the upper ranges of the 15% to 30% of total energy use.

OK, you say, "Now I am an energy using kind of person and I am exceeding my caloric intake. Oh my goodness, I am out of energy balance." Great! You will gradually lose fat and trim down. Muscle definition will evidence. You might begin to see your abs. If you reach your optimal weight, then you might just enjoy eating more to match your energy needs. Although rare in the United States, this is an interesting and desirable perspective, eating to keep up with your energy requirements.

The caloric intake side of the energy balance equation is simple and entirely under our control. Caloric intake is your total daily food intake, expressed in calories. Knowledge, the best prescription, will allow you to make informed, prospective choices about your diet. I urge you to be mindful about what you choose to eat.

Nutritional Considerations in Weight Management

The healthy individual maintains an energy equilibrium. Calories consumed as food balance calories needed for energy, and body weight remains constant. When the equilibrium is disturbed, by disease, gluttony, sloth-like sedentary existence, or hopefully, a well-planned exercise program, the result is a change in the body mass.

We know that 3500 calories of food ingested in excess of energy needs translates to one pound gained, and conversely, that 3500 calories spent in energy not answered in supply translates to one pound lost. A simple computation predicts the effect on body weight from imbalance in the energy equilibrium. **Consuming an extra 200 calories per day (one cinnamon-raisin bagel, plain;**

or daily cream in your coffee) in excess of energy needs results in a 20 pound weight gain in one year (200 cal x 365 days = 73,000 calories extra; 73,000 cal / 3,500 cal per pound = 20 pounds). Similarly, **spending an unanswered 200 calories in energy per day results in a 20 pound weight loss in one year.**

This is certainly great news, but did you notice I said one pound of weight? Most advertisers of gimmick machines will tell you 3500 calories equals one pound of fat. Do the math! One pound has 454 grams. Multiply 454 grams by 9 calories per gram of fat and we produce 4036 calories. What happened?

Passive weight loss turns out to be 75% fat and 25% muscle. A mass of fat requires one third of its weight in muscle for structural support. Now do the math. Muscle loss is 113.5 grams and fat loss is 340.5 grams. Multiply 113.5 grams by 4 calories per gram of protein (454 calories), and then add that to the product of 340.5 grams times 9 calories per gram of fat (3064 calories). Now it makes sense. Approximating 3500 calories per pound of weight loss agrees with the computed 3518 calories from protein and fat.

A word of caution arises. The 3500-calorie imbalance per pound of weight shouldn't occur precipitously. Let's understand why.

Our bodies have innate capacity to protect against large changes in internal physiology. Rapid temperature changes are met with cooling efforts like sweating or warming efforts like shivering. Climbing Mount Everest with less available atmospheric oxygen results in more rapid breathing. These are examples of short term, physiologic, adaptive and protective efforts. If we gradually immerse ourselves into the adverse conditions, other long-term adaptations occur. If we live in a cold environment, we may develop a bit more fat as insulation. If we live at altitude, physiologic changes occur in our lungs, hearts and red blood cell mass.

So it is with weight loss. With a slow approach to an environment of fewer calories, our bodies adapt with fewer emergency defenses. During a modest

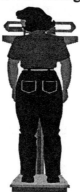

weight loss the body mobilizes fatty acids from stored fat and uses them as its major source of energy, regardless of what is eaten. This is the ideal result from dieting. Starvation (crash dieting) is another story entirely, as fat stores are protected at the expense of protein in muscle tissue. RMR decreases and starvation signals are broadcast on an emergency frequency from the brain. "Experts" recommend a one to two pound per week weight loss. **I say one pound**

per week, maximum. There simply isn't any rush. The longer the trip, the more you will see and the more you will learn.

What are normal caloric requirements if we are not concerned about gaining or losing weight? The sum of resting needs and activity needs, as well as the thermic effect of food defines caloric requirement. To estimate caloric requirements we compute each, then add all three parameters as follows:

Resting: Body weight (Kg) x 10 plus 900 (men)
Body weight (Kg) x 7 plus 800 (women)

Activity: Multiply resting needs by:

1.2 for sedentary persons
1.4 for moderately active persons
1.6 for very active people

Thermic effect of food: Add 100 calories

The total of resting, activity and thermic needs are your caloric requirements for the day to maintain your present weight. To calculate the calorie deficit needed to produce a one pound per week weight loss, do the following:

Subtract 500 calories from your daily needs for energy (500 calories per day x 7 days = 3,500 calories per week = 1 pound of fat, oops, of weight loss).

Example #1 – A moderately active 100 kg (220 pound) man has a daily requirement of: 100 x 10 = 1,000 + 900 = 1,900 x 1.4 = 2,660 + 100 = 2,760. Subtract 500 calories, producing a 2,260-calorie diet for a one pound per week weight loss. That's not too hard to take, is it? We can do more. What if we spend 200 calories per day in extra energy by exercising? Then we do not have to cut our intake quite as much. In the early stages of weight loss, we might lose weight just a bit faster than one pound per week. However you create it, a 500-calorie energy deficit per day is ideal for gradual, controlled weight loss.

Example #2 – Let's look at a 60 kg (132 pound) woman who wishes to lose weight. Follow the formula: 60 x 7 = 420 + 800 = 1,220 x 1.4 = 1,708 + 100 = 1,808. Subtract 500 calories and she has a 1,300-calorie diet to lose a pound per week. It's a bit more restrictive than that of the 100-kg man, but with a 200 calorie exercise program daily, then she has a 1,500-calorie diet. That's very palatable.

Specific nutrient needs in a weight loss diet parallel those of a well-balanced maintenance diet (20% fat, 15% protein and 65% carbohydrate). If you are doing strength training along with your diet, then increase your protein to 25% of calories. I see no need of any diet lower than 1,200 calories for weight loss, assuming associated exercise. A balanced diet and a minimum of 1,200 calories, provide adequate room for all nutrients, protein, carbohydrates, fats, vitamins and minerals. If you are unduly concerned about vitamin adequacy, take a good multivitamin.

Your weight management program only completes when you die. It is a life long effort. Obviously when you reach your goal of weight and body composition, the energy expenditure to maintain the new product is different than the needs of your previously obese state. Fewer calories in general will be required during maintenance than before the weight was lost.

With simple weight loss alone, energy requirements decrease. About 2/3 of the calorie decrease is due specifically to having less mass to support and 1/3 is due to loss of lean muscle mass. In the absence of strength training exercises to offset an attendant loss of muscle mass with fat loss, weight loss (or gain) is **75% fat and 25% muscle.** Remember, the 25% loss or gain of muscle is that amount of muscle needed to carry the additional fat mass. Obviously a strength-training program, designed to add muscle size and mass, when combined with a weight loss effort will attenuate the normal 25% loss in lean muscle weight.

With passive weight loss, RMR decreases 20 calories per day per kg of weight lost. Thus, a 20-kg weight loss is attended by a 400-calorie decrease in energy needs. Because we will have been foresighted in our weight management program, we will have exercised and maintained our lean muscle mass, our post weight loss caloric needs will be higher than the person who simply lost the weight without paying attention to maintaining muscle mass. We will remain active, too, necessitating a percentage more calories to fuel our body's needs. **Exercise is the variable that separates individuals who keep weight off from those who regain it.**

We are now in a position to "eat to live" rather than "living to eat." Mind set is critical. We have made a choice to lose weight, to exercise, to live a healthy, active lifestyle. The classic triad of diet, exercise, and behavior modification that has failed for so many "dieters" will work for us because we have taken active control of our lives. We have not been passive recipients. What is the difference? It is our **perception of control** that differentiates success and failure of the triad.

241

Yo-Yo Dieting Wreaks Havoc on the Weight-Energy Relationship

Some authorities believe that repeated cycles of weight loss followed by weight gain, the so called yo-yo dieting, may create a condition in which losing weight becomes increasingly difficult, and weight gain becomes quite easy and more rapid. It is hypothesized that weight loss results in a lowered resting metabolic rate (RMR), a protective adaptation by the body against starvation and death. Studies of cycling dieters, including wrestlers attempting to make weight limits, showed an average 14% decrease in RMR. Upon cessation of the "diet" and return to "normal" eating patterns (big mistake, because calorie needs are now lower due to the smaller body mass and diminished RMR) the weight loss is rapidly regained. Metabolic rates remain low for at least four to six weeks beyond the end of the "diet" period. Sometimes pre-diet RMRs are never attained, and the next attempt at dieting starts with one strike against the dieter, a lowered RMR. With the next diet RMR drops even further, again protecting against the physiologic perception of starvation, making weight loss even more difficult and regain so much easier and rapid. Often weight is gained in excess of pre-diet levels.

Studies also show that the risk of CVD is higher in yo-yo dieters than obese people of the same fatness who are not yo-yo dieters. The increased risk seems to be independent of associated factors such as high blood pressure. What, then, are the caveats?

First, dieting or weight loss is a serious undertaking and should be managed responsibly. Risks, other than CVD, lurk in the shadows of ignorance. Rapid weight loss in individuals predisposed to gallstones can precipitate gallstone formation and ignite gallbladder disease. Precipitous weight loss "eats" muscle and can threaten the integrity of the kidneys and the liver. The pedestrian dieter thinks that all weight loss is desirable, but the informed weight manager knows that handled improperly, weight loss can pose risks.

Second, prospective dieters should seek a diet that will be successful the first time, and offers the greatest chance of long term maintenance. That diet is one that promotes weight loss in a slow, but progressive fashion. Weight loss at a modest rate does not set off the body's defense alarms, and it allows the concomitant learning of new eating habits in the process, an essential component to long term weight management. Slow weight loss in the order of one pound per week is optimal.

Theories About the Etiology of Obesity

To better understand the nature of the weight-energy relationship, we may examine thoughts about how 30-35% of Americans may have become obese.

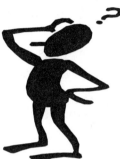

Theories about the etiology of obesity stuff the already plump academic research journals. I would like to introduce you to some of the most common theories, and toss out the oft-offered excuse that "my metabolism must be slow."

Genetics – Studies of twins and adopted children have led to clear recognition of a genetic contribution to obesity. Studies of adoptees have demonstrated a relationship of adult weight to the biologic parent rather than to the adopted parent. Learned behavior does appear to play a role, too. Heredity and environment interact to determine an individual's weight. The recognition of the role of genetics in weight determination has expanded society's view of obesity, so that psychological problems are no longer inferred as the root cause of obesity. Prevention programs and correction of obesity must be built upon a foundation of understanding of genetic prepotential.

Fat cell theory – The size and number of fat cells are two physiologic factors that may determine an individual's weight range. Fat cell numbers are primarily determined genetically. Fat cell replication occurs at certain times during fetal development and again during specific growth periods in childhood. In adulthood the number of fat cells remains constant, unless an overload stimulus is present that demands the production of increasing numbers of fat cells.

Although it had been formerly taught that the number of fat cells was determined at certain developmental growth periods and that number determined our fatness, we now understand differently. When existing fat cells become engorged to their maximum volume by fat storage, new fat cells are formed. The typical fat cell weighs about 0.5 ug and may increase to a maximum of 1.0 ug.

After all cells have reached their maximum size, and with continued positive energy balance (over-eating), new fat cells are formed, resulting in an increased total number of fat cells in the body. The number of fat cells that may be formed is virtually unlimited. Fat cells, once replicated are never lost, whether formed in-utero, in childhood or in adulthood; and we can get as fat as we wish.

Expansion of fat leading to obesity may result from increasing the size of each cell (hypertrophy), the number of cells (hyperplasia), or both. The normal fat cell cycle is from hypertrophy to hyperplasia, and then possibly to repeat itself. Consider a woman of 120 pounds and 25% body fat. She has 30 pounds of fat. If she gains 30 pounds more of fat, her fat cells will increase from 0.5 ug to 1.0 ug and be at their maximum weight. Beyond the 30-pound fat gain she will begin to make new fat cells.

Persons with large numbers of fat cells can only lose fat by decreasing cell volume to subnormal levels. If weight loss is great enough and cell size shrinks below the 0.5 ug size, the brain is stimulated to send out "starvation" signals and prompt eating behavior. For this reason previously very obese people have difficulty in maintaining their losses. The fat cells attempt to exist at sizes lower than normal fat cell size. Unfortunately, these persons face a constant barrage of "eat" signals from the undersized fat cells. With weight loss only cell size diminishes, not cell number.

Set point theory – One of the more recent theories conceives that a person's weight is the result of a biologically determined preset weight. Any alteration in weight from that point will result in a natural tendency to return to the original weight. Adherence to the set point theory could be very discouraging to persons attempting to lose weight because, if it is valid, long term weight loss and maintenance may be nearly impossible.

I feel that the validity of the set point theory lies in its description of the individual's current status of weight and energy balance. With small, incremental changes in weight over extended periods of time, a new set point may be reached at a lower weight level, with a new homeostasis established at that new level. The set point theory may be an expression of a body defense system, defending the body from rapid physiological changes.

Thyroid abnormalities – Although thyroid hormones are well known to play a role in regulating resting metabolism, and the thyroid has been implicated in animal models of obesity, it remains that precious few cases of obesity are thyroid grounded. Severe hypothyroidism, which is rather uncommon, is the only thyroid based cause of obesity, and it is easily treated with thyroid hormone replacement. So, if you gain weight, I am not going to buy your "under-active thyroid" excuse.

Impaired thermogenesis – Obese people spend less thermic energy to digest and process a similar meal as do their lean counterparts. Once obese, individuals have a lower thermic effect of food. As these individuals become progressively obese, their thermic effect of food becomes even lower. A "normal" caloric intake for these unfortunate people results in weight gain.

Neural theories of obesity – Are there brain centers that control eating stimuli? Most likely there are. It appears that those centers are in the hypothalamus, because experimentally produced lesions in hypothalamic centers induce eating behavior in laboratory animals, resulting in weight gain.

Hormonal feedback may play a role, too. Serotonin, a well known neurotransmitter found in the brain, has been proven to be a regulator of macronutrient preference in rodents. Carbohydrate intake stimulates insulin and serotonin release. Under normal circumstances serotonin suppresses desire for further carbohydrate. Obese persons, though, may have a deficiency in serotonin levels, resulting in increased appetite, especially for carbohydrates. Low serotonin levels have been associated with clinical depression, too. Could there be a connection between depression, obesity, and low serotonin levels?

Metabolic theories – Signals are sent to the brain before, during and after nutrient absorption. Information about nutrient absorption and concentration is relayed from the intestines to the brain by nerve impulses and by blood concentrations of nutrients. Multiple hormones play a feedback role in activating and suppressing appetite.

A theory of post absorptive regulation of food intake, specifically the desire to continue eating beyond the point of satiety, concerns the enzyme lipoprotein lipase (LPL). Normally, LPL regulates the rate of triglyceride deposition in fat cells. In obese persons LPL works overtime and efficiently, storing fat like there is no tomorrow, lowering serum triglyceride levels, stimulating the desire for more food. LPL's fat storage facilitation is even more pronounced in individuals who are fasting or losing weight.

What I have presented are theories based on scientific data. Whatever the origin of obesity, it remains indefensible that significant health risks accompany obesity.

Deleterious Effects of Obesity

Mortality – Three rather large prospective studies in 1959 and 1979 demonstrated that death rates increase as a function of body weight. The relationship is delineated by the J-curve of the graph below and illustrates an acceleration of the increase of death rates as weight increases towards morbid obesity (140% or more of ideal body weight). The lowest mortality ratios occur at body weights slightly below the average weight, about 90% of average body weight. What is the practical information from this data? Too thin or too fat and you are going to die. Slightly below normal is ideal.

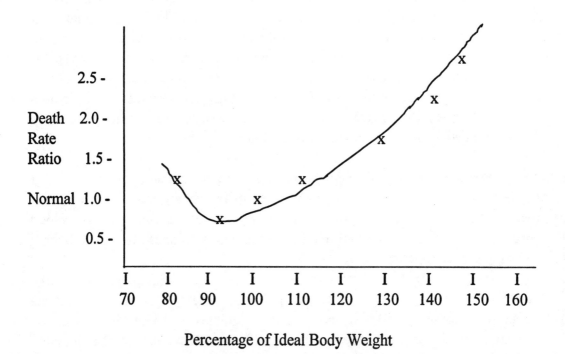

Percentage of Ideal Body Weight

The J-curve graph also holds true for the relationship between weight and chronic diseases such as diabetes mellitus, certain cancers, arteriosclerotic vascular disease, and gallbladder disease.

Obesity contributes to increased mortality through a complex array of adverse consequences, both metabolic and structural. Metabolic consequences include insulin resistance, high circulating insulin levels, high blood sugar, high cholesterol, high triglycerides, low HDL, high blood pressure, high uric acid (causes gout), and gallbladder disease. Structural consequences include orthopedic impairment, pulmonary difficulties and obstetrical and surgical complications.

Diabetes – Of all of the factors playing an etiologic role in the induction of Type II diabetes mellitus (non-insulin dependent diabetes mellitus), obesity is perhaps the most important. The risk of developing this disease more than doubles with each 20% of excess in body weight. You do not want diabetes or its complications, which include blindness, amputations, kidney failure, and increased risk of heart attack. Through proper weight management, it is estimated that 50% of the cases of Type II DM in the United States may be eliminated. Weight loss alone can restore blood sugar and blood insulin levels to normal in these individuals, therefore, weight loss is always the first effort in the management of Type II DM. To view the process from my perspective of prevention, this means that **50% or more of the cases of Type II DM never have to occur in the first place.**

Cardiovascular diseases – In the world famous Framingham Heart Study, obesity was proven to be an independent heart risk factor. That is to say that **obesity alone, aside from hypertension, high cholesterol, smoking, stress,**

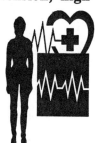

DM, and family history was a major risk factor in cardiovascular diseases. The risk from obesity is much greater for men than for women. The risk is greater for men and women under 50 years of age than in older people, although significant risk remains in the older population. As well, obesity is a strong predictor of risk for CVD in young adults. Among young people risks were 2.0 to 2.5 times the risk of a normal weight person.

The pathologic mechanism of increased risk in thought to be presented by atherogenic traits, including high cholesterol, low HDL, high blood pressure, and high triglycerides. Weight loss reverses all of these tendencies. Reduction of high blood pressure is well known after weight loss in obese persons. One study compared weight loss to anti-hypertensive medication and found favorable results with weight loss in HBP treatment. Weight loss in hypertension, like DM, is the initial step in management.

Gallbladder disease – Weight increase is the single most important risk factor for gallbladder disease among all of the other risks of gender, age, and parity (number of children). In autopsy studies the incidence of gallstones was 16% among men who were 20 pounds overweight. As much as a six-fold increase in risk is born by women who are obese.

Structural problems – Obesity has adverse structural consequences. The classic Pickwick Syndrome (from Charles Dickens', *Pickwick Papers*) is an example of someone who is so massive as to obstruct normal breathing mechanisms. Their work to breathe may increase four-fold over their normal work to breathe. The obese person experiences decreases in arterial oxygenation, as well as sleep apnea (periods of not breathing), snoring, and chronic fatigue.

Orthopedic concerns are significant. Although not related to mortality risk, osteoarthritis of major weight bearing joints, knees, and hips, is made much worse by carrying additional weight. The same arthritis responds nicely to weight loss. Respiratory difficulties also improve quickly with weight reduction. Even modest weight loss can ameliorate symptoms and risk.

Surgical risk – Surgical risk of mortality is two to three-fold higher for obese patients. This is not just headaches and nausea, it is postoperative infections, pneumonias, and pulmonary emboli – stuff that kills.

Grossly overweight, Dan Blocker, the actor who played the role of "Hoss" Cartwright on the television series Bonanza, died at age 43 from a pulmonary embolus after gallbladder surgery. John Candy, tipping the scales in excess of 300 pounds, never had the opportunity to have an operation for his cardiovascular disease. He died young of a massive heart attack. His surgical risk would have been sky high.

Benefits of Weight Loss

There are objective, statistically quantifiable, metabolic benefits of weight loss and less specific, less easily quantified subjective benefits. Although I have alluded to the benefits by describing the risks, let me list what you stand to gain from losing and managing your weight.

Objective benefits include:

1. Improved cardiovascular disease (CVD) risk profile
2. Normalization of triglyceride levels
3. Increase of HDL (good cholesterol)
4. Lowering of LDL (bad cholesterol)
5. Decrease or elimination of the need for drug treatment of hypertension and hyperlipidemia
6. Lowering of high blood pressure
7. Increased glucose tolerance
8. Increased insulin sensitivity
9. Decreased need for diabetes mellitus (DM) drugs
10. Decreased risk of gallbladder disease

Subjective benefits include:

1. Improved self image
2. Ease of movement
3. Facilitation of physical work

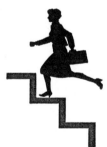

4. Greater enjoyment of sexuality
5. Improved appearance, much better "naked in the mirror" test result

Given the risks of obesity and the benefits of weight loss, a wise person will always choose losing weight to optimal levels. What are optimal levels? The Metropolitan Life Insurance Company judges optimal levels to be those associated with the lowest actuarial risk (lowest cost to the company). Is that a good enough measure for us? Is optimal a weight on the scale, or are other factors integral? Certainly, other factors weigh heavily on determining what is optimal for our health and wellness. Body composition is a critical factor, so let's look at the percentage of our bodies that are fat.

Percentage Body Fat

Fat is an essential structural component of our bodies. Integral in hormone synthesis, cell membrane structure, nerve sheath integrity, it's a significant potential energy source. Essential fat, that minimum amount necessary for certain specific anatomical and physiological functioning comprises about 3% of a man's body mass. Women's bodies have the same 3% as essential body fat but also have an additional 5% to 9% of sex specific fat. Body fat above the ground floor subsistence level is considered storage fat, and it is stored in fat cells for future use as energy and for use as insulation against cold.

Fat content of the body varies with age. At birth the human newborn is approximately 12% fat. An eight pound baby has about one pound of fat. The fat content and percentage increases rapidly during the first six months of life to 30%, and then the percentage drops to 18% when the child begins to walk. Puberty defines fat differentiation between men and women. Boys' muscularity develops in their post-puberty years while girls begin to deposit sex specific fat in the hips, buttocks, thighs, and breasts. At maturity men average 13% to 20% body fat while women average 20% to 25% body fat. Recall that these are statistical norms for sex groups, not upper and lower limits. Nor are they ideal or desirable levels. They are, in fact, statistical norms for a very fat country with rampant chronic diseases.

As we progress through our "maturing years" fatness increases gradually. The increase in fatness is not of physiologic or metabolic necessity but results mostly from inactivity and over feeding. A one pound per year increase in fat beyond age 35 is common in the United States. During this period the additional factor of minimal declines in resting metabolic rate exists, but decreasing RMR is a small contributing factor to weight gain. Unfortunately, because weight gain is so common in the United States, growing fatter with aging is considered normal.

Many doctors use an age-related sliding scale when determining risk from body composition. They may record the weight, but studies have demonstrated that less than half of physicians who observed obesity in a patient actually documented it in the medical record as a legitimate problem. Precious few doctors determine an individual's body composition.

Measurement of body fat percentage is important and should be done routinely to establish a record of trends. Is the body composition changing? Is the percentage increasing or decreasing with time? Currently, three methods for measuring body fat percentage give reasonable accuracy. The most accurate is hydrostatic or underwater weighing. Most doctors do not have a "dunk tank" available to them for this type of measurement. Mobile hydrostatic "dunk tanks" are available and make regularly scheduled stops at local health clubs. The cost of the test is about $20 when done by the mobile labs and represents a good value. By doing the test every six or so months and keeping your own records, it's easy to spot upward or downward trends.

Skin fold measurements taken with calipers at specific body sites, when summed and compared to a nomogram, allows practiced individuals to compute one's body fat percentage. Errors are inherent in this method depending upon where the measurement was taken, how the skin fold was secured and the experience of the tester. This is still a good test, and re-measuring the skin folds three times in succession tends to eliminate errors.

The newest method is an electronic gadget that measures electric impedance or infrared light transmission. Results are reported to be reasonably accurate and reproducible, although this is the least reliable of the three methods. These fancy instruments cost in the range of $3,500 and are not commonly available.

The easiest method to determine relative body fat is the "naked in the mirror test." Look critically at yourself in the mirror. The mirror doesn't lie.

Body Fat and Risk Status

Although we know that obesity carries increased risk of disease, we need some quantitative method to assess and express risk. Three indices give useful information about an individual's status for risk of disease with respect to body fat. The first two deal with total body fat and are essentially different ways of expressing the same thing. The third deals with the differential distribution of body fat. **Body mass index (BMI)** is an expression of body size standardized for individuals' variations in height, and bears a very close statistical correlation with **percentage body fat (PBF)**. **Waist hip ratio (WHR)** is an expression of the relative distribution of fat in the trunk compared to the hips.

We are well aware that increases of PBF correlate with increased risk for disease. As percentage of body fat increases or decreases, BMI reflects the change. Measurements of body fat percentages are available, but not as readily available as computing a BMI. BMI is computed by dividing your weight in kilograms (2.2 pounds per kilogram) by the square of your height in meters (0.0254 meters per inch). BMI is unreliable in very muscular men and diminutive women in its correlation with body fat percentage, a reason for keeping records of both BMI and PBF. In muscular men, BMI is a more accurate predictor of risk than is PBF, and in diminutive women, the converse is the rule.

The **distribution** of body fat is critical in determining disease risk. Abdominal obesity, termed android obesity (the "apple" shape) is more common in men than in women. Conversely, the hip and thigh obesity, termed gynoid

obesity (the "pear" shape) is more common in women. The greater the android distribution of fat, the greater the risk for CVD. The reason for the greater risk

from abdominal obesity is thought to be that abdominal fat is more easily mobilized and tends to be more atherogenic than hip fat. Trunkal obesity may be part of a general thoracic (including coronary arteries) deposition of fat. Waist hip ratios are determined by measurement of the greatest abdominal girth and dividing by the maximum hip girth. Adult men with WHR of 1.0 or more and women with WHR of 0.8 or more are at increased risk of diabetes mellitus, high blood pressure, cardiovascular disease, stroke and death. The higher the ratio the greater the risk.

I keep records of all three indices, BMI (body mass index), PBF (percentage body fat) and WHR (waist hip ratio). I favor the PBF as my staple measurement of trend. WHR, largely determined by genetics, is difficult to modify. When we lose fat from our bodies, we lose it homogeneously throughout our bodies. Unfortunately, spot reduction of body fat remains a myth. For this reason changing one's WHR is nigh onto impossible. If you discover risk based on WHR, don't be discouraged to paralysis. Control still rests with you. You may reduce your overall risk of CVD by reducing total body fat.

What are desirable numerical indices for body fat measurements? Remember, these are desirable numbers, not statistical averages. BMI should be under 27 kg/m2, preferably under 25 kg/m2. WHR in men should be under 0.8 and for women under 0.7. Percentage body fat should be less than 15% for men and less than 18% for women. These indices are well worth working for. I know of no short cuts, certainly not any pie-in-the-sky diet program.

What About all of Those Popular Diets?

Any diet that promises rapid results and large weight losses aren't worth your time or the paper they're written on. Nutritionally inadequate, scientifically unsound, useless and potentially dangerous, they do nothing to change eating habits, and weight lost is usually regained. Consider if you will, starvation, the ultimate diet, to demonstrate maximum weight loss potential. Then we will compare those potential weight losses to the "fourteen pounds in 10 days to 2 weeks" promises of fad diets.

If caloric needs for subsistence are 2,000 per day and that person eats nothing at all, save for water; his calorie deficit is 2,000 per day, 14,000 per week. We know that 3,500 calories is equal to one pound of fat (no, recall, weight). Dividing 3,500 into 14,000 results in a maximum 4-pound per week weight loss with absolutely no caloric intake. No greater weight loss is possible, or is it? Here comes some slight of hand.

Some quick fix fad diets do achieve initial weight losses that surpass the computed four-pound per week loss. How? Simple, an obligatory water loss, a diuresis, accompanies very low calorie diets. Starvation, or the near starvation of very low calorie diets produces complex biochemical changes resulting in ketosis, diuresis, and naturesis (loss of proteins, water and salt). The water loss in the early days of the fad, near starvation diets accounts for their claims of tremendous weight loss. Yes, it is water loss, not fat loss, and that water will be re-accumulated upon cessation of the diet. **The calorie deficit over time determines weight and fat loss.**

One type of diet commonly reappearing under different names is the low carbohydrate, high protein, moderate fat diet. Calories are usually low with 50 grams of carbohydrate (200 calories) and 120 grams of protein (480 calories) and some fat. The weight lost on this high protein diet results from the metabolic phenomenon known as ketosis, which in turn produces a diuresis, i.e., water loss. Dangers of this diet include renal damage, gout, hypoglycemia (low blood sugar), and electrolyte imbalance. Cardiac arrhythmias resulting from the imbalance of sodium and potassium have resulted in deaths from this diet.

Fad diets will tout a particular food or vitamin or magical combination thereof, or promote a timing sequence of eating certain foods. Others claim that weight can be reduced by diets that interfere with digestion or absorption without calorie restriction. These claims are scientifically untrue. My appreciation of these diets lies in their marketing, a masterful manipulation of the consuming public.

Part of the annual $40 billion effort to lose weight is spent on legitimate weight control programs. These programs are founded upon a modest restriction in calorie intake, most averaging 1,400 calories per day. Most have associated support and teaching. The philosophy of these programs is good, but weight loss is expensive per pound, and much of the weight is regained when the individual leaves the protection of the program. The downside of these programs remains that control is still not in the hands of the individual.

Diet Center, Jenny Craig, Nutri Systems and Weight Watchers International are among the legitimate modest calorie restriction programs. Offering exercise plans, but focusing on eating restrictions, most offer maintenance programs. Some offer a "financial reward" if weight loss is maintained. The token financial reward, however, is designed to keep you in their maintenance programs, where they continue to profit. These companies are in business to make money, and their money is made on selling prepackaged food, counseling, check visits, and memberships. Consider, too, that much of their money is made on recidivism, your returning for another go at it after having failed.

Recently popular very low calorie diets (VLCD's) still sell, but their popularity is waning. Oprah Winfrey's Optifast diet was widely publicized. She lost, she gained, end of story. Well, end of Optifast story. She did finally lose weight and maintained her loss by adopting a modest calorie restriction and exercise program. VLCD's work in the short run because they limit intake to a 600 calorie per day diet. Anyone will lose weight with such a severe caloric restriction. Most VLCD's include a decent amount of high quality protein to diminish muscle tissue loss that accompanies starvation. Complications are relatively few save for potential gallstone formation and kidney damage if you don't drink adequate water. One poorly publicized but very deleterious effect of VLCD's is the associated 20% decrease in RMR that may last for six to eight weeks following cessation of the diet. That is a big number and potentiates weight gain in the post diet period. It's an unacceptable downside of this kind of diet. A balanced energy restricted diet is without question the safest, sanest, most successful diet. It is the thinking person's diet.

How to Manage Your Weight and Body Composition

The key to managing any part of our lives is knowledge and awareness. So it is true with weight management. I have provided legitimate knowledge about weight and body composition management. Here are some techniques to implement that knowledge.

Consider your attitude and expectations – Are you ready to do this? Are you dealing with too many other details in your life to allow you reasonable expectation of success? Set realistic goals like eating better and taking control as opposed to a specific weight goal. The weight goal will come via the expectation of success. Look at your behaviors, your coping with lapses and successes. Use that information to help you expect and achieve success.

Create an energy usage diary – Energy usage comprises half of the energy balance equation. For two weeks keep a detailed diary of everything you do in a day that uses energy. Use the table of activity and sports energy requirements in the chapter on exercise to estimate the rate of energy usage for

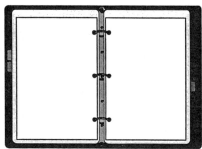

each of your activities. Include sleeping at 1.2 cal/min. Remember to adjust the rates of energy estimates for your weight (add or subtract 10% for each 15 pounds above or below 150 pounds). Compute your total use each day and compare that result with the estimate from the formula for calorie needs based on sex, weight, and activity level.

The practice of creating an energy diary promotes awareness about your energy expenditures on a moment to moment and a day to day basis. Your new found awareness will motivate you to change and may serve as a catalyst to change.

Keep a food diary – Keep a food diary of everything you eat for the first two to four weeks before you begin your weight loss phase. Record absolutely everything that goes into your mouth. The food diary proves a good look in your dietary mirror. What triggers your eating and your overeating? Look for patterns. Where are you consuming the greatest part of your calories?

Determine your body composition indices – Use any of the methods offered to determine BMI, PBF and WHR.

Keep records for trends – Don't ever forget the power of words on paper. Keep records of weight, BMI, PBF, WHR, calorie intake and expenditure, and any parameter you deem important.

Don't rush – This is a long, slow process, lifelong in fact. This is not a diet, it's a new way to eat, and it will take time to evolve into new healthier patterns of eating. Remember moderation. Do not crash diet.

Calculate your energy balance deficit – Establish an energy balance deficit of 500 calories per day, which equates to one pound per week of weight loss. Sit down and do the mathematical calculations. It's easy.

Men: Weight in kg x 10 plus 900; multiply by activity factor (1.2; 1.4; or 1.6) add 100 for thermic effect of food. Now, subtract 500.

Women: Weight in kg x7 plus 800; multiply by activity factor (1.2; 1.4; or 1.6) add 100 for thermic effect of food. Now, subtract 500.

Cut calories – Remember Sutton's Law. Go where the money is – banks. Start with cutting fats at 9 calories per gram and eliminate as much fat from your diet as possible. Examples are luncheon meats, marbled beef, whole milk products, cooking oils, margarines, toppings, sauces and commercial baked goods. Replace them with fruits, vegetables and complex carbohydrates.

Make dietary changes one at a time – Changing too much too quickly almost guarantees failure. How do you eat an elephant? One bite at a time. Take a week to adjust to fresh fruit instead of pastries as a snack or for dessert. The following week begin incremental changes in milk fat consumption, eventuating in drinking skim milk. You get the idea, but you must take the time to design your own diet. Doing it yourself rises as a critical part of the learning process.

Confine eating to planned mealtimes – However and whenever you eat, make it a conscious choice. Do not be a mindless muncher. Eating in a different location in your home can be fun and reinforce the idea of your being in control of your eating as long as you make the change mindfully.

Plan ahead – Plan meals one week, or one month, in advance and write out the menus on the calendar. Keep a calendar of the menus in plain sight in the kitchen. Stick to the planned menus. Use your file card system of recipes (see below) to make your job even easier.

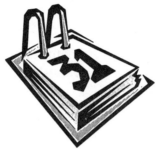

Simplify – Use some of the recipes in selected low-fat cookbooks. Be certain that they contain no more than 20% fat, with reasonable calorie content.

Develop a recipe file card system – For quick reference, keep a file system of recipes for your meal planning. I already suggested this in Chapter II on nutrition. It is your own Top Ten (or twenty) List.

Snack wisely – Make snacks low calorie items, like fruits, popcorn, or rice cakes.

Accept an occasional lapse – Keep those lapses only occasional. Enjoy the lapse and laugh at it, then carry on with your approach to new eating patterns. Do not do the guilt dance and do not have remorse at lapses. Record the lapse in your food diary for later review.

Practice awareness – Taste what you eat and pay attention to chewing. Put your fork down between bites. Appreciate what you are eating.

Incorporate exercise – Exercising uses energy and tips the energy balance equation even more in your favor. And (this is a big "and") exercise increases your chances of maintenance. In a study of dieting women in California who lost 20 pounds, 90% of them maintained the weight loss if they were regular exercisers. Powerful stuff, indeed! Exercise provides a psychological boost and sense of well being. It is a catalytic behavior that has carry over effect to other aspects of our lives.

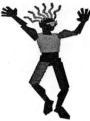

Aerobic exercise is an important adjunct to weight management, but strength training is equally critical. Strength training adds muscle mass, the biggest calorie burner in your body. Strength training also prevents the ratio of 75% fat and 25% muscle seen with passive weight loss, and shifts the ratio more towards 100% fat and 0% muscle.

Do not weigh often – Weigh yourself no more often than every two weeks. Be confident that you are changing your body. Pay attention to how you feel and look rather than what a set of scales reports.

Naked in the mirror test – In the privacy of your home, take a good look at yourself in the mirror, totally naked. What do you think? Are you making improvements? You can tell and the mirror doesn't lie either.

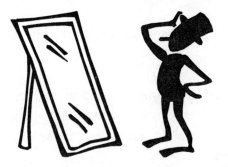

Sublimate – Substitute one activity for another. Recognize your desire to eat and choose some other activity. Take a walk, brush your teeth, or engage in a conversation when you have the desire to eat. Sublimation requires making a conscious decision and choice. By your consciously making the choice to engage in an alternate activity, you will be reinforcing your new behavior of eating less.

Relationships – Involve family members in your efforts. Communicate your intentions and ask for help, or at least ask not to be hindered in your efforts. Support is important for it is so hard to accomplish tasks alone in this world. Support groups are available, but remember the power in support groups comes from your seeking the group. You are in control. Contact your selected support individual or individuals, at least weekly in the beginning of your program, then perhaps biweekly. We are social animals and are happier when not alone. Happiness and satisfaction beget success.

Avoid extremes – Remember moderation. Never fast as a diet. Fasting is counterproductive and it teaches you misinformation. The best rate of weight loss is one pound per week. **One pound per week is 4 pounds per month, 26 pounds in six months and 52 pounds in a year.**

Behavior modification programs – Formal behavior modification programs are available through private counselors and from diet programs. I suggest that you are capable of modifying your own behavior.

Do not allow recidivism – Through your knowledge of the behavior modification process and the by fact that you perceive control of your life, you will avoid the pitfall of recidivism.

Read – Continue your education for a lifetime. Reading is valuable and inexpensive. I know of no substitute for reading. My routine solution for problems out of my arena of expertise is to find a book on the subject and read it.

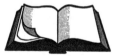

In your management of your weight and body composition, you will be learning a new way of living. The process is slow but valuable, much of the value coming from the very fact of the slowness. You will have more time to learn, to practice and to enjoy.

Post Script

I try to be a positive individual, and I am. I am positive that seductive and misleading advertising infuriates me.

The "Fat-Burning" Fallacy

Aren't we just the most gullible animals who have ever walked on this planet? Supplement sales are skyrocketing. Ab machines abound. Power Rider, Power Glider, Power Riser, Power Bar, Power Pacing, what's next, Power Puke?

Fitness gurus preach that the best way to exercise for weight loss is to perform long duration, relatively low intensity exercise, something in the vicinity of 60% of VO2 max. Exercise at this level uses about two-thirds fat and one-third carbohydrate as its fuels (see Figure 2, Chapter III). Although a sound principle of exercise physiology, TV infomercials, with their nauseatingly enthusiastic "experts," have picked it up and are using the principle as a marketing tool for machines that are allegedly "total body work out fat-burners." They "reason," if you exercise and burn primarily fat as the fuel, you will lose fat from your body. Errors of scientific law hide in their merchandising zealotry, leaving cash poor consumers with a useless piece of machinery.

If your interest is in aerobic fitness, legitimate exercise physiologists advise that exercise should be more intense, in the range of 70-80% of VO2 max. At this intensity the ratio of fuels used approximates one-third fat and two-thirds carbohydrate. If you intend to lose fat, according to the infomercial people and everyone else on the bandwagon, you should exercise low and slow for the two-thirds fat and one-third carbohydrate ratio. Confused and unenthusiastic, exercisers have left aerobics classes with a mixed-up message, "Take it easy and you'll slim down faster."

At first glance, the "total body work out fat-burner" is a tempting gimmick to fall for. Fat and carbohydrate are the two fuels for exercise, and the proportion of each used depends on exercise intensity. If you are sitting in your easy chair, the dog escapes and you run at top speed after him, you'll use mostly carbohydrate as fuel for energy. In fact, anytime you use maximum energy and breathe rapidly, your body relies mostly on carbohydrate as its energy source. If you walk or jog, your body will begin to call upon longer-term energy supplies, specifically fat. After about twenty minutes of moderate, 60% of VO2 max, exercise your body will begin to burn more fat than carbohydrate. So, yes, it is true that over a long slow work out you will burn more fat than carbohydrate. Walking for fifty minutes burns more fat than running for thirty minutes. A brisk walk burns one-third carbohydrate and two-thirds fat while a light run will reverse the ratio. So it seems logical to use and lose more fat by walking, right? Quite wrong! The answer is a bit involved.

The error of their thinking comes from the assumption that if you burn fat, you automatically lose body fat. This simply isn't so. No great advantage accrues from burning fat as a fuel if you target weight loss as your goal. **The only way to lose body fat is to eat fewer calories than you spend in energy.** If you don't eat fewer calories, your body will simply replenish the depleted stores of fat and carbohydrate (glycogen). Whatever your ratio of fuels spent as energy, eating enough calories to replace the energy spent assures replacement of both carbohydrate and fat stores.

What you eat after exercise makes a big difference, though. Consuming fifty grams of carbohydrate every two hours (four or five feedings) after significant exercise optimizes the rate of muscle glycogen replenishment. Normal replenishment rate approximates 5% per hour of glycogen stores, and the fifty grams of carbohydrate every two hours may increase that rate to 7% per hour. Selectively, the body will replenish muscle glycogen before storing calories as fat.

Post-exercise carbohydrate optimizes the process, but carbohydrate in excess of glycogen storage needs is always stored as fat. A post exercise fat diet will also replenish glycogen and fat stores, but at a slower rate, because dietary fat inhibits the process of muscle glycogen replenishment.

Aside from the "experts" errant application of the laws of nutritional biochemistry, they ignore laws of muscle physiology. Three rather critical principles of which the "experts" lose sight are: 1) Exercise below a threshold of 7.5 cal/min, or of less than 200 calories per workout, affords no aerobic training effect. Exercise on these machines may approximate 5 cal/min. No strength training effect is achieved either. 2) For a strength training effect, resistance must be great enough to limit repetitions to ten. Exercising on these machines requires repetitions in the hundreds. Aerobic training and strength training are "either-or" propositions, not simultaneous applications. 3) Weight lost in the absence of strength training is 75% fat and 25% muscle, a poorly advertised and relatively undesirable result. In their zeal to sell the "experts" dupe us into shifting our focus away from sound principles.

What should we focus upon? Calorie balance is critical. Spend more calories in exercise than you ingest, no matter what your fat/carbohydrate ratio intake and you'll lose weight. The wise exerciser gains other advantages, too.

Aerobic conditioning increases the number of mitochondria, effects an aerobic training response, and allows the individual to exercise longer. The body will also have a higher metabolic rate while it exercises, and for a period of time afterward. If you eat the same amount of food as usual with a higher energy usage rate, you will lose fat because the body always replenishes muscle glycogen before storing fat.

Strength training develops body muscle mass, a relatively "expensive" tissue to maintain with respect to energy needs when compared to fat. A pound of muscle burns 30-50 cal per day at its basal rate, compared with 2 cal per pound of fat per day. The greater ratio of muscle to fat requires greater energy supplies just to maintain the tissue. Some people fear that gaining muscle will add weight, but if so it is desirable weight. The well-developed muscle machine burns more calories at work and at rest.

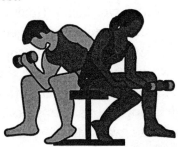

Emphasis should be on building and maintaining muscle, not fat-burning. As a muscle grows it needs increasing amounts of stored glycogen. This demand tips the balance towards glycogen storage at the expense of fat storage, assuming constant calorie replacement. A certain amount of fat is quite necessary and desirable, because it supplies the fuel for long term exercise. If we were to depend entirely on carbohydrate stores for energy, our exercise duration would be limited to two hours.

What are fat-burning advantages? Of course there are some, but the advantages are functional rather than cosmetic. Fat stores allow longer duration exercise, while conserving liver and muscle glycogen. That conservation assists rapid recovery from exercise. The metabolic cost of removing fat from storage, using it as a fuel for energy, but then restoring it with a carbohydrate diet offers advantage to the exerciser who wants to lose fat. Storing excess carbohydrate calories as fat uses 25% of the carbohydrate calories for the conversion to fat, compared to 3% of fat calories if fat is the replacement fuel.

So what are the final words? The final words are **EXERCISE** and **EAT RIGHT**! Exercise at whatever level will allow you to continue to exercise. You will spend calories and hopefully more calories than you take in. If so, you will lose weight. Increase exercise time and intensity, thereby increasing your aerobic training effect. Aerobic exercise increases basal metabolic rate, increases after-burn at levels greater than 70% VO2 max, and increases the anabolic (muscle building) process. Do strength training in addition to aerobic training to increase muscle mass. Replace calories spent with carbohydrate calories rather than fat calories.

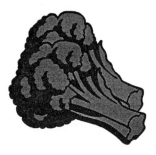

We love to discuss the minutiae as we vegetate on the sofa. We use alleged cerebral dilemmas as excuses for not exercising. The simple answer is to exercise, eat a high carbohydrate diet, and leave the minutiae out. Success is stacked in favor of the exerciser.

Under the Heading of: "He's Not Too Bright Sometimes ..."

The only person with whom I take free license of ridicule is me. Every so often it's just plain fun to laugh at my naivete or ignorance. Let me share this vignette with you in closing.

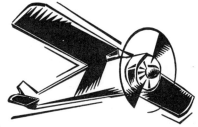

I love to fly and formerly spent loads of time at Chatham Municipal Airport on Cape Cod. One Saturday morning a photography company orchestrated a fashion photo shoot with the planes in the background. The obligatorily beautiful models sat in the lobby waiting for their turn to pose because October had brought unseasonably chilly temperatures.

One male model sat with his jacket off, revealing well-muscled and well-defined arms. Impressed by his arm definition I queried, "How did you get such cut arms?" He looked at me as if I had two heads and responded, "I lost fifteen pounds."

How dumb did I feel? I should have known the answer (actually, I did, but I wasn't thinking). Muscle definition, arms or abs, will only evidence if we remove the layer of fat that hides them.

Such simple and elegant truths await our discovery as we study how to *Get a Life!*

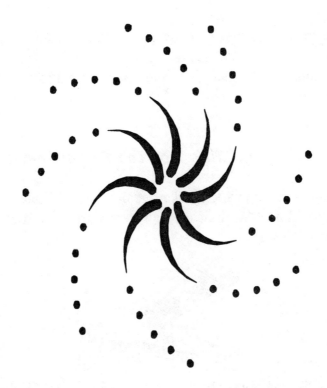

Chapter VIII

Vitamins Been Beriberi Good to Me

"Athletes are a gullible bunch, inclined to try anything to improve performance. And there are plenty of "snake oil salesmen" willing to sell a food or drug guaranteed to enhance performance .... Vitamin supplements will not improve the performance or health of people on an already adequate diet .... I still recommend vitamins in food over those contained in pills .... And, I do not endorse megadoses of fat or water-soluble vitamins."

❖

Brian J. Sharkey, Ph.D. Fitness and Health, 4ᵗʰ Edition

This chapter explains vitamins and minerals. It affirms the value of ingesting vitamins and minerals in the foods we eat. It examines antioxidants and offers evidence for their importance. It facilitates the ingestion of vitamins in the food we eat by providing you a top ten list of foods that contains all the vitamins and minerals we need. Still, this chapter ends with a recommendation of supplementation because of the ironic, yet irrefutable evidence of poor nutrition by a very intelligent and capable American population. We can do better folks. Come on, *Get a Life!*

Late in the 1980's, I received a phone call from a patient I had seen only once before. She lived on Nantucket Island, and I thought it curious that she was calling me in Chatham, Massachusetts, on the mainland. She came on the line, "Dr. Mees, I have a product that you can add to your practice, that you can sell exclusively and make a load of money. This will be the hottest product in recent years," she went on, "and you can make a lot of money. It's new. They're called antioxidants and you can make a lot of money."

"No, thanks anyway. I appreciate your calling to offer me the opportunity," I responded. I was being facetious without her recognizing it. Every multi-level marketing scheme uses the word, "opportunity," as their hook. So I tossed it back to her.

Since that time, I've received so many "opportunities" to sell products in my practice that it makes me dizzy to consider them all. They were all some form of vitamin or supplement. Unfortunately, we Americans don't perform well in our nutrition and vitamin arenas. However, I contend that with a mindful approach to our vitamin needs, we can easily *Get a Life, America!* without resorting to supplementation.

The fact that we medical types are susceptible to greed was driven home with sledgehammer emphasis at a recent American Medical Association Broadcasting Conference when a dotty, former "media doc" took the stage to declare that he had decided that "supplementation was a major solution to America's ills." Of course I now see his line of vitamins with his picture on the label in many of the "health food stores." I guess he seized the "opportunity."

Let's Create our Own Opportunity

I approach the topic of vitamins and minerals out of duty, and the subject of supplementation with a jaundiced eye. Vitamins and minerals, critical to life, deserve specific attention. Conversely, we oversell the concept of supplementation, shifting focus away from the Major League Players in Health and Wellness.

We should focus on vitamin content of foods, not vitamin content in a bottle. Vitamins and minerals are best consumed with the foods in our diets for two reasons. One, we receive additional benefits from foods like nutrition, water, and fiber. Two, by our consuming vitamins and minerals in food, we eat mindfully, aware of the content of our diets. Promoting awareness proves catalytic to other behaviors.

Allow me this "opportunity" to present basic vitamin information, more as a reference than as working information.

RDA's – Recommended Dietary Allowances

RDA's are standards set for the daily intake of various nutrients, the amounts considered to be adequate for most all healthy people to prevent deficiency states. First established in the 1930's, the RDA's are reestablished every five years. The experts, members of the Food and Nutrition Board and the National Academy of Sciences National Research Council, have combed the scientific literature to make these recommendations. After review of appropriate and available literature these scientists come up with a final "best guess figure" and then add about 20% as a safety margin.

Short-term ingestion of nutrients below the RDA will probably not put an individual at risk of nutritional deficiency. Eating well in excess of the RDA usually causes no problems either, because the body routinely rids itself of excess vitamins through the kidneys. People who take vitamin supplements in larger quantities generally produce "expensive urine."

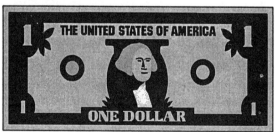

Caution is advised, though, with the fat-soluble vitamins. Not readily cleared by the kidneys and tightly bound in the fat stores, clearance may not be adequate, and toxicity, especially of vitamins A and D, may occur. Any vitamin taken in megadoses may overwhelm the physiologic process of clearance of the vitamin and produce toxicity.

Vitamins

Thirteen known vitamins are divided into two groups, water-soluble and fat-soluble. The four fat-soluble vitamins are A, D, E, and K, while the remaining nine are water-soluble, eight B vitamins and vitamin C. Some water-soluble vitamins are heat and light sensitive, and some can be easily washed away by water cooking. Most are not stored well in the body and need frequent replenishment. Fat-soluble vitamins, by contrast, are stored quite well in adipose tissue. Here's a quick run through of vitamins and minerals. Read it once and remember where it is in case you need to review.

Water-Soluble Vitamins

Vitamin B-1 (thiamine) is not stored well, thus deficiency becomes apparent rather quickly. Thiamine catalyzes the conversion of carbohydrate to energy. Thiamine deficiency produces beriberi. Good sources of vitamin B-1 are whole-wheat products, pork, liver, and peas. Flour and grain products may also be thiamine fortified. Adult RDA is 1.1-1.5 ug.

Vitamin B-2 (Riboflavin), similar to vitamin B-1, contributes to enzymatic reactions in the conversion of food to energy. Deficiencies result in dry scaly skin, cheilosis (cracks at the corners of the mouth), and hypersensitivity of the eyes to light. Long term deficiency may lead to cataracts.

Good sources of vitamin B-2 include meats, fish, milk, grains, and legumes. Due to vitamin B-2's sensitivity to destruction by light, food sources of vitamin B-2 should be stored in dark areas. Adult RDA is 1.3-1.7 mg.

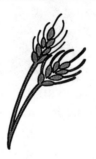

Vitamin B-3 (Niacin), usually eaten, may also be synthesized in the body. Similar to riboflavin, it plays a role in the conversion of food to energy. Niacin has been commonly used as a cholesterol-lowering agent for the past twenty years, but can have dangerous toxic effects in over dosage (liver damage, ulcers and hyperglycemia).

Niacin is available in foods such as liver, whole grains, and milk products. Adult RDA is 15-19 mg.

Vitamin B-6 (Pyridoxine) is required to help the body metabolize proteins, both the breakdown to amino acids and the synthesis of new proteins and muscle.

Pyridoxine is available in a wide variety of foods including meats, fish, nuts, legumes, vegetables, and whole-wheat products. Adult RDA is 15-19 mg.

Folic acid is essential for DNA metabolism and plays an important role in genetic functions like cell division and tissue growth. It's easily destroyed by oxidation, and as such, care should be taken in storage and food preparation.

Folic acid is readily available in liver, kidney, dark leafy green vegetables, fruits, beans, and peas. Adult RDA is 1.6-2.0 mg.

Vitamin B-12 (Cobalamin) is also important in DNA metabolism and assists in red blood cell formation and central nervous system maintenance. B-12 deficiency can result in pernicious anemia, an insidious and dangerous anemia. Vitamin B-12's reputation and function as an energy booster is unsupported by scientific evidence, any positive effect being that of placebo.

Primary sources of vitamin B-12 are from animal products like milk, eggs, fish, liver, kidney, and muscle meats. No plant sources of this vitamin exist. Adult RDA is 2 micrograms.

Pantothenic acid is essential for fat metabolism and associated processes like the synthesis of hormones and cholesterol. It's widely available in plant and animal foods, reported deficiencies having never been observed. Safe and adequate ranges are 4-7 mg.

Biotin aids in the formation of fatty acids and carbohydrate metabolism. It is available from a broad range of foods, but is also synthesized, like niacin, from microorganisms in the intestinal tract. Deficiencies are rare to non-existent. Safe and adequate ranges are 100-200 micrograms.

Vitamin C (Ascorbic acid), probably the most well known vitamin, was publicly popularized by Dr. Linus Pauling. We are not sure exactly how vitamin C works, but know it to be essential in the formation of the connective tissue, collagen. Collagen is a protein-based substance important for the growth and formation of teeth, bones, tendons, skin, and nails. Vitamin C is also integral in wound healing, infection resistance, metabolism of amino acids and folic acid, and the body's ability to absorb iron.

Varying factors may alter the need for vitamin C. Smoking, taking oral contraceptive pills, being stressed, and living in a hot environment all require greater vitamin C intake in those individuals. Commonly available in foods like fruits (especially citrus) and vegetables, vitamin C fortification is also frequent in foods. It's vulnerable to air and heat, so it's advisable to keep fruits with peels on, store vegetables in plastic wrap, and cook knowing that vitamin C can easily leech into water.

Megadose vitamin C can have deleterious effects. High doses may interfere with white blood cells and their ability to kill bacteria. It may inhibit copper absorption, create nausea and diarrhea, and interfere with diabetic urine testing. Adult RDA is 60 mg.

Fat-Soluble Vitamins

Fat-soluble vitamins (A, D, E, and K) are stored in the body's fat tissues until they are used. Little renal excretion occurs with fat-soluble vitamins. The storage, usage, and minimal renal excretion phenomenon increases the potential for vitamin toxicity if large doses are taken routinely.

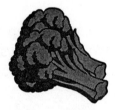 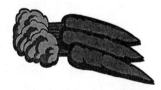

Vitamin A (Retinol) has multiple functions and wide ranging necessity in the body, affecting many different body cells. Deficiency produces abnormalities in skin and bone, respiratory system, urogenital, and gastrointestinal tracts. Vitamin A is essential to the integrity of the cell membranes and other barriers to bacterial invasion. Without vitamin A the body becomes more easily susceptible to infection. Vitamin A is most well known for its visual metabolic role, especially in night vision. Over ingestion of vitamin A may precipitate a yellow pigmentation to the skin, a relatively harmless and reversible condition, but long term supplements in high doses may cause fatigue, headaches, blurred vision, and in extreme cases, irreversible brain, bone, and liver damage.

Good sources of vitamin A are of both plant and animal origin. Animal sources include cheese, eggs, butter, chicken, and liver. Plant sources contain beta-carotene, a precursor to vitamin A. Ideal sources are yellow, orange, and some dark leafy green vegetables: carrots, cantaloupe, spinach, and broccoli. Some foods, like margarine, are fortified with vitamin A. Adult RDA is 1 mg.

Vitamin D is critical in the formation and maintenance of bones and teeth, for it aids in the absorption of calcium. Excessive vitamin D supply produces an exacerbation of vitamin D's normal effects, the enhancement of calcium deposition in the body tissues. That's fine for bones, but can be problematic if the calcium deposition begins to occur in soft tissues like heart, lung, and kidneys. That soft tissue deposition seems to be irreversible.

The best source of vitamin D for most of our population is vitamin D fortified milk. Other sources have too little vitamin D to supply the minimal needs. Curiously, vitamin D can be synthesized in our skin on exposure to sunlight. For many people, this is their primary source of the vitamin. Mild exposure of hands, arms and face for 10-15 minutes 2-3 times per week is adequate sun exposure for vitamin D synthesis in the skin. Adult RDA is 5 micrograms.

Vitamin E is still a bit of a mystery vitamin to the traditionalists. Anecdotal reports have lead to multiple uses of vitamin E. Ophthalmologists use it because they feel it may retard some of the chronic visual deterioration seen with aging. It has been used allegedly to enhance sexual desire. It has also been touted as a treatment for herpes simplex outbreaks. Vitamin E is also important in protecting the integrity of red blood cell membranes and thus helps preserve the red blood cell population.

It's available in vegetable oils, whole grain products, wheat germ, liver, nuts, and leafy green vegetables. Adult RDA is 10 mg.

Vitamin K, the clotting vitamin, is essential to the synthesis of at least 4 of the 13 essential proteins needed for the clotting sequence. Without it clotting is impossible, and minor injuries could lead to exsanguination. Vitamin K rich foods include liver, eggs, and dark green leafy vegetables. Adult RDA is 60-80 mg.

No matter who you are or what you do, recalling information about vitamins is difficult. Here are two solutions to the dilemma. One, remember where the information can be found in case you need it. Second, rather than trying to find foods to satisfy each vitamin requirement, let's produce a list of 10 foods and see what we receive in terms of vitamins.

Top 10 Foods for Vitamins

1) Chicken and fish – A, B-2, B-6, B-12 (fish), Biotin and Pantothenic acid
2) Whole grain breads and cereals – B-1, B-2, Niacin, B-6 and E
3) Dairy, eggs and cheese – A, B-2 (milk), Niacin, B-12, D (fortified milk), calcium
4) Legumes – B-1, B-2, Folic acid
5) Green leafy vegetables – B-1, B-2, B-6, Folic acid, C, E, K, Pantothenic acid, Biotin
6) Orange and yellow vegetables – A, C
7) Fruits – B-6, Folic acid, C
8) Potatoes – Potassium, C
9) Pasta – B-1, B-2, B-6
10) Beer and wine – B-1, B-2, Niacin, B-6, C (wine)

Selecting foods from the above list in various combinations covers all of our vitamin requirements. The list, although simple, allows for creativity and variety. None of the foods is high in fat and each of the foods (beer and wine possibly excepted) belongs in a healthy diet.

Minerals

Minerals are basic elements, right off the periodic chart, essential to cellular function and health. Some, called macro minerals, are required in larger amounts, while others, the trace minerals, are required in small quantities.

Three macro minerals have been included in the RDA's because the amounts necessary for the maintenance of health have been established. These are calcium, phosphorous, and magnesium. Three other macro minerals, potassium, chloride, and sodium, have varying requirements depending upon environmental conditions.

Calcium is essential to the development of bones and teeth. It seems that debate will never end about calcium supplements and their potential preventive effect against osteoporosis (thinning of the mineral portion of the bones). The RDA of calcium is 800 mg, and it is generally not recommended to take a supplement in excess of 1,200 mg. to 1,500 mg. High serum levels of calcium can be toxic, producing muscle spasms and possibly kidney stones. Calcium is most readily available in dairy products, especially milk, but also in yogurt (including

low-fat frozen yogurt), sardines, salmon, tofu, kale and broccoli.

Phosphorous complements calcium in the formation and maintenance of bones. It's also important in the formation of genetic material, cell membranes, and varying enzymes. Important as well in energy metabolism, phosphorous is abundant in meats and soft drinks. Deficiencies are rare. RDA is 1,200 mg.

Magnesium, a component of many enzyme systems, is particularly important in the normal functioning of nerve and muscle tissue. Deficiencies produce neurologic and muscular symptoms. Like so many of the vitamins and minerals, deficiency is rare because of magnesium's omnipresence in foods. Vegetables, grains, and legumes are major sources of magnesium. RDA is 350 mg.

Sodium, potassium, and chloride may be considered as a group because their common function is to maintain body fluid balance. Sodium is available in vegetables and animal foods, but the major supply is from the salt shaker on the dining table. Over use of the salt shaker often results in deleteriously high sodium intake in many people. Elevated serum sodium levels tend to attract water, expand blood volume and exacerbate high blood pressure. Decreasing sodium intake can reverse that process.

Potassium, less heavily ingested and primarily intracellular, does not cause similar blood pressure effects. Variation in potassium levels may have direct and severe effects on cardiac rhythms. Potassium may be over excreted by the kidneys in response to diuretic usage, but may be replaced by eating bananas or with potassium supplements.

Our knowledge about trace minerals is recent and as yet quite incomplete. We do know that they are essential to life, critical in cellular processes. RDA's have been established for four trace minerals: **iron, zinc, selenium, and iodine**. Five others are essential, but RDA's have not been established – copper, manganese, fluoride, chromium, and molybdenum. Other trace minerals like arsenic exist, but so little information is available that even safe and adequate levels are not available.

Iron is essential to hemoglobin formation. Zinc integrates the breakdown and utilization of carbohydrates and synthesis of proteins. Selenium assists proper heart muscle function. Iodine ensures thyroid hormone production. Copper is essential to hemoglobin synthesis, manufacture of collagen, maintenance of the nerve sheath, and proper cardiac functioning. Fluoride functions in prevention of bone loss and dental decay. Chromium assists insulin in regulation of blood glucose. Magnesium is involved in protein and energy metabolism, especially in nerve and muscle. Molybdenum (say that three times fast) is a component of many enzymes.

As with vitamins, information about minerals is tedious. Mineral deficiencies are rare in the United States, RDA's being easily satisfied with mindful attention to our dietary mix. Now that you have seen the traditional view of vitamins and minerals, let's address the question of supplementation with vitamins and minerals, dosages well in excess of the RDA's.

Supplements – Yes or No?

One hundred years has passed since the discovery that vitamin deficiencies were responsible for many common diseases. We know that niacin deficiency causes pellagra, vitamin C deficiency causes scurvy, vitamin D deficiency causes rickets, and thiamine deficiency causes beriberi. Relatively simple attention to these deficiency disorders proved that small amounts of specific vitamins in the diet were adequate to prevent the deficiency states. The United States government, through the USDA, has established recommended daily allowances (RDA's) of vitamins and minerals as 120% of the minimum requirement for prevention of deficiency states. So, in the past 100 years that has given us the industrial revolution, space travel, computerization of the world, two

World Wars, a plethora of antibiotics and drugs, the eradication of smallpox, organ transplants, and now AIDS; we also have RDA's for vitamins and minerals.

We are really making progress! Did you know that the RDA's sets the poverty level? The USDA computes how cheaply a family of four can get 100% of the USRDA's through food, then based on the premise that food constitutes one third of a family's budget, they multiply by three. Federal and state welfare allotments are based on these numbers.

Only recently, and fighting an excessively stubborn conservatism among scientists, medical types and government officials, a growing recognition is evolving that some vitamins may have important disease preventing and health promoting effects at doses higher than the RDA's. In the 1950's, Nobel Prize winning scientist, Linus Pauling, attempted to extol the benefits of Vitamin C as an anti viral agent, only to become the target of derision by the "establishment" of the scientific research community. We are so quick to judge. Forty years later

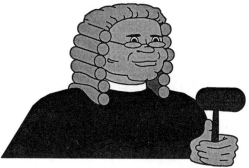

vitamin C has been discovered to possess significant antioxidant properties with vast potential health and wellness consequences.

We will now re-examine the group of vitamins known as antioxidants with a "modern eye." Are these vitamins the "right stuff" to make us healthier?

Antioxidant Vitamins – Theory of the Mechanism of Action

Potentially damaging compounds termed **free radicals** are formed by a number of processes in the body. These compounds are electrically charged and highly unstable molecules. The production of free radicals may occur in the liver, in the mitochondrial respiratory chain in skeletal muscles, or through the metabolism of fatty acids for energy. External environmental factors play a role in the creation of free radicals, too. Cigarette smoke, ozone, carbon tetrachloride and ionizing radiation appear to be toxic at least in part because of their free radical generation.

Free radicals, when released in controlled production by the body actually have a defensive purpose, to kill invading organisms and to offer some defense against cancer. However, the same free radicals when produced in excess or when augmented by environmental conditions can cause damage. Strenuous physical exercise can cause free radical mediated muscle cell damage. Free radicals can react with fatty acids to inhibit normal cellular enzymes, eventuating in cell damage. Free radicals can inhibit the formation of ATP (the currency of energy), damage DNA, and disrupt the integrity of the structure of complex carbohydrates.

Both intracellular and extracellular antioxidant systems exist within our body chemistry. Specific intracellular enzymes possess antioxidant properties. Extracellular vitamins also have antioxidant properties, specifically vitamins A, C, and E, as well as the mineral selenium. Estrogens have natural antioxidant properties, but some steroids like cortisone have pro-oxidant tendencies. Various foods like soybeans, garlic, and tea are reported to possess antioxidant properties.

In essence, antioxidants are enzymes, vitamins, or chemicals in foods that combine with and stabilize or neutralize the highly reactive, potentially damaging free radical, rendering it inert. Antioxidants appear to short-circuit the effects of free radicals before the chain reaction of cellular damage begins. Let's examine three of the processes in which free radicals are thought to induce damaging effects.

Free Radicals, Antioxidants and Disease Processes

Atherogenesis

LDL cholesterol in its un-oxidized form appears to be relatively inert. When oxidized, LDL becomes rapidly and intensely involved in the atherogenic process in the lining of the small and medium sized arteries. Oxidized LDL is able to bypass normal endothelial (the inner lining cells of the arteries) cellular defense processes and invade the subendothelial environs, initiating and perpetuating an inflammatory reaction. In response to the inflammatory reaction, the body sends cellular defenders to the site. The mobilization of the defenses causes damage to the lining of the arteries. Tiny defects in the normally smooth blood vessel wall lining allow the beginning of the atherogenic process (hardening of the arteries). These small defects, or rents, provide a wonderfully sticky foundation for the progressive accumulation of cholesterol, fats and calcium that grows into an atheromatous plaque.

Studies have shown a relationship between the susceptibility of LDL to oxidation and the severity of atherosclerosis. Undoubtedly, the genetic predisposition for the oxidative potential of any one individual's LDL determines, in part, his risk for cardiovascular disease.

While certain LDL's are more susceptible to oxidation, others carry goodly amounts of vitamin E, beta-carotene (a vitamin A precursor) and coenzyme Q, all antioxidants that may counteract or delay lipid oxidation. Vitamin C may intercept oxidants in solution before they attack the LDL molecule, thus affording additional protection from atherogenesis.

Considerable synergism exists among the antioxidants. Vitamin C helps restore oxidized vitamin E back to its original state (the antioxidant state). Vitamin C also maintains glutathione, a normally existing antioxidant in red blood cells, in its antioxidant state.

The research evidence favors cardio-protection in persons taking antioxidants, both in persons with and without existing vascular disease. While the evidence supports the use of antioxidants in prevention of CVD, these studies have not differentiated between good health habits (exercise, nutrition, stress management) and the specific role of supplementation.

Carcinogenesis

The complex nature of cancer makes atherogenesis seem simple. No one theoretical pathway has been proven as the cause of the chaotic cellular replication that is cancer. Many cancers, and just as many causes, are complicated by an overlay of differing degrees of genetic predisposition. We do have some evidence, however, that free radical damage may play a role in carcinogenesis.

These studies have corroborated a generally protective effect of the consumption of fruits, vegetables, and foods rich in vitamin C and beta-carotene against the development of many kinds of cancers. To what degree the antioxidant properties of vitamins are responsible for these effects remains unclear. It's certainly possible that persons who consume this type of diet may have other lifestyle behaviors that lower their risk of cancer.

The evidence from studies about antioxidants and their potential to affect carcinogenesis is controversial. Some studies support the hypothesis, some don't.

Some of the studies have even suggested an increase in cancers with antioxidant use. Let us for now accept that the jury is still out.

Age Associated Eye Disease

As with carcinogenesis, the jury is still out on the role of antioxidants in the prevention of age associated eye diseases. The incidence and prevalence of cataract formation, a cloudiness of the lens of the eye, increases with age to the degree that 45% of persons over the age of 75 will have senile cataracts severe enough to decrease vision and affect the quality of their lives. Oxidation may cause or be associated with cataract formation. As such, vitamins with antioxidant properties may prevent or delay the process of cataract formation.

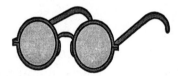

Epidemiologic evidence tends to support the role of antioxidant vitamins in prevention of age associated eye diseases. Combinations of vitamins C and E seem to afford the best protection. The inclusion of vitamin A, but moreover, foods rich in that vitamin, also provide protection. Other studies emphasize the balance of pro-oxidant and antioxidant molecules in the ocular environment as an important etiologic concern.

Macular degeneration, an incurable retinal deterioration resulting in progressive blindness in the elderly, was found to be 1/2 to 1/3 lower in prevalence among persons with higher serum carotenoid levels. Studies on the potential reversibility of macular degeneration are underway with cautious optimism.

Cautiously optimistic, that describes my position about antioxidant vitamins. I would place the emphasis on cautious.

Vitamin Toxicity

The preponderance of available evidence comparing the risk of the atherogenic process, carcinogenesis and age related eye diseases with the administration of antioxidant vitamins seems to be weighted in favor of the vitamins. Some studies have shown a threshold dose effect and a progressive dosage effect of antioxidant vitamins when matched against disease risk. But how high is high? When does dosage and protection become dosage and toxicity? Vitamin toxicity does exist and is relatively common considering that of the adult population, both active and sedentary, 40% to 50% rely on self-prescribed vitamin supplements.

Toxicity with vitamin A is easily the most dangerous. Symptoms include headaches, drowsiness, irritability and gastrointestinal irritability. Toxicity can occur at relatively low dosages and affect the live, growing part of our bones. Toxicity of vitamin E may present as diarrhea or fatigue, but large doses are usually well tolerated. Vitamin E may also potentiate the effects of the blood anticoagulant, coumadin. Vitamin C can increase iron absorption, and in the presence of copper or iron, vitamin C can act as a pro-oxidant. Like vitamin E, high doses of vitamin C rarely produce toxic effects. What is the lesson from this information? Don't take megadoses of the antioxidant vitamins, or of any vitamin.

Specific Antioxidant Vitamins

If antioxidant vitamins are beneficial, they must be **ACE's.** I am just providing you with a convenient method to remember the antioxidant vitamins (vitamins A, C, E and the mineral selenium). The antioxidant vitamins are presented here from their preventive perspective and for emphasis.

Vitamin A and carotene – Vitamin A actually refers to two different groups of substances. One form is retinol, or preformed vitamin A, found in dairy products and animal and fish meats. The other form is carotene, found primarily in plants, especially carrots and dark leafy vegetables. Current thinking is that the carotenoids (carotene) have the greatest antioxidant properties of the two groups. The message is to concentrate on eating your spinach and carrots.

Vitamin C – Vegetables and fruits (potatoes and citrus fruits, especially) contain the greatest concentrations of vitamin C. Smoking lowers vitamin C levels, and consequently smokers require a greater intake of the vitamin to achieve similar serum levels as non-smokers. Little is known about the mechanism of action of vitamin C, but epidemiologic studies support its role in the prevention of CVD, cancer, and age-associated eye diseases.

Vitamin E – Vitamin E occurs naturally in nuts and oils, but intake from these sources poses the burden of additional unwanted calories and fat. Synthetic vitamin E has only 74% of the activity of natural vitamin E, but provides equal antioxidant protection to LDL.

Vitamin E decreases platelet adhesion, thus decreasing the tendency toward and the risk of thromboembolic phenomena (clots, strokes and heart attacks). Vitamin E enhances immunity in elderly persons, and it may retard some of the age-related changes in the immune system. Vitamin E is thought to have some role in potentiating revascularization (improving the circulation to areas of compromised circulation) and thus may offer benefit to peripheral circulation difficulties, to healing of ischemic damage (heart attacks and strokes).

Selenium – Knowledge about selenium, like vitamin E, remains sketchy and anecdotal, but intriguing. It seems that the mineral, selenium, works most efficiently in concert with vitamin E. Together, they potentiate the maintenance of glutathione, a potent antioxidant itself. Facilitating the assimilation of vitamin E, selenium inhibits the oxidation of fats, and protects our body chemistry from environmental pollutants and heavy metals.

Selenium, found in the soil, transfers to plants and the animals that eat them. Human sources of selenium derive from those plants and animals. Readily available sources of selenium are fish, kidney, and liver. Vegetable sources include garlic, asparagus. and mushrooms. RDA is 60 micrograms, and toxicity becomes a danger at 1,000 micrograms.

Of epidemiologic interest is the fact that geographic areas of low selenium concentrations correlate with higher than normal cancer rates. One would think that facts like this will pique the interest of public health officials, spurring them to further investigations.

To Supplement or Not to Supplement ... Good Question

Should we or should we not use supplements? If not, the answer stops there. If so, then what and how much? I have never taken supplements and may never, but my recommendation is just the opposite. I recommend supplementation.

Personally, I choose not to take supplements because I practice the integration of the principles in this book. I integrate a mindful application of attitude, exercise, nutrition, stress management, and behavior modification with an enthusiastic participation in this world. I think that I have adequately covered the bases that I have selected for my life. It's highly unlikely that I will remember to take my vitamin A, C, E, and selenium every day for the rest of my life.

I keep an open mind and read current scientific literature. I do keep an open mind about other supplements like the current media darlings of chromium and L-carnitine. To date, I think that their place as supplements is only in states of deficiency. It may be possible that these chemicals do have a beneficial effect at peak levels of physical performance, but 99% of us don't operate at that extreme.

I remain a scientific Missourian curmudgeon, "show me" legitimate scientific research data. The research to date is insufficient to convince me that supplementation with amino acids and minerals makes a difference to our health. Conversely, the research on antioxidants is intriguing and seems to be much more clearly in favor of their use. However, I still question whether the antioxidant vitamins "work," or if they just restore us back to the physiologic position of function intended by Nature?

Let's remember that RDA's were developed to prevent deficiency states and deliberately do not reflect possible health promoting (health restoring?) benefits of vitamins. Therefore, RDA's have no role in determining vitamin use for optimization of health.

NHANES II, in a cohort of 12,000 persons surveyed, found that 17% had eaten no vegetables and 41% had eaten no fruit on the day of the survey. Additionally, only 25% of those surveyed had eaten a fruit or vegetable rich in vitamin A or C, and only 10% had satisfied the updated USDA recommendation of 5 servings of fruits and vegetables per day. This is irrefutable epidemiologic evidence of terrible nutrition in this country.

Researchers in the field of nutrition feel that modifying eating habits is more difficult than quitting smoking. Current studies suggest a societal trend back to more unhealthy diets, reversing some of the healthful gains of the past decade.

What to do? The answer is to change our lifestyles to optimal nutrition, but until we do, I favor supplementation. I include the following considerations in making my recommendation in favor of antioxidant supplementation:

1) Considerable benefit may be gained from the additional antioxidant vitamins even in healthy, "no present disease," persons based on epidemiologic evidence.

2) Although no long term studies of deleterious effects of antioxidants have been done, it appears that toxicity at moderate doses is not a concern. We shall keep our eyes open.

3) As individuals we have little control over environmental exposure to pollutants, to ionizing radiation, and to undeclared food additives that may potentiate the formation of free radicals. As a society, we do have control, but the control process is too slow to make a timely difference in our health risks.

4) Most of us are not living health lifestyles.

Julie Buring, an epidemiologist at Harvard University, when asked about antioxidant supplementation responded, "Look, if someone says to me, 'I'm taking vitamin E, do you think it will help?' My answer is, 'I don't think it will hurt. But, can I just run through your list of risk factors, because, for God's sake, don't tell me you are still smoking or that you are not watching your fat or exercising or that you are not eating a lot of fruits and vegetables.' Because all those things are much stronger at raising risk than vitamin E is at lowering it."

Let's talk about doses of antioxidant supplements. The RDA for vitamin C is 60 mg/d, for vitamin E 10 mg/d and none exists for beta carotene: My best current recommendations for antioxidant supplements are:

Vitamin C	500 mg twice daily
Vitamin E	400 IU twice daily
Beta carotene	20,000 IU daily
Vitamin A	1 mg
Selenium	50 - 200 micrograms daily

Spread the doses out throughout the day and, unless you are iron deficient, avoid taking antioxidants along with iron, as iron can counteract the antioxidant effect of the vitamins. But, remember, do what your mother told you to do, "Eat your fruits and vegetables and *Get a Life, America!*"

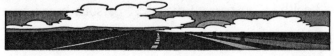

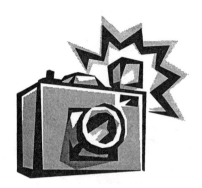

Chapter IX

Bringing All the Chickens Together to Take Their Picture

"Everybody's Crazy 'bout a Sharp Dressed Man ..."

❖

ZZ Top

My mother used to describe a difficult, multi-task job as, "Like trying to get a bunch of chickens together to take their picture." That's exactly what this chapter is about, accomplishing a difficult task, "taking the picture of the chickens."

This is a real "how" chapter. It addresses each previous chapter with the specifics of how to accomplish change in that discipline. Like education, it's a repeat and reinforcement of what we've learned so far. Now we're getting ready to practice what we've learned. Now we're really going find health, happiness, and love as we *Get a Life, America!*

The National Debt Theory of Living

Our national debt looms so large that we are unable to pay the interest on the principal. Hourly, we add interest to the principal, mounting an ever-larger national debt.

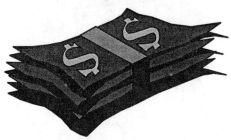

Similarly, many of us live our lives struggling to pay emotional and physical interest, only to find ourselves sinking deeper into "health debt." We don't exercise, we eat poorly, and we have no idea how to manage the escalating stresses in our lives. At best we struggle to survive. As our health declines, we have less and less "principal" upon which we may draw. Eventually, we bankrupt our system.

Health bankruptcy is unnecessary. By developing a prospective "investment schedule" of exercise, nutrition, stress management, and attitude adjustment we will garner wellness riches often beyond our expectations.

Lessons to Pass Along

In 1982 I attended a financial planning seminar, and I would like to share with you three lessons from that seminar. First, the professor, neatly groomed and nattily attired in a Brooks Brothers suit, presented himself quite well in an organized, clear, and concise manner. Second, he offered the "where are you now in your financial life, and where do you want to be at a specific time in the future" principle. Third, he concluded the seminar by warning that we would all go home, become engrossed in our lives and work, and make no changes in our financial management what so ever.

I remember his lessons as if I heard them only yesterday. Always be presentable and organized. Determine where you are now, choose where you want to be, and then chart your course between those two points. Beware of recidivism.

In each of the modalities of health and wellness, I want you to be well groomed ("sharp dressed"), to know where you are and where you want to be, to choose your course between the points, and to be aware of the potential pitfall of recidivism. Being "well groomed" is an external manifestation of your positive attitude. I will prompt your discovery of where you are, while you decide where you wish to be. I will assist you in charting your course. Your knowledge and understanding of the behavior modification process and the fact that your are in control of that process will eliminate your potential for recidivism.

Written records are a must, for an "idea or plan not committed to paper remains a wish." Purchase a multi-section loose-leaf notebook with loads of paper. Create the following sections, which parallel the chapters of *Get a Life, America!,* with a couple of additions:

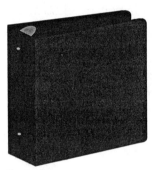

- Family history, (genetic tree)
- Attitudes and expectations
- Choices
- Behavior modification process
- Nutrition
- Exercise
- Stress and stress management
- Psychologic well being (depression?)
- Lipid profile
- Weight and body composition
- Vitamins and supplements
- Journal entries
- Self

I could provide you with a mindless, fill-in-the-blanks, chart for each of the above structural elements of health and wellness, but I think it's time for you to get your own life! If you have read the entire book to this point, I trust that you are committed to your good health. I believe that you want to be a mindful manager of your life. It's time for you to start drawing your plans, sawing your wood, driving your nails, and painting your walls.

Keep records of objective data on the right hand side of your ledger, and place any personal notes about that subject on the left-hand side. What is your motivation for changing that particular modality of health? How do you feel about it? Who will benefit from your making the change? Who is your role model for the intended change? Your conscious recognition of your emotions will assist your making changes successfully.

Plan to make changes in an incremental fashion, small and one at a time. Realize that the changes you make are to last for a lifetime. Realize, too, that you don't have to finish the first change before starting to make a second one, because implementing one change will potentiate the initiation and perpetuation of others. You may enter the process of change by choosing any one of the Major League Players of Health. Remember, though, that behavior change is of obligation, lengthy. Do not frustrate yourself by rushing.

Your integration of the modalities of health and wellness results from your simultaneous application of all of those complementary modalities. None of the modalities or principles is competitive or exclusive. The progressive application and marriage of each and all of the modalities eventuates in the final product, the state of grace we call wellness, the state of grace I call "getting a life!"

Family History

Establishing a family history provides genetic and behavioral data. Our genetic template provides relative risk information and a foundation upon which behavior change may erect growth. So, while the genetic limb of our family history offers insights to disease risk, the behavioral arm supplies grist for our mills of change.

How does one establish a family history? Ask your parents, their parents, your aunts and uncles, your siblings, and friends of the family. What do you ask? Ask about diseases (heart attacks, strokes, cancer, high blood pressure, diabetes), age at death, and cause of death. Ask about relatives' vocations, geographic locales, personalities, and number of marriages and divorces. Seek further information about the individual's world-view, philosophy, faith, communication style, level of responsibility accepted in the family, and attitudes and expectations. Ask, listen, and record.

Look at your family tree not only with an eye to physical traits, but especially with an eye to emotional traits. We have more control of the emotional traits than of the physical ones. Observation of your family tree does offer you information that is immediately useful. Have dysfunctional behaviors been passed from generation to generation? Does prejudice run in your family? Does your family communicate in a dysfunctional manner (90% of families do, so your chances are high)? Is anger an undercurrent of your family dynamic? Does your family have an entitlement mentality? Behaviors are learned, and as such, may be changed. You have total freedom to change any behavior that you identify.

Gather all of the pertinent information available, then address your answers to the question, "Where are you now in your family?" Write your responses in your notebook under the following suggested headings: age, position (son, daughter, father, mother), education, marriage, children and grandchildren, vocation, responsibilities to family, communication style, living accommodations, disease risks, and family roadblocks to potential change.

Make entries on the left-hand side of your ledger about your attitude with respect to your position. How do you feel about your defined position? Do you feel satisfied, bored, trapped, with no way out? Do you sense dissonance, but are not sure why? Do you definitely want to change for the better?

With a well-defined understanding of where you are, decide where you want to be, and when you want to be there. Where do you want to be with respect to family size, children (or not), geographic locale, vocation, living accommodations? Could you be a better husband or better wife? Could your communication style be improved?

When do you want to arrive at your chosen goal? Be realistic, behavior change takes a minimum of two years. Can you accept that? Could you set interim mini-goals along the way?

Review your understanding of the behavior modification process. Do you have the capacity, awareness, etc? If your answer is yes, then start to address, "How do you get there?" Recall the common denominators to changing.

- Commit to paper
- Draw up a plan
- Sign a contract with a witness
- Ask for help
- Use your daily team for support
- Establish rewards
- Practice

Greeting the millenium, your family genetic tree defines your genetic template and affords you no freedom of modification. In the near future, that circumstance may change with the advent of genetic manipulation. Careful scrutiny of your heritage will reveal valuable health and wellness information. Does your lineage exhibit genetic traits that would be best ended with your

generation? Does your family have a high rate of early deaths from heart disease? Do you want to burden your progeny with that concern? Does diabetes run in your family? Is that a sentence you would give to your children?

The generational compulsion to repeat may have given you a bad set of genes, but you retain the right to choose whether or not to perpetuate the mindless seeding of bad genes. I want you to think about having compassion for your children and for their children. Out of your "right to have children," do you wish to sentence those children to an unhealthy existence or a guaranteed early death? The choice remains yours, not mine and not society's. If you choose to take the risk of producing a child with a high probability of disease, then you must be willing to accept the responsibility that attends your choice.

Choice–"Beyond the Five-Second Rage, it's all Choice"

The concept of choice is critical to our success in making changes in our lives. Making changes in our lives requires our consciously choosing to do so. Choice is always available to us, but it isn't free. We pay the cost of choice by accepting the attendant responsibility.

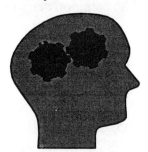

One of the biggest and most important choices you have already made is to have chosen health and wellness, to have chosen *Get a Life!* It's one of the smartest choices you will ever make, because the return on investment assures positive growth of health principal.

Attitudes and Expectations

I contend that attitudes and expectation, in the light of genetic potential, are essential elements of health and wellness. We will not achieve what we do not conceive. Attitudes and expectations come free for the choosing. We're not obligated or destined to repeat the attitudes and expectations of our families. Since our future successes depend upon our attitudes and expectations, we must examine them in the full light of day.

What is your attitude now? Is your attitude optimistic, defeated, ambiguous, empowered, out of control, positive, or negative? What are your expectations? Are your expectations of success, failure, embarrassment, and mediocrity?

What are your choices of attitudes and expectations for your future? They are anything you can imagine. Take some time with this section and let your mind run. No limits restrict your choices of attitudes and expectations.

What attitudes did you choose? What expectations did you choose? When would you like to have your chosen attitudes and expectations? You may have them immediately. You may own them in two years.

Behavior Modification Process – Change Your Heart

In general, and in specific reference to your intended behavior change, always address the question, "Where are you now?" Look now, specifically at the behavior modification process. Do you understand the process? Do you understand the process as it applies to you? Do you accept the process? Do you need to review the chapter? Where are you in the flow of the process? With those questions answered on paper, proceed to the next question.

Where do you want to be? Allow me to suggest that you want to be facing forward, in the direction of positive completion, and proceeding toward the goal of a new behavior. If you can't answer that question as I suggested, I would advise that you review and focus on your capacity and awareness. Renewed focus on the earliest parts of behavior modification may re-motivate you to your goal of changing.

When? This is entirely up to you, but the sooner you start, the sooner you will make your intended changes.

How? Use the process as explained in the chapter on behavior modification mindfully. See yourself proceeding through the stages of capacity, awareness, external motivation, internal motivation and execution. Commit to paper, draw up a plan, get a witness, ask for help, reward yourself, and practice.

Nutrition – What's Eating You?

Where are you now? How do you find out? Keep a food journal for three or four weeks, computing the following information about your daily diet: total calories, fat calories, saturated fat calories, carbohydrate calories, protein calories, vitamin and mineral adequacy, distribution of calories (from fat, protein and carbohydrate), fiber, and water intake.

Make entries in your notebook about how you feel, physically and emotionally with respect to eating. Notebook entries promote awareness about your psychology of eating. Give yourself credit for the good dietary behaviors that you already practice. You may be closer to your goal than you thought.

Where do you want to be? You want to be eating a diet that provides **65% of calories from carbohydrate, 15% of calories from protein and 20% of calories from fat.** You want to be eating high fiber foods, consuming large volumes of water and obtaining good vitamin intake, well above the RDA's. You desire to be eating a variety of foods and willing to try new foods. You desire to be eating to survive, rather than surviving to eat.

How do you establish a program of good nutrition? Remember the basic principles – commit to paper, draw up a plan, sign a contract, ask for help, use rewards, and practice.

Write your own plan utilizing the knowledge that you have gained in reading the section on nutrition. Remember that good nutrition is a catalytic behavior. Create your own file card system of menus that meet the defined parameters. Share your nutritional information among members of your family. You may modify the information presented in *Get a Life!* to met your specific needs, but make the modification thoughtfully.

I am not leaving you high and dry, but please realize that the most valuable and resilient behaviors are those created of our own efforts. You must put in some time and effort, because I can't *Get a Life!* for you.

When do you want to reach your goal? Start whenever you choose and then progress. When you want to reach your goal is entirely up to you. Set interim mini goals. Remember the two year stewardship for behavior change.

Exercise – Use it or Lose it

Where are you now? What is your aerobic capacity? How do you measure it? You may estimate it by reviewing your recent activity level (inactive – low; good level of activity – medium; very active, athletic – high), or you may use the walk a mile as fast as you can test (Appendix).

How is your strength? How do you measure that? Go to a health club and determine what weight allows you to do ten repetitions of a particular exercise. That weight is two thirds of your maximum. Do not attempt a maximum lift initially because of a high injury potential for untrained muscles. List the weights for each of the fourteen exercises listed in the exercise chapter of *Get a Life, America!*

How flexible are you? Play with your body to determine your flexibility. Can you touch your toes with straight legs? Do it gently. Can you scratch your back? Can you sit lotus style?

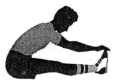

Where do you want to be? You might consider being stronger overall with better aerobic capacity. Are you training for a sport? Do you want to take part in a weight loss campaign? Perhaps you want gain muscle mass for appearance, improve your metabolism of fats, or become more flexible.

How do you get there? Do some more planning. Use the exercise prescription blank in the exercise chapter to assist your planning. Commit your plan to paper in your notebook.

Stress and Stress Management–Remember the Tiger

Where are you now? You may be so stressed that you don't know how to begin. Begin by eating the elephant. Take a stress test questionnaire and pay attention to the score. Review for bodily expressions of stress (headaches, high blood pressure, backaches, changes in intestinal habits, fatigue). Ask members of your first team if they notice any signs of stress in you (we are always the last to know). Identify the sources of your stress. Is the source your perception of an event or your perception of yourself? Write down your findings.

Where do you want to be? You might consider being less stressed, more in control, more energetic, happier, at less risk for stress related diseases, or more productive.

How do you accomplish that? Remind yourself that **stress is perception**. Remind yourself that **you have choice**. Remind yourself that **choice gives you control.** Review the chapter on stress for the available modalities for coping with stress. Work with all of the modalities available to you for discovery and execution of your plan. Continue recording all of your thoughts and discoveries on paper. Commit your plan to paper. Use the behavior modification process.

When do you want to have better coping abilities? Better stress management is entirely your choice, and you may begin immediately. Benefits of your efforts begin to accrue with your making the choice to better manage your stress.

Psychologic Well Being – Look Out for the Black Dog

The biggest problem with our emotional well being is lack of awareness of how we feel, the "where are you now." Your subconscious, but judicious and bulldogged use of ego defense mechanisms may cloud clear vision of your emotional health. And, you may be ignorant of how you feel because you don't ever ask. Where are you now? Are you happy? Are you depressed? Do you have any idea? Do you sense dissonance? Why? What else can you do? Take a screening test and pay attention to the results. Canvas members of your first team; ask their opinions of your emotional health.

Where do you want to be? If you are satisfied with your emotional well being, that is great. At least you have asked the question. If you are depressed, do you want to be happier, or does your depression serve you in some manipulative way? If your goal is happiness, then choose happiness.

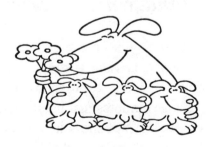

How do you achieve happiness? Happiness, like stress, is largely perception. Because depression feeds on ignorance, creating awareness is paramount in combating depression. Create awareness by the methods listed in the chapters on behavior modification, stress, and depression. Your problem will be half solved. The remainder of your charge is to use the knowledge gained in the chapter on depression to chart your course out of the Bermuda Triangle of Depression. If you feel that professional help is in order, do it now. Do not wait. Act upon your analysis of your needs.

When? I will give you the same answer. It's up to you. Make the choice.

Lipids – It's a Matter of Fat

In order to determine the present status of your lipid profile, fast for twelve hours and then donate a sample of blood for analysis. The parameters of interest to you are total cholesterol, HDL, LDL, triglycerides, and the total cholesterol/ HDL ratio. Instruct the laboratory technician that you want those and only those indices.

With the results of your lipid profile in hand (where are you now?), you may plan where you want to be and how to get there. Of course, we all aspire to the desirable ranges (total cholesterol under 200, HDL over 60, LDL under 130, triglycerides under 200 and ratio of total cholesterol to HDL of less than 4. Genetics may not allow all of us to reach those desired environs. I promise you that you can be better, but how much better is up to you.

Achieving better indices is relatively simple. Choose to take responsibility for minimizing fat (especially saturated fat) and cholesterol intake. Eat smart, get lean, don't smoke, drink only moderately, and monitor your lipid profile as you deem necessary. Allow yourself two to three months to effect the initial changes in your lipid profile.

Body Composition and Weight Management – Eat to Live

Where are you now? First, keep an energy use diary for two weeks to graphically demonstrate your caloric needs. What else do you need to know? What is your weight? What is your WHR (waist hip ratio)? What is your body fat percentage? What is your BMI (body mass index)? What is your daily caloric requirement? Use the formula to determine yours, then compare it to your energy use diary product. What is your daily caloric intake? What is your daily energy output above basal levels? How active are you?

Where do you want to be? Review each of the above parameters and make a conscious choice. Do you want to lose weight? Do you want to change your body composition? Do you want muscle definition to show? That will result from fat loss.

How do you get there? All of the above parameters are directly related to body composition, and we control our body composition. Remember that weight loss in the absence of strength training exercise is 75% fat and 25% muscle. For this reason, always combine an exercise program with dietary restriction. Plan a 500-calorie per day energy deficit for a one pound per week weight loss. The deficit should be a combination of increased expense from exercise and decreased expense from diet. You plan and draw up the schedule.

When? Changing body weight and composition is obligatorily slow. Good things take time. Have fun during the change.

Vitamins and Supplements – Beriberi Good

Vitamins and minerals are essential to life, catalysts to the metabolic process. Without them, we die. If that is the case, then we had better rush out and get all we can, right? Wrong! Vitamins and minerals, although essential, are but one of the integral components to health and wellness. Any modality of health and wellness when applied in excess may put us at risk. Vitamins are no exception.

Where are you now? Your present position with respect to vitamin and mineral adequacy may be difficult and tedious to determine. One method to determine your adequacy is to include vitamin and mineral content in your food journal. This practice encourages awareness while it educates you about vitamins and minerals. Another method is to assume that you are among the legion of

Americans who are nutritionally deficient. Either method will substantiate that 90% of us need to improve our nutritional habits.

Where do you want to be? I propose that you want to be eating a diet that provides all your vitamins and minerals in the food you consume, and that the diet provides quantities well in excess of the RDA's.

How do you accomplish that goal? If you have completed the nutrition section, you have already succeeded. Some may debate that statement and offer that additional health gains may be achieved by additional vitamins. While I cannot deny the possibility, I will re-warn you about the potential toxicity of megadose vitamins. The choice of supplementation lies with you.

I maintain that the greatest benefits to health and wellness are to be garnered from integrating the Major League Players like genetics, attitudes and expectations, nutrition, exercise, stress management, etc. Ninety-eight percent of health and wellness lies within the purview of these big league players. Use them first, get your 98%, and then if you desire, fiddle with the remaining 2%.

Journal Entries

Journal entries are for your edification. Any idea, discovery, success, failure, or emotion deserves its location on paper. They are yours, why not keep them? Bond them to paper for posterity. Read your entries periodically. Journaling allows you to track your trends of self-growth. Journaling allows you to "talk" when there is no one to listen. Journaling allows you to be honest and assertive in your communication, and it gives you a venue for practice. I highly recommend journaling.

Self

I recommend including a section entitled "self." All of *Get a Life, America!* is about you. The fact that an entire book is dedicated to the improvement and maintenance of you is not enough. Nothing in this world is more important to you than you. It is not selfish to consider ourselves first, it's our responsibility. If we are to be integral and contributing members of society, then we must participate from a position of strength, not a point of weakness.

Periodic Review

Once you have established your notebook, periodically review it. For every change that you are attempting to accomplish, initially review it weekly and then review it every two weeks for the first two months. Monthly review will suffice thereafter. Review takes only a minute to ask the basic question, "How am I doing in my effort to change? Do I need to make any course adjustments?" If not, that's fine. If so, make them. Write your changes down on paper.

After six months of thinking, planning, executing and recording you will begin to feel comfortable in your evolution. Don't stop the process, for your behavior isn't yet cemented. Practice your new behavior. Practice makes perfect.

Be Alert for Recidivism

None of us is perfect, and we may expect to make mistakes. The earlier we recognize the mistakes, the easier the mistakes are to correct. If you see yourself sliding back into old habits, immediately review where you are and where you erred in the behavior modification process. How is your capacity? Are you aware? Have you resurrected old ego defense mechanisms to cloud your vision? Have external motivators changed? Have you given ownership of the problem to someone else? Is you plan obsolete? Have you abdicated your responsibility for control? Ask these questions and answer them honestly. If necessary, retreat and repeat some of your steps.

When a baseball player hits a home run, they must touch all of the bases for the run to count. When you change a behavior, you must "touch all the bases" in the process for the behavior to become yours.

Do the Full Monty – Go the Full Two Years

At the end of two years, wouldn't you rather reflect on that time with the pride of accomplishment, than to realize you still wallow in a familiar quagmire? It's your choice.

As you build your health to wellness, I would like to remind you of the power of catalytic behaviors. Catalytic behaviors potentiate and facilitate the integration of other behaviors into your whole health and wellness framework. Choose them freely and well.

Don't forget that Nature abhors a vacuum. Create an artificial void in your life by eliminating an unhealthy behavior, then allow it to fill with your healthy choice.

Remember to eat the elephant one bite at a time. Watch your progressive attention to each of the parts dissect a seemingly insurmountable whole. If you run the film reel backwards, you may experience the progressive summation of the parts to create the whole.

Understand the power of integration of the principles of health and wellness. The process of synergy creates a whole, larger than the sum of the parts. The individual application of exercise and of nutrition cannot approximate the beneficial result of their marriage. Add to this family, the integral principles of attitude and expectations, stress management, body composition management and emotional well being, and you will achieve the higher state of grace of health called wellness.

Yes, do the Full Monty, spend the full two-year stewardship of behavior modification. You'll *Get a Life!*

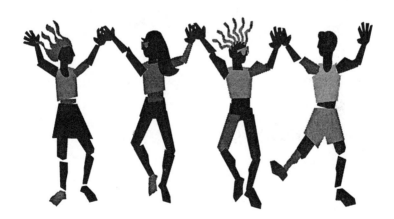

Author's Note:

The first of many times that I "finished" *Get a Life, America!,* I sat in review. That was maybe two years before this time I "finished" *Get a Life, America!* I had originally written it as an educational manual for any individual wishing to improve his or her healthy lifestyle.

Although "finished," something was lacking. After meditating about the missing piece, I discovered that I had neglected the health of our country. So began another time-consuming, research-laden, but personally-empowering journey to pioneer methods for our nation to *Get a Life!*

An after-thought, but a good thought, hence the final chapter of *Get a Life, America!* Read on McDuff. Here's the last piece of the pie.

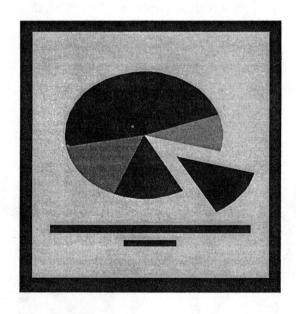

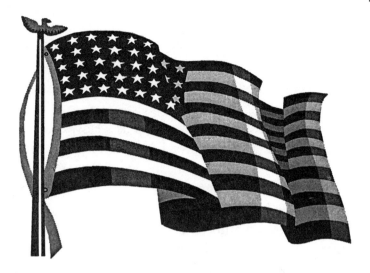

Chapter X

Get a Life! America!

"The health of the people is really the foundation upon which all their happiness and all their powers as a state depend."

❖

Benjamin Disraeli

"I haven't done as much writing as I wish. I've been more involved in doing. People ask, When are you going to write your autobiography? and Are you keeping records of all you experiences? I invariably say, No, I don't have time. I'll worry about the writing later. I'm worried about the doing now."

❖

David Satcher, MD,
Then, head of CDC in Atlanta, now United States Surgeon General,
from a 1977 interview.

So far, we've talked about how to change you. Now it's time to face the nation. As Dr. Satcher urgently implores, "Now it's time to **do**."

How do we change society's unhealthy behaviors? As a New York City literary agent and Harry, a patron at the coffee shop, challenged me, "How are you going to get people to exercise who don't want to exercise? How are you going to motivate me to change?"

This chapter addresses those questions. How do we motivate the unmotivated? This chapter speaks of broad-spectrum health education. It presents some unique and visionary ideas for education and change. Like what your ask? How about putting healthy messages on milk cartons, opposite the pictures of missing children, a metaphor for missing information and education. What about placing healthful messages on billboards?

In motivating a nation to change, we take lessons from the master marketers and market the concept of health and education like we're running for public office. We can offer rewards for healthy behaviors. How about granting a tax credit for good health?

In closing, I ask for your help. This is a huge job, and together, one bite at a time, we can eat the elephant. We can *Get a Life, America!*

Let's Do It!

To *Get a Life!* for our nation, I propose a multifaceted interventional program, instituted society wide. We will establish **(1) interventional teaching programs** at select target sites along a time continuum from birth to old age. Coincident with this broad spectrum teaching effort, we will initiate a **(2) marketing campaign** to sell the idea of health and wellness as a desirable product, to sell it like we're running for public office. Meanwhile, we shall encourage and nurture the development of a **(3) positive modification of society's attitude about health and wellness**.

At one time I thought it most prudent and reasonable to focus our teaching program on one segment of our society, concentrating our efforts there. I held that our children were the most important resource in the country and deserved our primary attention. I reasoned that we could do a "hard sell" on them, support healthy behaviors and allow (trust and hope) them to carry these behaviors, attitudes, beliefs, and expectations forward with them throughout their lives.

I still affirm that children are our most important resource. I have realized, however, that the single shot approach will not work. The single shot approach will fail because the sedentary inertia of the remainder of society steadfastly resists our every positive step. Any improvement we might make in our children would be buffered, dampened, or eliminated by unthinking, blind resistance from the adult community who "knows" (or at least they "know" what they have always done, right or wrong).

We must implement a broad-spectrum approach to educating all ages of our society, lest we have some groups dragging others back to square one. Each educational endeavor must be tailored for the abilities, learning level, interests, and amount of resistance (unlearning and relearning) of the intended target group.

Great resistance to changing our societal attitude about health and wellness hides in the deep recesses of the generational compulsion to repeat, but we cannot shrink in fear of that monster. So, too, we cannot wait for a cumulative societal pain, or threat to our survival, to initiate change. Let's begin now.

We must first create a societal awareness of the need to change by employing catalytic behaviors for change. We must develop a marketing campaign to make IBM, Microsoft, and Coca-Cola jealous. We will change society's attitude and market the idea of health and wellness, getting a life, inexpensively, with great public involvement and support; for better health begets increased production, economic growth, and lower costs to society for medical care. Everyone wins and no one loses.

I do not promise a population of programmed super humans. Rather, I propose that we move our collective state of health from one position on the scale of wellness to a higher one. As we learn and become adept at health and lifestyle management, we will step up the scale again in the future. Our national health, taking societal baby steps similar to those we took as individuals in our getting a life, will accrue exponential benefits.

Before we proceed to the specifics of the program, lets take a glance back over our shoulders to understand why past efforts to create better health for our society have failed. The industrial revolution facilitated many of the advances in medicine, but coincidentally tossed new health risks in society's pathway. More sedentary, more gluttonous, and more stressed in the latter part of the twentieth century, we face self imposed risks and diseases associated with those changes; specifically, heart disease, lung disease, strokes, and cancer.

Previous efforts to create a healthier public arrived in the form of edicts from upon high. Proclamations from governmental bodies that we as a society should exercise more, eat better, and lose weight trumpeted from the sterile, granite edifices in Washington D.C. Many of us maintain a wary distrust of the government and its covert motives, and therefore, implicitly distrust the message.

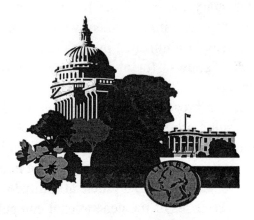

The message told us **what** to do, but said nothing of **how** to do it. The governmental health agencies who dictated the edicts never enlisted us in the decision making process. We became passive recipients, not active participants. To effect legitimate change, individuals must be actively involved, with the perception that they have control and the prerogative to make choices.

How many of us have heard of *Healthy People 2000*? Not many, I assure you. How can the government's program to improve health and have 60% of us exercising by the year 2000 work if we have not even heard of it? Poor advertisement and essentially no ongoing support mechanism doomed *Healthy People 2000* from the start. We can't choose something we don't know about.

What we do know, however, affirms that government and organized medicine err in their perspective about health. "Fix the broken part, don't be mindful of preventive maintenance." How could such a wasteful government as ours be expected to think with a conserving mentality?

If we ask for prevention, we are asking too much of them. The government mentality for prevention hasn't evolved yet. Organized medicine, a bit different from government, with the capacity to conceive the idea of prevention, stubbornly resists enlightenment because steadfast inertia and profit motive from illnesses mold their attitudes. As a society, we have unconsciously bought into the party line, the "fix-it" mentality. That attitude has demanded bad health in the past, and that attitude must change.

I hate to be mercenary, but what rewards have been offered to society for better health habits. None. What incentives? None. If we truly want to change our society's health, then we must toss out a few carrots as motivational incentives.

Some organized efforts, however, have worked, and we must acknowledge them. Immunizations and antibiotics play major roles in eliminating deaths from infectious diseases. Life expectancy increased significantly with their development and use. The development of sophisticated diagnostic and surgical techniques allowed some people to live when they surely would have died had they been living in the early twentieth century. Recently, we have reached a plateau in survival rates. An opportune time for individuals to make a difference, we can increase survival rates and improve quality of life with the institution of our societal intervention program.

Why will our program work when past attempts have not? Here are some reasons:

> **Commitment** – We commit to the principle of prevention, and we will sell it like we're running for public office.
> **Involvement of individuals** – We reach out to individuals, invite them to join us, and integrate them in the process of national change.
> **Broad-based approach** – We do not limit our appeal to one or two groups. Purposeful and wide spectrum, our appeal invites an entire population.
> **Everyone wins** – No one loses, for no risk confronts us.
> **Choosing to change societal attitudes and expectations** – We emphasize that society has choice, the freedom to choose its attitudes and expectations.
> **Create rewards for individuals and for society** – We will establish financial and social incentives, and we will give loads of "atta-boys" for our successes.
> **Documentation** – We shall document efforts and results on local and national levels. Remember the power of words committed to paper.
> **Marketing campaign** – Rather than my complaining about the successes of deceitful marketers selling worthless products to a gullible public, I propose that we employ their time honored techniques and sell a legitimate product, societal health and wellness.
> **Our societal perception of control** – When we perceive as a society that we do have control over our collective lives, we are empowered to accomplish anything we desire.
> **Maintain a persistent presence** – We can't expect a nation to change if we're not obviously present and supportive each step of the way.

Health Education Across America

Education is the best provision for old age.
❖
Aristotle

Let's keep this timeless advice foremost in our minds as we journey through the ages of educational potential. Now, we'll get to specifics. What are our targeted groups for teaching intervention?

Teaching Mothers During Pregnancy

Expectant mothers radiate beauty. Their pregnancy symbolizes renewal and opportunity. Great anticipation, expectation, and hope accompany the birth and development of every child. What better time to blend with the hope, enthusiasm, and joy that attends this event and offer information that will increase the chance for that child's success in a rather imposing world. What expectant mother doesn't want her child to be healthy and to have the advantages she might have missed? Eager to help her newborn, motivated, and receptive to learning, expectant mothers hunger for information.

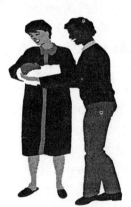

What information is most important to the mother-to-be? The necessity of **physical and verbal human contact** with the infant leads the list by far. More than anything else, this mother to child contact affords a child the sense of security, security to last a lifetime. Without the contact, however, the child develops insecurity, also to last a lifetime.

Information about **nutrition** sits second on the list. We must teach not only nutritional information for the infancy of the child, but also eating habits for the life of the child. We need to impart the message that a child carries habits of eating, habits learned in childhood, throughout her life. Let's get it right at the start, avoiding the necessity to change habits later in life.

With obesity running rampant on our city streets and country roads, mothers-to-be should understand that obese children become obese adults. The greater number of fat cells produced at specific developmental stages of the child predisposes to an obese adult. No parent should allow his or her baby to be fat. Unthinking and unkind parents sentence children to a lifetime of fighting the "battle of the bulge" because those parents ignored good health practices.

A critical component of good health, **exercise** in the form of physical motion should begin early in the lives of our children. Mothers should be encouraged to carry their new child for walks, to stroll her in the park, to bounce her on their knees. Show her child motion as a normal part of its life.

New mothers should be aware that they become their child's principal **role model,** especially during the child's critical developmental years. The behavior she demonstrates to her child, not what she says, but what she does, sends the strongest message. The new mother may show her child the joy, enthusiasm, and importance of good health practices in her life. Then we trust the generational compulsion to repeat to work in a positive manner, passing along healthy behaviors.

It seems reasonable that we ask mothers to share **physical contact, nutrition, exercise and attitude** with their children. What a great start for our children! Where, though, do we have the opportunity to impart this healthy lifestyle information to the mothers?

During each check-up at her obstetrician, the new mother may be provided with a quiz – questionnaire to assess her nutritional, exercise, and attitudinal knowledge. The five or ten minutes that the nurse uses to check blood pressure and weight affords ample opportunity for sharing two or three nutritional and exercise pearls. Educational reading material may be provided for the next visit's quiz. The material, gathered from a standard textbook of nutrition, bears directly on the present and future health of her child. Now, rather than being a passive recipient of obstetric care, the new mother becomes integrated into the process of caring for herself and the new child. Actively involved in learning, eventually, she will teach her child. Active participation in a team or process motivates and empowers the new mother.

Pre-delivery "La Maze" type classes have traditionally focused on preparation for labor and delivery. Does labor and delivery, certainly important, but generally a four to twelve hour process, command the entirety of a course? What about the rest of our lives? What about mom's nutrition? What about the child's nutrition? Here lies a vast teaching opportunity and a wonderful forum for dialogue.

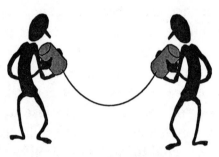

Dialogue, one of the most powerful teaching tools ever created, begs you to employ it. The ancient Greek philosophers taught by dialogue. We can, too. Dialogue encourages participation by the student. Through stimulating a student's talking and questioning, dialogue becomes a catalyst to learning.

Are you aware of any adult education program directed at pregnant women? Have you ever found a course with the theme specific to child rearing and development? I haven't, and I wonder why not. Community colleges and university extension programs could offer these courses as a community service. In doing so they would receive invaluable public relations benefits. They might also offer a prototype course, prospectively addressing issues like communication, husband and wife relationships, health, how to handle disagreements, and how to parent.

What fertile fields we have to cultivate in teaching new mothers about the health and wellness of their child. We have only just begun, yet our teaching opportunities blossom like flowers in spring.

Teaching Children in their Earliest Formal Schooling Years – Nursery School, Grades 1,2,3

Nursery school through grade three provides a period of progressive transition from teaching by demonstration to teaching didactically. Here, planned simple teaching vignettes may add impact to the teaching message set by example. We impart *Get a Life!* education to these young people in a fun, interactive, noncompetitive atmosphere.

"Let early education be a sort of amusement;
you will then be better able to find out the natural bent."

❖

Plato

The first experiences of a child away from his home, if positive, evoke good feelings about everything she has been exposed to, including healthful information. Although we counter some previously learned negative home habits, we reassure ourselves that the habits are new enough to be easily modified. The brains of these young "diamonds in the rough" are not so full as to resist new ideas and information.

What is important to a child at this age in his life? Teachers, fun, movement, play, recess, lunch, new friends, moms, dads, and pets are some of the important parts of a growing world to young children. Let's attempt to make good use of everything available from that list in teaching our children good health habits.

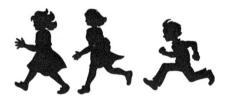

Teachers become significant role models, opportunistically ideal candidates for demonstrating desired behaviors. For children, anything fun tends to be accepted and repeated. Movement, fun and natural to children, erupts without hesitation. Children greet lunchtime with eager anticipation, "What's for lunch? Is it soup yet? Wednesday, Prince spaghetti day!" New friends become part of their socialization. Desiring "acceptance" in a social group, the child learns the importance of accommodating accepted social norms. If being active and eating well is a social norm, the child espouses that norm. Moms and dads may be asked at parents' meetings to support and reward their child's healthful habits at home. "Pets," you say, "what can they do?" Involvement of a child in the exercise and nutrition care of a pet mirrors and reinforces those same modalities for the child. OK, we have some good teaching tools, opportunities, and resources, but what do we want to teach?

Let's begin with teaching and reinforcing the **joy of movement** of our bodies. What mechanical marvels our bodies are. Let's use them and watch ourselves as we do. Recess, a great place for movement, should locate a fair distance from the school building, necessitating a three-minute walk to get there. Encourage random activities like throwing balls, jumping rope, swinging, and broad jumping. Do not make running a requisite. Focus only on movement. Walking is fine, run if they wish. The teacher, active as any of the students, plays role model. Make bodies move and faces happy.

Integrate movement in class. Tell stories by dancing or mime. Do not encourage interpersonal competition. Everybody wins. Always reward participation in movement, paying special attention to hesitant individuals. Encourage them, then reward them. Emphasize, too, the importance of achieving strong muscles. Record a collage of movement of the class from recess to classroom, from arrival at school to leaving school. Use video cameras to record each child's accomplishments, then play the video for the class.

Plant the seeds of **social confidence** in the earliest school years. The growth and future development of a child's social confidence depends upon how well we care for her early development. We nurturers of our children must be cognizant of our responsibility to support their social confidence. We must recognize and support any initiative towards social confidence at this age. The later ability of an individual to choose her attitudes and expectations, indeed to choose her pathway through life, relies on her social confidence.

"Good nutrition begins .... where?" It begins wherever we choose. It can begin at home, at school, or at a friend's house. Let's manage what we "show and tell" about nutrition at school, because we don't have as much control over nutritional "show and tell" at home or away at a friend's house. Work with the school's food service staff to provide the 65% / 20% / 15% ratio of total calories obtained from carbohydrate, fat, and protein, respectively. Make the food attractive and appealing. Various pieces of artwork featuring fruits, vegetables and whole grains, should adorn cafeteria walls. Refrain from putting a printed message on the pictures. Exhibit other artwork like an eagle soaring or a cheetah running, and allow the student to draw his own conclusions.

Encourage children to bring "home lunches" that are healthy. These brown bag lunches should include fruits, vegetables, and whole grain products. Seize the moment to teach what is a fruit, what is a vegetable, and what is a source of whole grains.

Do not chastise bad eating behaviors, but quickly reward or praise good ones. The message disseminates rapidly. Reward especially any initiative or involvement of the student in his nutrition planning or execution. Reinforce a "can do" attitude of any student.

Teachers must maintain a positive attitude about healthy behaviors, constantly being alert for manifestations of positive behaviors in the children. Teachers should reward positive behaviors immediately with verbal praise, for public verbal praise is one of the most sought after rewards for young children. Give it freely and often.

I would have the teacher eat with the class. Unobtrusive, but in plain sight, teachers should exhibit their own good choices of nutrition and their enjoyment of the food.

As the children progress through grade two and into grade three, increasing opportunity for didactic teaching avails us. Didactic teaching reinforces behaviors developed by mimicry. Teach basic nutritional information, like what foods are carbohydrates, what foods are proteins, and what foods are fats. Introduce the concept that food provides energy and that our bodies store excess food as fat. Emphasize the philosophical principle of "eating to live rather than living to eat." We can integrate these pearls of getting a life into the reading program of the students. Yes, let's write inviting storybooks that incorporate these principles.

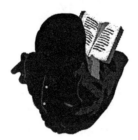

What about games? Kids love games. Let's create games that teach about getting a life.

One may argue that we overload an already stressed academic curriculum by adding such information. I understand and agree partly, but counter that a healthy, happy school environment can accomplish yeoman's work.

I also contend that society disrespects teachers, demeans them, and pays them poorly. Yet, we ask so much of them. I appreciate teachers and thank them in advance for their dedication. As a teacher and role model, if you are able to redirect the course of a single student towards a healthier lifestyle, you have more than accomplished your charge.

Grades 4 through 8

The initial teaching effort at all levels of intervention above the nursery – grades 1,2,3 level will differ from subsequent ones because we must first establish a basic foundation of information at all levels. At the upper school levels in future years the sophistication of our approach elevates, predicated upon prior knowledge and habits.

Grades 4 – 8, with their higher level of didactic teaching potential, allow a more direct approach. We may present young people in the age range of 9 – 13 with simple, logical information about healthy habits and lifestyles, encouraging their participation in those behaviors.

The dedication of one to two hours per week of teaching time provides foundations in anatomy, physiology, nutrition, and early concepts of stress management. An opportune time to introduce the concept of **stress and its management,** we will teach healthy coping techniques rather than ignore or support maladaptive behaviors.

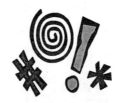

Of course we will work with the cafeteria crew to continue to provide and demonstrate the **65 / 20 / 15 ratio of nutrients in meals**. We will continue to serve the food in a pleasant and attractive manner. Providing good nutrition at school remains our primary goal, but our demonstrating daily examples of good food selection and preparation assumes equal importance. Demonstrating food preparation as a hands-on classroom activity adds impact to our message.

Continued presentation of artwork themes, still central to our efforts, suggests an interesting project that creative teachers may employ. Photograph students in motion or in the act of some positive behavior and then display that photograph on the classroom, hallway, or cafeteria walls. Again, allow no captions, no printed messages, just the photo. Involve the students in taking photos, too. Keep movement and exercise consistently in focus, verbally rewarding any individual initiative towards them.

Team sports evolve during this period, a wonderful occurrence for those participants. Remember to encourage the participation in individual sports like golf, track, aerobics, dance (jazz, ballet, ballroom) for girls, boys, and teachers, because more students participate in these activities than in team sports. Here waits an opportunity for an enthusiastic and creative physical education teacher, to shine in coordinating a school-wide physical participation program.

Physical activity should not be limited to school time. Logic demands the institution and facilitation of after school movement programs. Encourage the students to involve their parents in activities at home, too.

Students in grades 4 – 8 have developed the mental capacity to become integral in the planning of healthy lifestyles. During the didactic program, ask the students for their ideas about exercise or motion programs, meal planning, and methods for coping with stressors. For homework, the student could write a simple meal plan, establish exercise goals, or develop a dance or mime expression for stress management.

The more we involve a student in the process of developing healthy behaviors the more likely he will adopt the behaviors. I suggest that we integrate students in various "administrative" tasks like meal planning with the cafeteria staff, meal planning as part of math class (computing caloric needs and how to satisfy the needs), or planning a school wide exercise program with the physical education department. By involving students in the planning process we expose them to the problem solving dilemmas that we all face daily, as well as demonstrate to him the advantages of team solutions. Integration into the planning process instills an individual and collective responsibility for developing healthy habits.

Continue the theme of responsibility with the introduction of student record keeping. Students keep records of planning programs, successes of the programs, and trends of those programs. Students maintain their own records in the form of journals. Remember the awesome power of words on paper.

Speaking of awesome power, **peer pressure and the individualization – conformity paradox** begin to play important roles in the lives of these young people. How do we use these significant behavior molders to our advantage? **Being healthy has to be cool,** while being unhealthy must be uncool. "Nothing is stronger than cool," quotes Albert Fonzarelli (the "Fonz") of *Happy Days*.

We cannot coerce or create "cool" over night, but we can facilitate its evolution through operant conditioning. The choice of behavior must be the student's choice, and if we alertly reward it, we will see the behavior repeated. Of course we will work very hard to "stack the deck" by providing an environment in which the students are prone to good choices. Behavior developed in this manner stands much stronger, perceived as the result of the individual's free choice.

Teachers remain as role models for healthy behaviors. Gradually, they assume a less obvious position to the class, allowing for and encouraging the autonomy of the students. The teacher should not disappear into the teachers' room or teachers' dining area, for good, healthy lifestyle behavior should always be on display.

We request **continued involvement of the parents**. Through their support of good behaviors at home, parents play a vital role in the conditioning process towards health and wellness. We achieve the presence and assistance of parents through groups like the Parent Teacher's Association, using the PTA forum to share our philosophy and plans for developing healthy lifestyles for our students. Teachers and parents must work in concert, a necessity, lest we as teachers work our fingers to the bone at school, only to have our efforts sabotaged at home by counter-current messages. PTA meetings will always be a forum for sharing of ideas among parents, teachers, and administrators.

An interesting test, taking away the formal program of lifestyle, health, and wellness practices for two weeks, quietly and without warning, will provoke reactions. Observe the reactions and behaviors of the students. Do they miss it? Do good behaviors predominate, or not? After the period of two weeks, talk about that two-week hiatus. Valuable dialogue, providing insight for possible modifications of the program, results. We must always be amenable to modifying our presentation.

If a wellness philosophy integrates in the school day among students, teachers, and administration, then the repetition of the behaviors reinforces and cements those philosophies and behaviors. It comes down to practice .... reward .... practice .... reward ..... (time) .... success for life .... *Got a Life!*

High School

Here lies a wondrous opportunity for success, fun, and enlightenment. These students are young adults, and I would recommend meeting them and treating them as such in our common effort to discover and adopt good living habits. They will teach us as much as we might teach them, maybe more. Not so long ago, each of us walked in their shoes.

Yes, we rebelled against authority, values, and traditions, and we probably did some dumb things in the process. Possibly we engaged in some self-destructive behavior, but what fun it was to grow up. Aware or not, we were allowing ourselves the freedom of exploration, thought, and expression.

Unfortunately, society tells us to put a lid on that kind of freedom, and most of us acquiesce. I suggest that we keep the lid off and revel in the freedom together.

An opportunity to **encourage communication**, high school provides the ideal environment. Encourage communication among students, between students and teachers, and between students and parents. High school students have loads to say. We must be good listeners for them, encouraging their talking and discovery, providing a forum for that purpose. Certainly, didactic teaching of good health habits centers our program, but the cultivation of "self" in the individual rises paramount. The ideas they formulate, the habits they develop, the philosophies they own, will most likely last a lifetime.

Specific communication skills may be introduced and practiced. **Assertive communication is the ultimate goal.** The concepts of honesty, love, and compassion blend quite well with assertive communication and assertive behavior. Stress them. Practice them. Assertive communication often prevents stressful situations.

Introduce the concept of **charity**, that the value of the gift is in the giving. In a civilized society, all of us who can, should give. Because one chooses what one gives, we present the concept of charity in word and deed, and then allow the students to make their own final judgment.

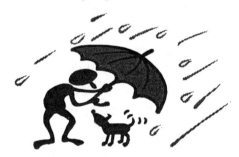

A time for the introduction of ideas and concepts, followed by the practicing of those ideas and concepts, we introduce the concepts of **awareness, choices, attitudes, and expectations.** Such powerful tools to grant individuals so early in their lives, sadly, many people never know these tools exist.

Student involvement in planning and implementation of nutrition and exercise programs has become *de rigeur,* the roots of the concept planted in grades 4 – 8. Students may manage the exercise and nutrition portions of the schools as class projects.

Begin to involve the **students as role models** and teachers for the younger students. Acknowledge their position and importance as role models and as present contributing members of society. Stress the importance of self-sufficiency and self-maintenance as basic traits for being an integral member of society.

An ideal time to teach in dialogue-style a class about life, parenting, being a mate, being a citizen; a prototype class of this sort should be routinely integrated in all schools' curricula.

Phenomenally tumultuous years, emotionally and physically, for all of us who pass through, high school tests our coping capacity. Stresses occur, magnify, explode, destroy, or so it seems. **Stress recognition and stress management** philosophies and techniques become part of our curriculum. Because early recognition of stress and training in coping techniques is essential to healthy lifestyles, we will teach and practice prospective training, not retrospective patching.

High school prepares the student to fledge from the protective nest of home and familiar surroundings. Whether she chooses the working world or college is of no consequence, she assumes the status of independent.

College Years

College marks the beginning of the ages with the greatest potential for deterioration, physically, emotionally, and behaviorally. Our structured support system through grade school and high school has been wrested away from us as if someone took our favorite security blanket. College can be a very naked feeling. Conversely, a time period equally fertile for the development and maintenance of health and wellness, what we make of the opportunity determines our success.

The potential for deterioration lies in three areas. One, the individual, out of his "nest" and on his own, may not have established firmly rooted health habits. His choices of behavior may be unconscious, random, and sub-optimal. Two, time and schedule management can become defeating. The individual focuses on schoolwork, often to the exclusion of self. The college academic challenge, substantial and sometimes overwhelming, always with more reading, writing and thinking to be done than can fit into any twenty-four hour period, looms like rain clouds over our heads. We must learn to apportion the time for academics and time allotted to ourselves. In this environment we are often not mindful of the importance of developing and sustaining one's self. Without a happy, healthy self, we cannot assure success in any arena. Three, an absence of readily available organized athletic programs places individual responsibility squarely on the shoulders of the student for seeking out exercise venues. Sad news results as we join the 90% of adults who do not exercise and suffer the deleterious health consequences of a sedentary lifestyle.

I propose that colleges offer an elective course, taught by one of the school's best, most enthusiastic teachers. Rapidly, the most popular course on campus, it covers the text of *Get a Life, America!*, with additional sections on parenting, marriage, sexuality, career counseling, and the individual choice – responsibility relationship. Our population screams for such didactic teaching, because people do not absorb functional life skills by exposure and experience. Will we learn science, Shakespeare, mathematics, good English, and foreign languages by casual life experience?

Selling good healthful behaviors to college students challenges the most astute marketer. Accepting that challenge, we should work with food service personnel to provide choices of healthy foods, and then advertise those foods aggressively in the eating facilities. Post information about grams of fat in food and calorie content in prominent view. Grams of fat in food provides information, but moreover, it proves a catalytic stimulus for the student to think about what he selects to eat. Make salads, fresh fruits, and grain products readily available. Present them attractively, in plain view, not like Mc Donald's who displays salads in small, out-of-the-way, unattractive, refrigerated cases. Think like a supermarket manager, locating these items so obviously that one almost trips over them. Place a suggestion box prominently for student input of ideas about nutrition. Open dining facilities to light and brighten them with artwork on the walls. Always keep in mind that we desire to "sell" good nutrition to college students.

We must encourage and facilitate exercise in college. Gymnasiums and athletic facilities decorate the campus landscape, yet with a paucity of the students using them. How do we change that? Open athletic facilities 24 hours, 7 days per week. Make them user friendly, with healthy snack bars, and a comfortable place to congregate.

Let's also make use of role models. The administration and professors must demonstrate a consensus of opinion that exercise is good and desirable. The administration, role models for the students, must exercise in full public view. Routinely remind professors and administrators of their responsibility as role models. Their daily behaviors must reflect good lifestyle choices. Students could be engaged to critique the effectiveness of the professors' behavior choices.

Grant some academic credit towards graduation for a student's achieving and maintaining an active lifestyle throughout college. Grant four credit hours of study for maintaining desirable body composition, aerobic fitness, and strength through four years at the school. This program, entirely voluntary, provides a strong incentive with four hours of credit.

Allow no driving on the interior academic part of the campus, forcing walking, blading, or biking where-ever one travels. Apply this rule to the teaching staff, too. Advertise hiking and outdoor clubs and activities. Make them affordable. Encourage students to seek additional courses of study to compliment healthy habits. After all, what do we have if we don't have our health?

College, perhaps the most memorable years of our lives, assumes a pivotal position in our developing healthy lifestyles. Potentially, a make or break experience, I suggest we deem it a "make" experience.

Work Environment

An environment more maliciously destructive to good health and wellness than college is that of the workplace. This hellhole for health deserves special consideration and attention. Gratuitous lip service has been paid to creating a healthy working force, but with precious little application of immediately available programs for improving the health of employees.

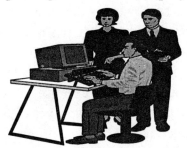

I propose self-sustaining "in-house" health and wellness programs with incentives and rewards for employees. Exercise facilities should be present and available in every business employing more than 300 employees. The figure of 300 employees defines the minimum membership to sustain a small private health club facility. Businesses with fewer than 300 employees may contract with established health clubs or form a consortium club on their own.

Dining facilities in these businesses should provide the same good nutrition as do our ideal colleges. Publish the food content and composition in an effort to educate the consuming employee. Place it obviously. Catalytic information that stares back at us while we select our food proves hard to miss and hard to forget.

Weekly seminar-type teaching sessions will be offered on a variety of health and wellness topics. Employees may be given that hour off, with pay, to attend the session. Granting pay for one session per month, twelve sessions per year, accrues to one and one half days of pay per employee. The health benefit to the business of increased productivity and lessened use sick time more than covers the expense for the seminar.

In a similar gesture as I proposed for college students, I suggest bonuses for employees who maintain their health. The bonus incentives, either monetary or time off with pay, support a happier, more productive work force. In a healthy environment everyone wins.

Adult Education Programs through University Extension, Community College and Service Organizations

Adult education programs, available in nearly every community in the country, or within comfortable geographical proximity, rest as untapped health and wellness resources. These programs publish course schedules twice yearly, for fall and spring semesters. Some centers run summer classes, too. Most of the classes meet in the evenings, once or twice weekly. Availability and location make them user friendly.

Some adult education programs already offer classes on healthy lifestyles and I applaud their foresight. I want more. I want more classes, more variety, more teaching about integration of healthy principles. I want omnipresent repetition, because practice makes perfect.

I applaud any person's attempt to learn about getting a life. Take one class, then sign up for another. We must beat the drum slowly and steadily. We must encourage taking a series of classes with overlapping and mutually supportive themes. Our continued presence in the adult education program, over time, supports behavior change. Our stable presence in the program assists individuals through the critical and obligatory "two-year stewardship" of behavior modification. Only after this lengthy rite of passage does new and real behavior belong to them.

Obviously, I cannot teach all of those classes, even though I would love to do so. Who will teach? Any good teacher, committed to healthy lifestyles, may contribute his expertise. Recently, however, a number of colleges have begun to offer "Health Education" as a major study. These recent grads will be a fine asset to our cadre of teachers. The course material isn't esoteric or difficult. The

317

difficulty comes from the fact that we are asking people to make changes in their lives. For that task we need enthusiastic "sales" teachers. I have always held that an excellent salesperson makes a good teacher, "selling" their information to a hopefully interested audience.

Nursing Homes

Now I pose an interesting point to ponder, one that many of us purposefully avoid. Nursing homes have become a holding station wasteland for a large segment of our population. Many people have been put there, against their wishes, out of their families' sight and responsibility, "just waiting for the funeral." The very obvious societal message that we no longer value this population group reinforces that same perception in the senior's mind. It seems obvious to me and to others that we waste a very valuable human resource in our nursing homes. These people, with experience, opinions, and life stories to tell, our mentors, whom we have allowed to deteriorate, often unnecessarily, raised us. Thanklessly, we tuck them away and forget about them. Significant collective rehabilitation potential wastes under the roofs of our nursing homes.

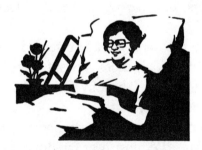

Nursing home patients need more **exercise, human compassion, and touch.** Even nursing home patients who have "never" exercised will benefit from increasing demands on their muscles. Eighty and ninety year-old muscles respond equally well to exercise as do twenty and thirty year-old muscles. Certainly, limitations like arthritis or damage from a previous stroke may present as hurdles. But, we can view those hurdles as low hurdles as easily as high hurdles.

Begin by asking the body parts to move, those parts that haven't been doing much in recent years. With staff assistance, we may institute a general strength-training program. Use small hand weights for resistance training while the person sits. Safe and effective, the upside rehabilitation potential is remarkable.

Occupational therapy, a fancy name for providing something for these patients to do with their hands, eyes, and minds, carries critical import. Unfortunately, like exercise, it takes a back seat to changing bedpans and passing out mind-numbing medications. Every patient, the slightest bit able, should be presented with the challenge of occupational therapy. We need to provide routine mental stimulation, lest they lose more mentation than they already have lost.

The human interaction necessary in implementing an exercise program donates inestimable value. These poor lost souls starve for regular human contact, verbal and physical. With exercise, compassion, and touch, functional improvement will amaze even veteran observers. With reasonable personal attention and the application of exercise, some patients may become independent enough to live outside of nursing homes. Perhaps they can return to the status of being a contributing member of society.

Of course we must remain cognizant of the threat that rehabilitation of patients poses to the nursing home industry. For each client that we manage to liberate, the industry loses $50,000 to $60,000 of gross income annually, a huge loss. Viewed from the payer's perspective, rehabilitation produces a gain of $50,000 to $60,000 for each patient freed from the bondage of the nursing home, a huge gain.

The patients' families could use that money to care for their relative at home. Some of the money freed by rehabilitation might be directed to research on the prevention of illnesses or be given to deserving social programs for the less fortunate in our society.

Corporate Programs

I believe in the theory of trickle down behavior. It works in families and I believe it works in the business environment, too. If we can teach the managers of large corporations the principles and practices of health and wellness, and if we motivate them to exhibit those behaviors, then we will have "in house" role models for the employees of the corporation.

I propose the presentation of weeklong health and wellness seminars to the management of corporations. Every two weeks after the seminar, for the next two months, we will meet as a group for one morning. That meeting will be to discuss problems, to present new ideas, and to reinforce the behavior changes of the managers in our group. After two months, the frequency of the reinforcement meetings will fall to once monthly. These meeting will continue for two years and may eventually be run by the members of the group. The long-term design of the group becomes a self-sustaining reinforcement vehicle.

Each week a new group of managers will be invited to participate in the weeklong seminar and then to join in the long term group sessions. The seminar groups will be purposely kept small to guarantee individual attention. The principles presented in the sessions will be those of *Get a Life!* We will expand on some of the ideas and ensure that each individual understands how to implement the principles into his life. Dialogue, one of the most effective teaching tools, will ensue, creating a lively discussion environment.

The evolution from recipient to participant, from student to manager, from seminar to self-sustaining group, decreases the potential for recidivism. The group learns a process, takes control, and teaches others.

Central Health and Wellness Facility

My dream for twenty years has been to create a central health and wellness facility, a fun place to teach people how to *Get a Life!* I am getting closer, in large part because I have committed my ideas to paper. Nothing could please me more in a professional sense than to be able to teach, demonstrate, and live the principles of health and wellness at a common location.

"Health spas," plush, pompous and plentiful, equate to nothing more than an expensive two week back rub. Few, if any, plan to obviate recidivism. Most deal with the recidivism problem by encouraging revisits to their facility. Why not? The spa makes more money on each revisit. Why should they teach long term success when they make money on revisits?

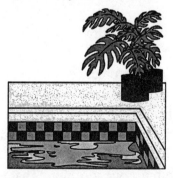

I want an education center to teach for present and lasting successes. Interestingly, Gerald Celente, writing in his book, *Trends 2000,* foresees the regular development of "universities" that will teach an aging population how to achieve and maintain health. That's us, folks. We will provide an inside look at behavior modification. We will require that individuals take responsibility for the management of their lives. Only through an individual's understanding the process of change and his perceiving that he is in control of his life, may he avoid the quicksand trap of recidivism. Continued support of his behavior change and of his practicing the behavior integrates to avert failure. We will provide that support and encourage his practicing his new behavior.

Our support systems will include follow-up phone calls, mailed questionnaires, as well as teaching the participants how to organize their own support teams when away from the "mother facility." Our focus on avoiding recidivism, along with a genuine commitment to teaching will differentiate our facility from the run-of-the-mill spa.

The concept of health and wellness is not new. In fact, the movement is well entrenched. How wonderful, because a lot of people are already involved and more are becoming involved daily. I envision our central facility as a meeting place where the researchers in our field to gather to share information.

Certainly, always a topic of discussion, the choice, development, and nurturing of attitudes and expectations challenges our dialogue. I eagerly anticipate a round table discussion of this subject with enthusiastic minds.

Campaign to Change Societal Attitudes and Expectations

How do we accomplish the task of changing societal attitudes and expectations about healthy living? How do we change the attitude from the "let it break, then fix it" perspective to the "let's take care of what we have been given" view. The same process of behavior modification functions as well on a societal level as on an individual level. We can use **catalysts** to speed up the process just as we did for the individual.

Without the conscious and conspicuous introduction of catalysts, I fear that we would never live long enough to witness societal change to healthier behaviors. We cannot afford to wait for evolutionary motivation to change, the threat of extinction, or a societal collective perception of pain, lest we become dinosaurs in the tar pits.

How do we use catalysts to initiate awareness of the necessity to change? Let's do what corporations do, **choose a spokesperson.** Who would be a good spokesperson for our message that "health and wellness is good and desirable?" I speak for our cause. Through my writing, speaking, teaching, and practicing wellness principles, I do influence the people that I am able to reach.

We need more than just me. Any individual who chooses to become involved in the process will affect those around him in a positive manner, more by what he does than what he might say. I have always known that I have a positive effect on people that I meet, and in retrospect, that aspect of my personality was an important factor in my choice of a career in medicine. Again, pivotal in my choice to teach about health and wellness, I don't have a monopoly on this trait. It avails to anyone. We may all choose to have positive, supportive effects on those around us. I suggest that we start by choice as catalytic individuals and develop a legion of catalytic personalities.

Healthy Role Model Program

This is huge! I propose that we seek prominent people to be **role models** as well as spokespersons. Approach them and coach them for this specific purpose. Charge them to exhibit how they lead their healthy lives. Ask them to teach us good behavior by example. Show us the successes that good healthy behaviors produce. Target prominent people with high visibility profiles, people we know and think we can trust.

January 1998 witnessed the inauguration of Surgeon General David Satcher, MD. When questioned about his vision for the future of the health of the United States, he thought for a moment and calmly responded, "I'm well known for my dedication to education about nutrition and exercise. That will be a priority. And I want all members of the public health corps to serve as role models for healthy living."

Donna Shalala, Secretary of Health Education and Welfare, has written extensively about the importance of role modeling healthy behaviors. I admire their dedication to the principle of role modeling healthy behaviors, but talk is getting cheap. It's time to start the ball rolling and create healthy role model programs across the country.

Select visible persons in the federal, state, and local government. In enlisting individual senators, governors, and representatives of our choice, we could entice these "soldiers" to join our cause by explaining that their adoption of a healthy lifestyle will not only benefit their personal health, but also the health of their campaign for reelection. Include prominent members of service organizations and professions, as well as educators and clergy. Believing in the trickle down theory of behavior, we have the power to initiate the process of changing public attitudes by placing selected people in public view to demonstrate what we want the public to emulate.

Some seemingly obvious choices carry a downside. Bill Bradley, United States senator from New Jersey, former athlete with Princeton University and the New York Knicks, and Rhodes scholar, could be a leading spokesperson for health. Sadly, he immersed himself in his career, became sedentary, and grew fat. There's still hope for Mr. Bradley, though. He retired from the Senate to pursue writing, teaching, and public service television. Now, as a presidential contender, the service mentality exists for his participation in our movement.

Bill Clinton sits in the most public position in our country, with a great opportunity for setting an example of a healthy lifestyle. Is he a good example when he jogs publicly with his too-short-shorts accentuating poorly toned thighs? No, certainly not. Then, adding insult to injury, he retires to his favorite cheeseburger haunt. He would send a better message if he wore a conservative sweat outfit, walked on a regular basis, ate fruit, and lost weight.

Bill Clinton, the consummate political animal, able to recover from political and personal jeopardy by putting a positive spin on his circumstances, can do the same with his health. He could announce that he will lose 30 pounds in 30 weeks, will begin a routine walking program, will adopt a 65 / 20 / 15 diet, and will practice assertive communication with the public. Well, three out of four isn't bad.

Police, from chiefs to patrolmen, school principals, firemen, ministers, and local businessmen could all serve as positive role models, stimulating awareness of healthy behaviors. How do we enlist their services? Go through the front door and ask them.

I have often considered the military as a potential peacetime resource for a multitude of tasks. Why couldn't we put them to use building and rebuilding the infrastructure of our country? Why can't we enlist their help as role models for health? Fit, alert and capable, the military integrates well into our society as good role models. Our invitation would give them a greater sense of purpose, especially in peacetime.

Let's seek senior citizens who exemplify healthy lifestyles and herald their successes. Willard Scott might look for octogenarians and nonagenarians who lead active lives and showcase them to the public, rather than focus on someone who just happened to have the genes and luck to make 100.

Spokespersons and role models for our cause sit ready at the wait, willing and able to contribute. What other advantages avail our drive to modify social attitudes and expectations?

Let's "Go Hollywood"

The Surgeon General's report on the adverse effects of smoking appeared first in 1969. Surprise, surprise, "Smoking is bad for us!" During World War II cigarettes were standard issue for our fighting men. Were we so ignorant in 1942 and enlightened by 1969? I don't think so. Between 1942 and 1969 and the ten years thereafter, little changed in our smoking behavior. Only when Hollywood began to portray smoking as socially unacceptable, through film messages and through the individual behavior of actors, did smoking behavior in the United States began to decline. I offer to you that **Hollywood** and **the media** hold powerful influence over society. Combined, Hollywood and the media may be the strongest, most influential body for initiating behavior change in a short period of time.

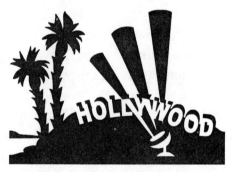

Let's ask them to help us in our quest to promote better social attitudes, expectations and practices for good health. I do not propose making a movie about Valerie Vegetarian. Rather I ask that they consciously plant some characters in movies, and portray them as healthy people who eat well and exercise regularly. A healthy lifestyle, not the main theme of the movie, is just how that particular character lives. He could be some high powered lawyer-type who practices meditation, exercises regularly by schedule for 45 minutes, eats a low-fat diet, and still competes as a complete corporate rat. Subliminal themes of healthy lifestyles could be woven throughout exciting story lines.

The timing for sending a message of health and wellness is now. As a society, we are primed and receptive for a message of healthier attitudes and visions, but as yet, we lack the motivation and knowledge to proceed of our own free will. Until we realize that we have the freedom of choice, we shall remain passive and malleable little lab rats, susceptible to Hollywood's influencing our opinions and thinking. I want all of us to realize that we do have free choice, but until we do realize that fact, let's use whatever means we can to change our collective consciousness.

Our heroes, actors and actresses could be living, demonstrative examples of health, a "this is how it's done" approach. Then we as the public, having near obligatory tendencies to copy, play "monkey see, monkey do," and emulate their philosophy, thinking, attitudes, and behavior.

Hollywood has taken our vision of the "ideal" woman from Marilyn Monroe and Jayne Mansfield, through Bridget Bardot, Twiggy and Kate Moss, to Julia Roberts, Sally Field and Jody Foster. I like the current trend, pretty women with brains and a sense of humor. The leading men presented to us have evolved from the cigarette puffing Edward G. Robinson and Humphrey Bogart, through cerebrally vacuous pretty boys like Rock Hudson, to elite testosterone-laden athletes, like A-a-a-a-nold, and finally to their present offerings of Tom Cruise, Tom Hanks and Robin Williams. Again, I like the present, men with intelligence, humor, and humility.

The current icons of Hollywood seem to have developed a decent and compassionate world-view, the world-view being a prerequisite for their contributing to society. Would these present actors, actresses, directors and producers help our cause?

I would love to have Paul Newman's support. He has surely passed the test of time in so many respects; health, charity, acting, marriage, and racecar driving. Such a credible spokesperson and role model, if only I could enlist his aid to utter some words in the direction of the collective health of the nation.

Hollywood constitutes a major part of our national media, but not the only part. Radio and television news and sports coverage offer fertile fields for health promotion. Anyone whose voice travels across the airwaves has the opportunity to offer ideas, philosophy and support for health and wellness.

Who Else?

I don't want preaching as much as the offering of living examples of healthy changes. Don Imus smoked. He suffered a collapsed lung from emphysema and subsequently was operated upon to remove part of his lung. He did quit smoking (I think, I hope), and he chronicled the whole event on the radio, even broadcasting from his hospital bed via the phone. If public sharing of his experience influenced just one person to stop smoking, I applaud Imus for his efforts. Don Imus did not preach about the evils of smoking, he lived them for us. Don is among the legion of people who choose to have a positive effect on the people around us.

Prominent television and radio personalities can all participate. Oprah did by losing weight. Rush Limbaugh also did, by losing weight. Regis Philbin participated by having coronary by-pass surgery and then sharing his experience with us. Dan Rather participates by sharing his sense of humor on *Late Night* with David Letterman. Humor, essential to survival in a stressful world, deserves broad venue.

Did Walter Cronkite ever smile or laugh? He must have to survive so well, but he must have done it off camera. When he was delivering the news, a sense of humor wasn't in style. Walter Cronkite, now in his retirement years, narrates some wonderful public information television. I would love to encourage him to join our crusade for good health. Wow, just think of it, Walter Cronkite, perhaps the most believable person in television history, sending a message of health.

What about sports figures? Public icons, could they spread the message? Unfortunately, they excel at sending messages of greed, selfishness, and drug use. In spite of the plethora of negative press that athletes earn, some individual sports heroes have maintained a position of credibility, and do send powerful messages. I like the message that the Professional Golf Association sends, that of individual responsibility and charity.

What could be better? Gary Player, Jack Nicklaus, and Arnold Palmer have all recently acknowledged the importance of attitude and physical training in prolonging their participation in a sport and profession they love. Gary Player and

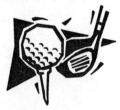

Jack Nicklaus, in particular, speak of their ability to modify and select better attitudes that help their performance. How do they accomplish the task of choosing better attitudes? Their conscious choice and subsequent practicing cements their attitude over time. These delightful gentlemen, ambassadors of the great game of golf, may serve as ambassadors of healthy lifestyles.

You already know that I aspire to ambassadorship. I have already seized the opportunity to present our message via the media. Host and creator of the *Get a Life!* radio show in Phoenix, I present educational shows about prevention and I solicit guests with related messages. In the near future, I will host a television show dedicated to health and wellness. Just as with *Get a Life!* the radio show, I will use the medium as a didactic teaching forum and as a forum for dialogue. Guests will be selected to exemplify lifestyle change successes. Guests from the health and wellness profession will keep us abreast of research breakthroughs and of alternative ideas for achieving wellness. As we present the best current available information on health and wellness, our visible presence will reinforce the public evolution towards our goal of a healthy population.

Nationwide Marketing Campaign for Health and Wellness

Why should we have a marketing campaign? What are we marketing? We market an idea, a philosophy, an improved and healthier lifestyle, better life, longer life, increased productivity in the workplace and at home, greater individual incomes, and increased corporate incomes. Consequently, we sell lower health (sick) care costs to the country, to individuals, to corporations, and to the government.

I do not envision our marketing as a blitz of television advertisements, but as a publicly demonstrative, hands-on approach to health and wellness. **Providing work site health promotion facilities, with the time and directions to use them,** leads our campaign. Many corporations have already provided the hardware, but have neglected the teaching portion. Expeditiously, we will change that error. We will lead our horses to water and help them drink.

We must offer dynamic, didactic, continuing, **health and wellness teaching programs** for employees. In doing so we provide education and support during the health and wellness evolution of the individual employee.

We mandate **routine rewards.** Corporations should offer financial rewards for maintaining good health and job attendance. Recording trends of certain parameters like non-usage of health insurance, work attendance, stability of body composition, aerobic performance capacity, and strength maintenance over time may monitor good health. Financial rewards, good motivators in business, may be granted to those employees who meet the healthy trend parameters.

327

It would be wrong to think we could mete out some penalty for poor performance in health. Not my philosophy or direction, negative and judgmental messages fail. We wish only to reward the positive, for rewarding the positive emerges as a much stronger conditioner of behavior than punishing the negative. Everyone can make improvements, and I am here to lead the cheers for their successes.

Aside from the demonstrative marketing of employee wellness programs, I suggest that we seek out businesses and organizations that could give us some free advertising. Perhaps we could join forces with them and "scratch each others' backs."

Companies with health related products to sell, already in the marketing fray, unfortunately, focus more on selling products than on developing healthy lifestyles for their employees. I do understand the profit motive, and I think that we might be able to blend our message with their products. I do not propose that we sell products. We will use their products as a vehicle for our message. We must exercise excellent judgment in choosing products to which we can attach our message. Our credibility is our lifeline. We can not allow it to be severed.

Fortuitously positioned as windfall winners from an improvement in society's health, insurance companies eagerly anticipate our success. Since their business pays for ill health, the less they pay out for illness, the greater their profits. Would it make sense to assume that insurance companies will reduce premiums if illness and usage of sick care facilities decline? A precarious assumption, but I predict that they will reduce premiums. The percentage reduction in premiums may not equal the percentage drop in sick care payments, but that's OK. I accept their increased profit margin in exchange for their playing an integral role in our marketing campaign for *Getting a Life, America!*

Who spends the most money on advertising, by far, of any "business" in this country? The answer – the United States military, Army, Navy, Marines, Air Force and Coast Guard, outspends on television, radio and printed advertisements any other business in this country. Would they consider sending healthy messages in their advertising time? Why not? They advertise education, career development and travel. Why not advertise good health? Perhaps their marketing minds haven't thought of it.

Perhaps charities haven't either. Although founded in principle to combat disease, charities like the American Heart Association, the American Cancer Society, the American Diabetes Association, the National Kidney Foundation, and the United Way might be cajoled into sending messages of health, messages quite a bit different than treating diseases. Isn't achieving and maintaining health as valuable as doing research on the causes of diseases and treating those diseases?

Create Societal Rewards

Aside from the marketing and sales efforts, we must think about rewarding good behavior and rewarding behavior modification by our society. The government writes freely and frequently about our failures to achieve health as a society. The fact that we are getting fatter not fitter is a theme common to epidemiological studies. Although factual, these studies simply toss failure in our faces. That negativity, counter-productive to our attempting to achieve better health, could with equal enthusiasm become positivity.

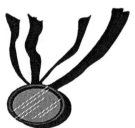

Reports that chronicle a decrease in cardiovascular disease encourage the public. We need more "atta-boys" from government agencies, educational research facilities, and from businesses, for even our small victories. What, after all, does a child seek from his parent, an employee from his employer, a population from their governors? It's praise. It goes a long, long way.

Physical and monetary rewards formulate part of our marketing plan, too. These rewards could take the form of a gift, bonus, or additional vacation time from businesses, or a tax credit from the IRS for good health. Just imagine, the IRS offering us a tax credit for good health.

Where Does the Money Come From and Who is Going to do the Work?

Having alluded to solutions about the funding of our project and how to provide the labor market for a rather large task at hand, I know that without financial support we fail. With it, we are free to pursue our stated goals. Making money is not our objective, improving health is. So, let's view finances as a tool to allow us to do our job, and let's use Sutton's Law to find the money. Willie Sutton, renowned bank robber, when captured and queried why he robbed banks, replied, "That's where the money is."

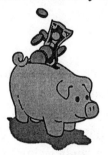 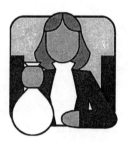

In a manner of speaking, let's rob a bank. Where are large pools of money that might be partially reapportioned in our direction? Who among those "pools" is likely to benefit financially from joining us?

❖ Large corporations who shoulder the lion's share of the burden for paying the obscene health care (sick care) costs of their employees would gladly contribute. Intuition suggests that a healthier work force will result in decreased sick care costs, freeing a large portion of that money pool for use elsewhere. Intuition is nice, but test market proof becomes a better sales tool. We accept the responsibility to provide the corporations with reasonable assurance of their economic advantage in contributing to our program.

❖ Corporate advertising budgets, necessarily gargantuan, provide an ocean of economic opportunity. With the competition among corporations to sell products, wouldn't it make sense for a corporation to create good public relations as part of their advertising campaign? From whom would you be most likely to purchase products, everything else being equal, Company A who has a reputation for social awareness, or Company B who is known to have none? I suggest that corporations "advertise" by making it known that they have joined in our effort to create a healthier society.

❖ Insurance companies, granite-solid financial institutions, may assist in creating a healthier population, while we assist them in achieving bigger profit margins. We ask only for some financial support.

❖ Charitable groups and organizations have loads of money. Good sense dictates the prevention of heart disease, cancer, diabetes, and renal disease. Wouldn't (shouldn't) any of these charities have interest in supporting a program directed at prevention? If I were their director, I certainly would.

❖ Individuals and small businesses pay significant insurance premiums. All tolled, the premiums represent a large dollar figure. We are unlikely to convince a large number of these individuals or small businesses to support our efforts financially, but perhaps a representative of this segment of society might be amenable to our campaign. Consider approaching the American Association of Retired Persons or the Independent Business Association with our ideas.

❖ I will always maintain that America has an entrepreneurial spirit and humanitarian philosophy. Enough money rests in private hands to support our entire effort. We will never get it unless we articulate a good message and ask for help.

Where do we select our labor force? For the school programs, we use the teachers already there, and many of the newly graduated health educators. Apply the Hermit Crab Concept of business; use what is already in place, as the hermit crab uses the shell of other crustaceans as his new dwelling. We will work with the schools and teachers to develop the curriculum based on a health and wellness philosophy.

In the adult education programs, we use teachers who might have retired, but who maintain interest in healthy lifestyles. With our principal thrust as education and behavior modification, we can enlist a cadre of teachers and train them at their locales, or better yet, at our central facility.

In the final analysis, I propose the creation of a multipurpose facility and then future satellite facilities for the teaching and support of healthy behaviors. How do we start? Where do we start? I am starting by thinking, reading, and writing. I have progressed to speaking to groups about the problems and proposed solutions. I cannot and do not plan to be alone in this effort. I need and solicit your help and ideas. Write to me at:

Leonard R. Mees
c/o Sabec Publishing Company
P.O. Box 82545
Portland, OR 97282-0545

Divided we Fall – Together we Win

How do we follow to provide ongoing support? The establishment and continuation of teaching programs creates a support network. The progressive involvement of large numbers of people continually adds to our foundation. A central "mother" facility will supply additional nurturing functions. New ideas, generated from increased numbers of people becoming involved in the program, serve to cement divergent concepts in a cohesive unit.

We've been working on creating healthier lifestyles for the last quarter century, at least. At best we're only started. But it's a great start. Join us. Give me your ideas, or write to the Surgeon General with your suggestions.

The seeds of the philosophy of national health and wellness have been planted. With nurturing support and patient practice of healthy behaviors we may harvest untold bounty. Together, we all may *Get a Life, America!*

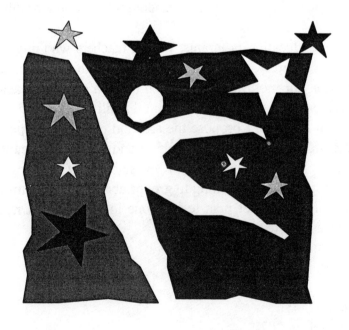

Appendix

Aerobic Fitness Tests

1) How Active Have You Been Lately Test

Perceived activity level	Fitness level
Working hard every day to point of profuse sweating	High
Active; play tennis and golf three times weekly	Medium
Sedentary; go to work then home to watch television	Low

2) <u>Walk a Mile as Fast as You Can Test</u>

Measure a mile on a car odometer or use a treadmill with distance readout. Walk the mile as fast as you can, then calculate your fitness level according to the chart.

<u>Time (minutes and seconds)</u>

	<u>Men</u>	<u>Women</u>
<u>Excellent</u>	under 10:15	under 11:30
<u>Good</u>	10:16 – 12:00	11:31 – 13:30
<u>Average</u>	12:00 – 14:40	13:31 – 16:00
<u>Fair to poor</u>	14:41 – 16:30 (or more)	16:01 – 17:40 (or more)

Burn Out Inventory

Review your past six months. Have you noticed changes in yourself or in the world around you? Consider the office, your family and your social world. Allow about thirty seconds for each question, then give your best answer. Assign a number from 1 (for little to no change) to 5 (for a great deal of change) to indicate the degree of change you perceive.

_____1. Do you tire more easily? Are you fatigued rather than energetic?

_____2. Do people annoy you by telling you that you don't look so good?

_____3. Are you working harder and harder and accomplishing less?

_____4. Are you increasingly cynical and disenchanted?

_____5. Are you often invaded by a sadness that you can't explain?

_____6. Are you becoming forgetful? (appointments and personal items)

_____7. Are you becoming increasingly irritable? Are you more short-tempered? Are you disappointed in the people around you?

_____8. Are you seeing close friends and family members less frequently?

_____9. Are you too busy to do even routine things like make phone calls?

_____10. Are you suffering from physical complaints? (aches, pains, frequent colds)

_____11. Do you feel disoriented when the activity of the day ends?

_____12. Is joy elusive?

_____13. Are you able to laugh at a joke about yourself?

_____14. Does sex seem like more trouble than it is worth?

_____15. Do you have very little to say to people?

Burnout Inventory Key

0 - 25	Doing fine
26 - 35	There are things that you should be watching
36 - 50	You are a candidate for burnout
51 - 65	You are burning out
65 and up	You are in a dangerous situation which places you in severe jeopardy of physical and/or emotional illness

Emotional Inventory

The following is a list of words that may or may not apply to how we feel. Proceed through the list and place a check by the words that apply to you. Then take the words that you have checked and place them in either of two columns, positive or negative. Count the number of words in each column and compare the positives and the negatives.

agitated	dislike	hostile	pleasure	vulnerable
aggravated	dismal	hysterical	pride	warm
aggressive	disappointed	impulsive	rage	weary
alienated	disconcerted	inadequate	rapturous	
alone	disgust	inconclusive	rejection	
alarmed	dreary	inertia	regrets	
altruistic	dawn	indecisive	remorse	
anger	elated	inferior	resentment	
anxious	envy	irascible	sad	
assertive	euphoric	irritated	satisfaction	
antagonized	excited	jealousy	self pity	
aroused	exhausted	jovial	sensitive	
animosity	faith	joy	shame	
bewildered	flat	jubilance	sorrow	
bitter	flight	kindness	suspicious	
bored	fright	lonesome	sympathy	
blue	frustrated	low	tense	
comfort	frivolous	melancholy	terror	
confused	grief	manic	threatened	
cheerful	growling	morbid	turned off	
dazed	grouchy	nervous	turned on	
defensive	guilt	overwrought	unselfish	
dejection	happy	panic	withdrawn	
delight	hate	passive	wavering	
depression	hopeless	perplexed	worthless	
despair	horror	playful	worry	

Determining Your Nutritional Health

Read the statements below. Circle the number in the yes column for those that apply to you. For each yes answer, score the number in the yes column. Total your nutrition score.

	YES
I have an illness or condition that made me change the kind and/or amount of food I eat.	____2____
I eat fewer than two meals per day.	____3____
I eat few fruits or vegetables, or dairy product	____2____
I have 3 or more drinks of beer, liquor or wine almost daily	____2____
I have a mouth problem that makes it hard for me to eat.	____2____
I don't always have enough money to buy the food I need.	____4____
I eat alone most of the time	____1____
I take 3 or more different prescribed or over-the counter drugs a day.	____1____
I have lost or gained 10 pounds in the past 6 months, without trying.	____2____
I am not always physically able to shop, cook and/or feed myself.	____2____
TOTAL	_____

Total Your Nutrition Score. If it is:

0 – 2	Quite good. Recheck in 6 months.
3 – 5	You are at moderate nutritional risk.
6 or more	You are at high nutritional risk.

Healthy Nutrition Score

Here is another screening test with a different twist. Answer each question to the best of your ability and memory. Then add all of the points for your total score.

	1	**2**	**3**	**4**
Type of fat or spread I use at the table	Butter	Stick Margarine	Soft Margarine	None
Type of fat I usually use in cooking	Butter Lard	Shortening	Vegetable oil	Corn, Safflower oil
Total number of eggs used in a week	More than 6	4 - 6	3 - 4	2or less
Kind of milk drank or used on cereal	Don't use milk	Whole or Low-fat (2%)	Low-fat (1%)	Skim (1/2%)
Number of times each week I eat cheese	More than	Once daily once a day	4 - 6 times a week	3 times or less
Number of times each week I eat meat	More than once a day	Once daily	4 - 6 times a week	3 times or less
Number of times each week I eat fish or poultry	Don't eat it	Once	2 - 3 times	4 times or more
Method I add salt to food or cooking	Always add	Cooking & at table	Cooking only	None

Number of times each week I eat salted snacks	Daily	3 - 6 times	2 times	Once or less
Number of times each week I use convenience foods	Daily	3 - 6 times	2 times	Once or less
Number of servings each day of fruits and vegetables	None	1 - 2	2	4 or more
Number of servings each day of grains or starches	One or less	2	3	4 or more

Scoring:

12 – 20	Risky!
21 – 30	Could be better
31 – 40	You're trying, decent
41 – 48	Superb!

Anger-In Personality Screening Test

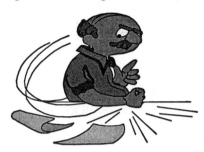

Both men and women increase their risk of first heart attack, second heart attack, and sudden death by covering a seething anger with a placid exterior. Dr. Robert S. Eliot found an alarming risk of sudden death in "hot reactors" who were also "anger-in" personalities. Take this screening test to see if you qualify. Choose one response for each question.

1. A teenager speeds past with a radio blaring heavy-metal music.
   - A. I begin to understand why teenagers can't hear.
   - B. I shout after him.
   - C. I don't respond, but feel my fury rise.

2. Someone is speaking to me very slowly.
   - A. I listen and nod encouragement.
   - B. I finish his or her sentences.
   - C. I say nothing and get irritated.

3. I am stuck in a traffic jam.
   - A. I turn on the radio and daydream.
   - B. I switch lanes back and forth, trying to get an advantage.
   - C. I sit helplessly and fume.

4. A friend ridicules something I've done.
   - A. I ask him or her to help me improve.
   - B. I immediately criticize back.
   - C. I change the subject, pretending I didn't notice.

5. I'm fighting with my spouse or lover.
    A. I try to stay calm, helping us get through it.
    B. I raise my voice, stomp around, or throw a shoe.
    C. I'm so furious I say nothing and leave the house.

6. I recall a bitter family conflict.
    A. The memory feels like water under the bridge.
    B. I immediately call up someone in my family and revisit it.
    C. I am enraged again for hours.

7. Someone is hogging the conversation at a party.
    A. I move on to another group.
    B. I make a quip to let him know I think he's a jerk.
    C. I smile blandly, thinking how much I despise him.

Answer Key:

A. If you answered A four or more times, you do not anger easily. You are cool.

B. If you answered B four or more times, you rate high in aggression. This is only positive if it allows you to vent frustration without hurting others. Usually, others become victim to your fallout, and in the long run you will alienate those around you.

C. If you answered C four or more times, you rate high in hidden anger. You place yourself at high risk for heart disease and sudden death. Take your score as a suggestion that you find assertive methods for venting you anger. Even in situations where control eludes your grasp, search for some way to release your anger with grace. Try humor, try understanding, try forgiveness.

Test Your Job Stress

As you read the descriptions of stressful job conditions listed on the left-hand side of the test, think back over the past month. Decide how much each factor has been a source of stress to you and assign it a number; 3 for severe, 2 for moderate, 1 for little and 0 for none. When you have finished, add each column and then total the columns. Check your results with the descriptions at the end.

	severe (3)	moderate (2)	little (1)	none (0)
Too many tasks or responsibilities	_____	_____	___	___
Workplace bleak, uncomfortable, Depressing	_____	_____	___	___
Physically difficult or hazardous. work conditions	_____	_____	___	___
Conflicting or competing Demands	_____	_____	___	___
Boring or repetitive tasks	_____	_____	___	___
No opportunity for advancement	_____	_____	___	___
No room for creativity or personal Input	_____	_____	___	___
Long hours or too many days without break	_____	_____	___	___
No input to decision affecting my work	_____	_____	___	___
Difficult commute	_____	_____	___	___
Deadline pressures	_____	_____	___	___

Many organizational or task changes	_____	_____	_____	_____
Confused or unclear expectations about tasks	_____	_____	_____	_____
Too many people telling me what to do	_____	_____	_____	_____
Job insecurity due to cutbacks or Changes	_____	_____	_____	_____
Office politics	_____	_____	_____	_____
Don't like my job	_____	_____	_____	_____
Ethical problems with my work	_____	_____	_____	_____
Unrealized expectations from my job	_____	_____	_____	_____
Loss of commitment or dedication to work	_____	_____	_____	_____
Inadequate salary	_____	_____	_____	_____
Conflict with coworkers or Supervisor	_____	_____	_____	_____
Job doesn't use skills or abilities	_____	_____	_____	_____
Inadequate resources to get job done	_____	_____	_____	_____
Things are changing too fast	_____	_____	_____	_____
TOTAL	_____	_____	_____	_____
GRAND TOTAL		_____		

Scoring

1 – 12 Optimum Performance. I you score within this range, you cope well with your job. You have allowed room for additional stressors should they occur.

12 – 25 Steady Performance. Indicative of effective performance in most situations. Job stress hasn't yet pierced your armor.

25 – 40 Strain. You experience frequent difficulty and sense of feeling overwhelmed or drained. Try to lessen the stressors of your life and job before you melt down.

Above 40 Breakdown. You experience severe difficulty, impaired functioning, and extreme distress. Stress on the job takes its toll on your mind and body. If allowed to continue, the stress damage could become permanent (e.g. heart attack). You must make changes.

Glossary

Accommodation – the body's process of changing; those changes required to adapt to a new environment.

Adenosine triphosphate (ATP) – high energy compound produced by the metabolism of carbohydrate and fat, used as energy supply for muscles; energy currency

Aerobic – in the presence of oxygen

Amino acid – the building blocks of proteins, 22 in number; 13 non-essential (made by the body), 9 essential (available only through diet).

Anaerobic – in the absence of oxygen

Anaerobic threshold – the exercise intensity above which lactic acid begins to accumulate in the blood; all energy production above this threshold produced anaerobically.

Antioxidants – compounds that neutralize free radicals

Atherosclerosis – narrowing of the arteries by cholesterol build-up

Behavior modification – the process by which we learn new behavior skills

Body mass index (BMI) – an expression of body size standardized for individuals' variations in height; bears close correlation with percentage body fat

Calorie – a unit of heat energy; used to measure energy available in foods and energy used in exercise.

Catalytic behavior – any behavior that potentiates the development of another behavior.

Carbohydrate – Simple (e.g., sugar) and complex (e.g., potatoes, rice, beans and corn) that the body uses for energy; stored in the liver and muscles as glycogen; excess stored as fat

Carcinogenesis – the tendency to cause cancer

Cholesterol – essential fatty substance found in nerves and other tissues; excess amounts or unusual kinds associated with atherosclerosis

Cholesterol profile – a measurement of total cholesterol, HDL, LDL, and triglycerides

Conditioned response – a learned automatic behavior

Depression – profound emotional disturbance with fatigue and decreased affect; Winston Churchill's "black dog"

Dissonance – a sense of psychological unsettledness; an emotional itch you can't scratch

Enzyme – a catalyst (facilitator) to a biochemical reaction

Fast twitch muscle fiber – muscle fibers that contract quickly; energy produced by anaerobic metabolism

Fat (lipid) – essential energy source, stored for future use when excess calories are ingested; the primary fuel for aerobic energy production.

Fat-soluble vitamins – vitamins A, D, E, K

Fitness – the combination of strength, aerobic endurance and flexibility

FIT Principle – the formula for successful aerobic training; a combination of Frequency, Intensity and Time

Flexibility – the range of motion through which the body part can move.

Free radical – electrically charged, potentially damaging molecules, products of various metabolic and environmental processes

Generational compulsion to repeat – the mindless repetition of behaviors from generation to generation

Get a Life, America! – a metaphor for making healthy lifestyle changes, for achieving health, happiness and love.

Glucose – a molecule of six carbons, the energy source circulating in the blood.

Glycogen – the storage form of carbohydrate

High density lipoprotein (HDL) – a carrier molecule that takes cholesterol from sites of deposition to the liver for metabolism; inversely related to heart disease, it's the good kind of cholesterol.

Homeostasis – the natural tendency to maintain the emotional and physical body in a functional state of balance

Jacks or Better – that's what you have to have to open in poker; it's a metaphor for having some ability to play the game of life.

Lactic acid – a by-product of glycogen metabolism; high levels in muscle inhibit muscle contraction and inhibit enzyme activity.

Legumes – vegetables that come in a pod; e.g., peas, lentils, beans

Lipoprotein – a combination of fat and protein designed to carry fat through a watery medium

Lipoprotein lipase – an enzyme that regulates the rate of fat deposition in fat cells.

Low density lipoprotein (LDL) – the fraction of the cholesterol that attaches to arterial walls, causes narrowing of the artery; the bad kind of cholesterol

Metabolism – energy production and utilization process

Mitochondria – tiny sub-cellular structures; the site of aerobic energy production

Motor unit – motor nerve and the muscle fibers it feeds

Muscle fiber types – fast twitch are fast to contract, but fatigue quickly; slow twitch contract more slowly, but are fatigue-resistant.

Nutrition – provision of adequate energy in the form of calories, as well as needed amounts of fat, carbohydrate, protein, vitamins, minerals, and water.

Obesity – excess body fat.

Potentiate – to assist or make an event more likely or easier

Protein – organic compound formed of amino acids; makes us muscle, hormones and enzymes.

Recidivism – failure to maintain an intended behavior change.

Recommended dietary allowances (RDA) – the minimum daily amount of a vitamin needed to prevent deficiency disease plus 20%

Resting metabolic rate – expresses energy required for breathing, heart activity and general cell functioning.

Saturated fat – a fat maximally "saturated" with hydrogen (hence also called "hydrogenated"); usually solid at room temperature; stimulates the liver to produce cholesterol

Slow twitch muscle fiber – muscle fibers that contract more slowly, but are resistant to fatigue; energy provided primarily by aerobic metabolism.

Strength – ability of a muscle to exert force

Synergy – two processes combining to form a whole greater than the sum of the parts

Thermic effect of food – energy used by the body to process food

Thermic effect of physical activity – energy used in activity

Training stimulus – the type of exercise that elicits the desired adaptation to training

Training zone – the heart rate zone within which training is likely to produce the desired effect.

Warm-up – a pre-exercise activity designed to increase muscle temperature.

Water-soluble vitamins – all B vitamins and vitamin C

Weight training – progressive resistance exercise using weight for resistance.

References

General:

Allen, R.G. (1983). *Creating Wealth.* New York: Simon and Schuster.

American Heart Association. (1984). *American Heart Association Cookbook.* New York: David Mac Kay Company, Inc.

Benson, H. (1975). *The Relaxation Response.* New York: Harper and Row.

Blair, S. and Kohl, H. (1988). Physical activity or physical fitness: Which is more important? *Medicine and Science in Sports and Exercise.* 20, 58.

Borg, G.V. (1982). The Borg Scale for rate of perceived exertion. *Medicine and Science in Sports and Exercise.* 14, 377-387.

Brown, B.B. (1981). *Stress and the Art of Biofeedback.* New York: Bantam.

Califano, J.A. (1994). *Radical Surgery.* New York: Random House.

Carper J. (1988). *The Food Pharmacy.* New York: Bantam.

Centers for Disease Control. (1978). Protective effect of physical activity on coronary heart disease. *MMWR.* 36, 426-430.

Chopra, D. (1993). *Ageless Body, Timeless Mind.* New York: Crown Publishers, Inc.

Clark, N. (1990). *Sports Nutrition Guidebook.* Champaign, IL: Leisure Press.

Cooper, K.H. (1981). *The New Aerobics.* New York: Bantam.

Cooper, K.H. (1988). *Controlling Cholesterol.* New York: Bantam.

Cousins, N. (1976). *Anatomy of an Illness as Perceived by the Patient: Reflections on Healing and Regeneration.* New York: E.P. Dutton.

Cousins, N. (1989). *Head First, the Biology of Hope.* New York: E.P. Dutton.

Eliot, R.S. (1986). *Is It Worth Dying For?* New York: Bantam.

Eliot, R.S. (1988). *Stress and the Heart, Mechanisms, Measurements, Management.* Mount Kisco, New York: Futura Publishing.

Gershoff, S. (1990). *The Tufts University Guide to Total Nutrition.* New York: Harper Perennial.

Hanan, M. (1990). *Consultative Selling.* New York: ANACOM.

Hilfiker, D. (1985). *Healing the Wounds.* New York: Pantheon Books.

Kabat-Zinn, J. (1990). *Full Catastrophe Living.* New York: Dell.

Kramer, P.D. (1993). *Listening to Prozac.* New York: Viking.

Kramsch, D.M., Aspen, A. J., Abramowitz, B.M., et al. (1981). Reduction of coronary artery atherosclerosis by moderate conditioning exercise in monkeys on an atherogenic diet. *New England Journal of Medicine.* 305, 1483-1489.

Laurence, L. and Weinhouse, B. (1994). *Outrageous Practices.* New York: Fawcett Columbine.

Mc Dougall, J.A. (1985). *Mc Dougall's Medicine, A Challenging Second Opinion.* Clinton, New Jersey: New Win Publishing.

Mendelsohn, R.S. (1979). *Confessions of a Medical Heretic.* Chicago: Contemporary Books.

Moloney, K. and the Staff at Canyon Ranch. (1989). *The Canyon Ranch Health and Fitness Program.* New York: Simon and Schuster.

Murray, R.K., Granner, Daryl K., Mayes, Peter A., Rodwell, Victor W. (1993). *Harper's Biochemistry.* Norwalk, Connecticut: Appleton and Lange.

Ornish, D. (1982). *Stress Diet and Your Heart.* New York: Holt, Rinehart and Winston.

Ornish, D. (1990). *Dr. Dean Ornish's Program for Reversing Heart Disease.* New York: Ballantine.

Ornish, D. (1993). *Eat More, Weigh Less.* New York: Harper Collins.

Paffenbarger, R. S. (1978). Physical activity as an index of heart disease risk in college alumni. *American Journal of Epidemiology.* 108, 161-172.

Paffenbarger, R.S. and Hale, W.E. (1975). Work activity and coronary heart mortality. *The New England Journal of Medicine.* 292, 455-464.

Paffenbarger, R.S., Hyde, R. and Wing, A. (1986). Physical activity, all-cause mortality, and longevity of college alumni. *The New England Journal of Medicine.* 314, 605-613.

Paul, S.P. (1991). *Illuminations: Visions for Change, Growth and Self-Acceptance.* San Francisco: Harper.

Piscatella, J.C. (1987). *Don't Eat Your Heart Out.* New York: Workman Publishing.

Pritikin, N. (1984). *The Pritikin Program for Diet and Exercise.* New York: Bantam.

Raichlen, S. (1995). *Steven Raichlen's High Flavor, Low Fat Vegetarian Cooking.* New York: Viking.

Reader's Digest. (1988). *Great Recipes for Good Health.* Pleasantville, New York: The Reader's Digest Association, Inc.

Selye, H. (1978). *The Stress of Life.* New York: Mc Graw Hill.

Sharkey, B.J. (1990). *Physiology of Fitness, 3rd. Ed.* Champaign IL: Human Kinetics Books.

Skinner, B.F. (1983). *Enjoy Old Age.* New York: Warner.

Sorenson, M. (1993). *Mega Health.* Ivins, Utah: National Institute of Fitness.

University of California at Berkeley, Wellness Letter. (1993). *The Wellness Lowfat Cookbook.* New York: Rebus.

University of California, Berkeley, Wellness Letter. (1991). *The Wellness Encyclopedia.* Boston: Houghton Mifflin.

Weil, A. (1995). *Spontaneous Healing.* New York: Alfred A. Knopf.

White, T.P. (1993). *The Wellness Guide to Lifelong Fitness.* New York, Random House.

Nutrition:

Behan, E. (1986). Pasta perfect. *American Health.* 6/86, 101-104.

Clark, N. (1992). Power breakfasts. *Women's Sports and Fitness.* 1/92, 18-19.

Clark, N. (1995). Energy bars, are these fast fuelers for you? *The Physician and Sports Medicine.* Vol. 23, No. 9, 7-8.

Densford, L.E. (1985). Heart-healthy haute cuisine. *Rx Being Well.* 5/85, 29-35.

Dolnick, E. (1993). Beyond the French paradox. *Hippocrates.* 1/93, 62-71.

Green, H. (1990). In Northern California, a new cuisine is born. *Fine Dining, a Guide for Physicians.* 6/90, 3-9.

Hirsch, J. (1987). Taking charge. *Rx Being Well.* 5/87, 13-15.

Houze, P. (1986). Sun coolers. *American Health.* 7/86, 90-99.

Jacobi, D. (1994). Dressing up salad. *American Health.* 3/94, 100-102.

Kleiner, S.M. (1995). Nutrition on the run. *The Physician and Sports Medicine.* Vol. 23, No. 2, 15-16.

Levy, F. (1983). Sumptuous summer desserts. *Bon Appetit.* 6/83, 66-78.

Long, P. (1990). Cholesterol city. *Hippocrates.* 9/90, 37-45.

Lynden, P. (1985). California cuisine. *American Health.* 9/85, 63-67.

Ness, J. (1986). The art of recipe modification. *Rx Being Well.* 5/86, 15-19.

Paulsen, E. (1986). Sweetness and light. *Rx Being Well.* 1/86, 22-29.

Ricketts, D. and Mc Quillan, S. (1994). Perfect pizza. *American Health.* 3/94, 83-88.

Schrambling, R. (1992). Into the lite. *Hippocrates.* 4/92, 49-53.

Schrambling, R. (1993). Ethnic light. *Hippocrates.* 9/93, 59-71.

Seligson, S.V. (1993). Diary of a demanding diner. *Hippocrates.* 6/93, 53-58.

Shockey, G. (1990). Near perfect pasta. *Women's Sports and Fitness.* 4/90, 20-22.

Webb, D. (1989). 39 Tips for top nutrition. *Working Mother.* 7/89, 66-68.

Weiner, L. (1990). Meal makeovers. *Working Mother.* 2/90, 102-115.

Zarrow, S. (1992). 12 Secrets of peak nutrition. *Men's Health.* 4/92, 72-73.

Exercise:

Barksdale, B., Estes, E.H. and Segal, M. S. (1991). Getting your patients to exercise. *Patient Care.* 12/91, 115-125.

Barry, H.C. and Rich, B.S.E. (1993). How exercise can benefit older patients. *The Physician and Sports Medicine.* Vol. 21, No. 2, 124-140.

Bartels, R.L. (1992). Weight training: How to lift and eat for strength and power. *The Physician and Sports Medicine.* Vol. 20, No. 3, 233-234.

Caldwell, F. (1985). City parks: Untapped resource for fitness. *The Physician and Sports Medicine.* Vol. 13, No. 7, 120-133.

Chambers, M.J. (1991). Exercise: A prescription for a good night's sleep? *The Physician and Sports Medicine.* Vol. 19, No. 8, 107-116.

Clark, N. (1991). How to gain weight healthfully. *The Physician and Sports Medicine.* Vol. 19, No. 9, 53-54.

Cooper, K.H. (1990). Prescribing exercise as a means of reducing coronary risk. *Illustrated Medicine.* Vol 5, No. 5, 1-15.

Couzens, G.S. (1992). Personal trainers: A formula for fitness? *The Physician and Sports Medicine.* Vol. 20, No. 11, 130-140.

Coyle, E.F. and Coyle, E. (1993). Carbohydrates that speed recovery from training. *The Physician and Sports Medicine.* Vol. 21, No. 2, 111-123.

Fletcher, G.F. (1993) The value of exercise in preventing coronary atherosclerotic heart disease. *Heart Disease and Stroke.* 5/93, 183-188.

Frontera, W.R. and Adams, R.P. (1986). Endurance exercise: Normal physiology and limitations imposed by pathological processes. *The Physician and Sports Medicine.* Vol. 14, No. 9, 108-121.

Gauthier, M.M. (1986). Can exercise reduce the risk of cancer? *The Physician and Sports Medicine.* Vol. 14, No. 10, 170-178.

Gibson, S.B., Gerberich, S.G. and Leon, A.S. (1983). Writing the exercise prescription: An individualized approach. *The Physician and Sports Medicine.* Vol. 11, No. 7, 87-110.

Hoerr, S.M. (1987). Counseling obese adolescents. *The Physician and Sports Medicine.* Vol. 15, No. 7, 201-202.

Humphrey, D. (1988). Strength and endurance of the lower arm muscles. *The Physician and Sports Medicine.* Vol. 16, No. 12, 157-158.

Jones, T.F. and Eaton, C.B. (1995). Exercise prescription. *American Family Physician.* 8/95, 543-50.

Kasch, F.W., et. al. (1988). A longitudinal study of cardiovascular stability in active men aged 45 to 65 years. *The Physician and Sports Medicine.* Vol. 16, No. 1, 117-126.

Kasch, F.W., et. al. (1990). The effect of physical activity and inactivity on aerobic power in older men. *The Physician and Sports Medicine.* Vol. 18, No. 4, 73-83.

Kavanagh, T and Shepard, R.J. (1990). Can regular sports participation slow the aging process? Data on masters athletes. *The Physician and Sports Medicine.* Vol. 18, No. 6, 94-104.

Koszuta, L.E. (1987). Can fitness be found at the top of the stairs? *The Physician and Sports Medicine.* Vol. 15, No. 2, 165-169.

La Porte, R.E., et. al. (1985). Physical activity or cardiovascular fitness: Which is more important for health? *The Physician and Sports Medicine.* Vol. 13, No. 3, 145-157.

Levin, S. (1993). Does exercise enhance sexuality? *The Physician and Sports Medicine.* Vol. 21, No. 3, 199-203.

Levin, S. (1993). Women in sports medicine. *The Physician and Sports Medicine. Vol.* 21, No. 2, 167-174.

Mc Cleary, K. (1992). The no gimmick weight loss plan. *Hippocrates.* 1/92, 83-85.

Powell, K.E. (1985). Workshop on epidemiological and public health aspects of physical activity and exercise. *The Physician and Sports Medicine.* Vol. 13, No. 3, 161-168.

Ramotar, J. E. (1990). The art of safe walking. *The Physician and Sports Medicine.* Vol. 18, No. 10, 36-37.

Rippe, J.M. (1986). Walking for fitness. *The Physician and Sports Medicine.* Vol. 14, No. 10, 144-159.

Rogers, C.C. (1985). Of magic, miracles and exercise myths. *The Physician and Sports Medicine.* Vol. 13, No. 5, 156-166.

Rosenstein, A.H. (1987). The benefits of health maintenance. *The Physician and Sports Medicine.* Vol. 15, No. 4, 57-68.

Safran, M.R., Garrett, W.E., Seaver, A.V., et. al. (1988). The role of warm-up in muscular injury prevention. *American Journal of Sports Medicine*. 16 (2), 123-129.

Schatz, M.P. (1991). Walk your way back to health. *The Physician and Sports Medicine*. Vol. 19, No. 5, 127-128.

Schatz, M.P. (1992). Exercises you can take to work. *The Physician and Sports Medicine*. Vol. 20, No. 1, 165-166.

Schatz, M.P. (1993). Boosting abdominal strength without back pain. *The Physician and Sports Medicine*. Vol. 21, No. 4, 153-154.

Schelkun, P.H. (1992). Exercise after angioplasty: How much? How soon? *The Physician and Sports Medicine*. Vol. 20, No. 3, 199-203.

Sharp, D. (1994). The quitter's exercise plan. *Hippocrates*. 5/94, 54-61.

Sheehan, G. (1986). Write that down! *The Physician and Sports Medicine*. Vol. 14, No. 6, 56.

Sheehan, G. (1991). Health risk appraisals. *The Physician and Sports Medicine*. Vol. 19, No. 5, 41.

Sheehan, G. (1991). Less is more. *The Physician and Sports Medicine*. Vol. 19, No. 1, 21.

Sheehan, G. (1991). Running away from smoking. *The Physician and Sports Medicine*. *Vol*. 19, No. 6, 55.

Sheehan, G. Sports medicine renaissance. *The Physician and Sports Medicine*. *Vol*. 18, No. 11, 26.

Simon, H.B. (1989). Physician-al fitness: Setting an example. *The Physician and Sports Medicine*. Vol. 17, No. 10, 45-48.

Slavin, J.L. (1986). Calorie supplements for athletes. *The Physician and Sports Medicine*. Vol. 14, No. 11, 201-203.

Sparling, P.B. (1984). Physiological determinants of distance running performance. *The Physician and Sports Medicine*. Vol. 12, No. 3, 68-77.

Stamford B. (1990). Strength vs. endurance. *The Physician and Sports Medicine.* Vol. 18, No. 10, 105-106.

Stamford, B. (1984). Weight training principles. *The Physician and Sports Medicine.* Vol. 12, No. 3, 195.

Stamford, B. (1985). A "stitch" in the side. *The Physician and Sports Medicine.* Vol. 13, No.5, 187.

Stamford, B. (1985). Predicting your aerobic fitness. *The Physician and Sports Medicine.* Vol. 13, No. 3, 183.

Stamford, B. (1986). How do muscles work? *The Physician and Sports Medicine.* Vol. 14, No. 10, 208.

Stamford, B. (1986). To walk rather than run. *The Physician and Sports Medicine.* Vol. 14, No. 3, 296.

Stamford, B. (1987). Building bigger muscles. *The Physician and Sports Medicine.* Vol. 15, No. 6, 166.

Stamford, B. (1987). Exercise and the common cold. *The Physician and Sports Medicine. Vol.* 15, No. 2, 197.

Stamford, B. (1987).What is target heart rate? *The Physician and Sports Medicine.* Vol. 15, No. 1, 214.

Stamford, B. (1988). When to eat and exercise. *The Physician and Sports Medicine.* Vol. 16, No. 1, 184.

Stamford, B. (1991). Exercise for a fast burn. *The Physician and Sports Medicine.* Vol. 19, No. 11, 151-152.

Stamford, B. (1992). Keeping cool during hot-weather workouts. *The Physician and Sports Medicine.* Vol. 20, No. 6, 167-168.

Stamford, B. (1992). When workouts are a gas. Exercise and the digestive system. *The Physician and Sports Medicine.* Vol. 20, No. 11, 163-164.

Stamford, B. (1993). Muscle cramps, untying the knots. *The Physician and Sports Medicine.* Vol. 21, No. 7, 115-116.

Stamford, B. (1993). Tracking your heart rate for fitness. *The Physician and Sports Medicine.* Vol. 21, No. 3, 227-228.

Strauss, R.H. (1993). Sex, health and exercise. *The Physician and Sports Medicine.* Vol. 21, No. 3, 3.

Strovas, J. (1984). Seniors walk away from sedentary life. *The Physician and Sports Medicine.* Vol. 12, No. 4, 144-149.

Van Camp, S.P. and Choi, J.H. (1988). Exercise and sudden death. *The Physician and Sports Medicine.* Vol. 16, No. 3, 49-52.

Wilmore, J.H. (1986). Body composition. *The Physician and Sports Medicine.* Vol. 14, No. 3, 144-162.

Work, J. (1990). Exercise for the overweight person. *The Physician and Sports Medicine.* Vol. 18, No. 7, 113-122.

Work, J.A. (1990). Healthy people 2000. *The Physician and Sports Medicine.* Vol. 18, No. 11, 31-32.

Stress and Stress Management:

Agras, W.S. (1983). Relaxation therapy in hypertension. *Hospital Practice.* 5/83, 129-137.

Altschuler, K.Z. (1983). Stress management: State of the art. *Patient Care.* 7/83, 88-163.

Benson, H. and Caudill, M.A. (1984). Relaxation techniques for managing hypertension. *Primary Cardiology.* 9/84, 137-144.

Brodsky, M.A. and Allen B.J. (1989). Stress, cardiac arrhythmias, and sudden death. *Practical Cardiology.* Vol. 15, No. 7, 49-55.

Brown, S.J. (1994). Before getting angry, count to two times the risk of heart attack. *Family Practice News.* 5/94, 14.

Carney, R.S. (1983). Clinical applications of relaxation training. *Hospital Practice.* 7/83, 83-94.

Carpi, J. (1993). Relieving the strain of stress. *Medical World News.* 5/93, 22-31.

Conrad, E. (1990). Let Laughter Ring. *Working Mother.* 2/90, 40-47.

de Paolo, R. (1984). How to reduce stress in your practice. *Physician's Management.* 1/84, 114-127.

Duncan, D.E. (1994). Compassion fatigue. *Hippocrates*, 4/94, 35-41.

Eliot, R.S. (1987). Stress and the heart: Measuring and evaluating reactivity. *Illustrated Medicine.* Vol. 2, No. 3, 1-16.

Engler, A. (1993). When silence makes sense. *Hippocrates.* 4/93, 30-32.

Freedman, D.X. (1983). When stress requires a management plan. *Patient Care.* 2/83, 14-29.

Ganong, W.F. (1988). The stress response, a dynamic overview. *Hospital Practice.* 6/88, 155-171.

Goldman, B. (1992). Smart looks. *Hippocrates.* 9/92, 21-24.

Goldman, B. (1994). The essence of attraction. *Hippocrates.* 4/94, 66-68.

Hales, D. (1990). 8 Stress busting strategies. *Working Mother.* 9/90, 60-61.

Hall, S.S. (1992). Cheating fate. *Hippocrates.* 4/92, 38-45.

Halpern, S. (1986). Good vibrations. *Women's Health.* 2/86, 21-25.

Hand, D. (1992). Nightmare personality. *Hippocrates.* 9/92, 72-76.

Hearn, W. (1993). Getting a grip. *American Medical News.* 3/93, 41-45.

Huyghe, P. (1992). Voices from inner space. *Hippocrates.* 3/92, 19-20.

Jabs, C. (1990). Relax, seven ways to be a happy, stress-free parent. *Working Mother.* 1/90, 56-60.

Jaret, P. (1992). Dark clouds, silver linings. *Hippocrates*, 2/92, 34-39.

Jaret, P. (1992). Mind over malady. *Hippocrates.* 9/(2, 27-37.

Kabat-Zinn, J. (1982). An outpatient program in behavioral medicine for chronic pain patients based on the practice of mindfulness meditation: Theoretical considerations and preliminary results. *General Hospital Psychiatry.* 4, 33-47.

King. T.M. (1984) Stress and medical practice. *The Female Patient.* 9, 90-104.

Kriegel, R. and Kriegel, M. (1984). "Type C" behavior and your career. *The Executive Female.* 9, 22-25.

Lawren, B. (1992). Mind over body. *Living Well.* 4/92, 77-80.

Makihara, K. (1991). Death of a salaryman. *Hippocrates.* 5/91, 34-43.

Mc Kay, D.A., et. al. (1985). Social supports and stress as predictors of illness. *The Journal of Family Practice.* Vol. 20, No. 6, 575-581.

Murphy, P. (1984). Office stress: Is a solution shaping up? *The Physician and Sports Medicine.* Vol. 12, No. 12, 114-118.

Neimark, J. (1989). Lift your spirits. *Working Mother.* 10/89, 20-24.

Nelson, A-M. (1987). Stress center preaches cool down for hot reactors. *Saturday Magazine of the Scottsdale Progress.* 2/87, 22-25.

Nieman, D.C. (1989). Exercise and the mind. *Women's Sports and Fitness.* 9/89, 53-57.

Okun, S. (1992). Facing your future. *Hippocrates.* 4/92, 28-31.

Pacelli, L.C. (1990). Mike Ditka and stress or ... the case of the exploding coach. *The Physician and Sports Medicine.* Vol. 18, No. 2, 126-130.

Parkerson, G.R., Broadhead, W.E. and Tse, C-K. J. (1995). Perceived family stress as a predictor of health related outcomes. *Archives of Family Medicine.* 3/95, 153-160.

Pfifferling, J.H. (1992). A profession assailed by pressure. *Medical Tribune.* 7/92, 22.

Poppy, J. (1990). She rubbed me the right way. *Hippocrates.* 10/90, 26-30.

Rosch, P.J. (1983) Effects of stress on the cadiovascular system. *Physician and Patient.* 11/83, 29-44.

Rowntree, R. (1994). Joining forces. *Hippocrates.* 3/94, 42-47.

Seligson, S.V. (1993). Time's up. *Hippocrates.* 4/93, 34-40.

Shahady, E.J. (1993). Physician stress: How to avoid burnout. *Consultant.* 6/93, 16-22.

Sheehan, G. (1989) Laughter and the love of friends. *The Physician and Sports Medicine. Vol.* 17, No. 9, 58.

Shelton, S.K. (1990). Surviving coming home. *Working Mother.* 11/90, 104-107.

Sherman, C. (1994). Stress: How to help patients cope. *The Physician and Sports Medicine.* Vol. 22, No. 7, 66-75.

Skelly, F.J. (1994). Stress busters. *American Medical News.* 10/94, 23-25.

Taylor, R. B. (1987). What are the best ways to handle stress? *Physician's Management.* 5/87, 153-167.

Thornton, J.S. (1984). The Iowa family stress clinic: A model for management. *The Female Patient.* 9, 67-68.

Turbo, R. (1987). Stress and disease: Cellular evidence hints as therapy. *Medical World News.* 1/87, 26-41.

Wallis, C. (1983). Stress: Can we cope? *Time.* 6/83, 48-54.

Zimmer, J. (1985). The pleasure of giving a great massage and getting one in return. *Health*. 4/85, 50-68.

Depression:

Akiskal, H.S., Jensvold, M.F., Kramer, P.D., Paist, S.S. and Potter, W.Z. (1994). The wise use of psychiatric drugs. *Patient Care*. 11/94, 82-117.

Hales, R.E., Rakel, R.E. and Rothschild, S. (1994). Depression: Practical tips for detection and treatment. *Patient Care*. 11/94, 60-80.

Hurley, D. (1995). Quick depression checklist unveiled. *Medical Tribune for the Family Physician*. Vol. 36, No. 3, 1-6.

Kelly, M.J. (1991). Strategies for diagnosing and treating depression. *Medical Update, Brigham and Women's Hospital*. Vol. 3, No. 8, 1-5.

Monahan, T. (1986). Exercise and depression: Swapping sweat for serenity. *The Physician and Sports Medicine*. Vol. 14, No.9, 192-197.

Nicoloff, G. and Schwenck, T.L. (1995). Using exercise to ward off depression. *The Physician and Sports Medicine*. Vol. 23, No. 9, 44-58.

Rush, A.J., et. al. (1994). Depression: Serious, prevalent, detectable. *Patient Care*. 2/94, 30-87.

Stuart, M.R. and Lieberman, J.A. III. (1994). Finding time for counseling in primary care. *Patient Care*. 11/94, 118-129.

Cholesterol:

Alexander, W. (1995). Lowering cholesterol does pay off. *Patient Care*. 3/95, 23.

Berger, H. (1985). Hyperlipoproteinemia. *Primary Cardiology*. 5/85, 109-128.

Blake, G.H. and Triplett, L.C. (1995). Management of hypercholesterolemia. *American Family Physician*. 4/95, 1157-1166.

Bullock, C. (1995). Soy protein has profound effect on lipid levels. *Medical Tribune.* 6.95, 14.

Clark, M. (1988). Controlling cholesterol. *Newsweek on Health.* Winter 1988, 16-20.

Connor, W.E. (1987). Diet and hyperlipidemia. *Lipid Letter.* Vol. 4, No. 4, 1-4.

Corti, M-C. (1995). HDL cholesterol predicts coronary heart disease mortality in nolder persons. *JAMA.* Vol. 274, No. 7, 539-544.

Feldman, E.B. and Kuske, T.T. (1988). Lipid disorders: Diet and drug therapy. *Modern Medicine.* 56, 60-71.

Goor, R. (1988). A new approach to dietary management of high blood cholesterol. *Medical Management Dymanics.* Vol.6, No.1, 3-9.

Gotto, A.M. (1987). Hypercholesterolemia: An assessment of screening and diagnostic techniques. *Modern Medicine.* 55, 28-44.

Gotto, A.M., La Rosa, J.C., Naito, H.K. and Stone, N.J. (1989). Hyperlipidemia: A complete approach. *Patient Care.* 2/98, 34-50.

Grundy, S. (1994). Guidelines for cholesterol management: Recommendations of the national cholesterol education program's adult treatment panel II. *Heart Disease and Stroke.* 5/94, 123-129.

Grundy, S.M. (1985). Diet and hypercholesterolemia. *Cardiovascular Medicine.* 1/85, 39-52.

Guinard, M. (1988). Castelli on cholesterol: Treat by the numbers. *Cardiology World News.* 10/88, 22

Gwynne, J.T. (1988). The metabolism and function of HDL in reverse transport of cholesterol. *Lipid Letter.* Vol. 5, No. 3, 1-4.

Jones, P.H. and Gotto, A.M. (1987). Hyperlipoproteinemia: Risk assessment and dietary management. *Consultant.* 11/87, 126-150.

Jones, P.H. and Gotto, A.M. (1989). Gauging patient's risks and instituting dietary control. *Consultant.* 3/89, 130-163.

Karpen, M. (1988). Toughening goals for cholesterol levels. *Cardiology World News.* 10/88, 23.

Kasim, S. (1987). Cholesterol changes with aging: Their nature and significance. *Geriatrics.* Vol. 42, No. 3, 73-82.

Kottke, B.A., et. al., (1986). Apolipoproteins and coronary artery disease. *Mayo Clinic Proceedings.* 61, 313-320.

Kuritsky, L. (1994). Dyslipidemia: Drugs, diet, and common sense. *Hospital Practice.* 8/94, 40-44.

Kuznar, W. (1993). High cholesterol: Should you routinely screen and treat otherwise healthy young adults? *Modern Medicine.* 61, 15-18.

La Rosa, J.C. (1994). Easy-to-digest answers to your patients' questions about diet and cholesterol. *Modern Medicine.* 62, 36-42.

Laino, C. (1995). Treating even mildly elevated cholesterol cost-effective. *Medical Tribune.* 4/95, 7.

Levine, G.N., Keaney, J.F. and Vita, J.A. (1995). Cholesterol reduction in cardiovascular disease, clinical benefits and possible mechanisms. *The New England Journal of Medicine.* Vol. 332,No. 8, 512-521.

Long, P. (1994). A town with a golden gene. *Hippocrates.* 2/94, 50-61.

Mandelbaum-Schmid, J. (1994). Are we addicted to fat? *Hippocrates.* 2/94, 28-29.

Mc Gowan, M. (1994). The effect of life-cycle and exogenous hormones on the female lipid profile. *The Female Patient.* 19, 31-40.

Miller, V. and La Rosa, J.C. (1988). Hypercholesterolemia in women: What are the special considerations? *The Female Patient.* 13, 22-32.

Naito, H.K. (1986). The clinical significance of apolipoprotein measurements. *Journal of Clinical Immunoassay.* Vol. 9, No. 1, 11-20.

National Cholesterol Education Program. (1993). Second report of the expert panel on detection, evaluation, and treatment of high blood cholesterol in adults. *National Institutes of Health.* 9/93.

National Cholesterol Education Program. (1991). Highlights of the report of the expert panel on blood cholesterol levels in children and adolescents. *U.S. Department of Health and Human Services.* 1991.

Rifkind, B.M. (1988). Cholesterol treatment today. *Practical Cardiology, Special Issue.* 5/88.

Smith, D.A., Karmally, W. and Brown, W.V. (1987). Treating hyperlipidemia, Part I: Whether and when in the elderly. *Geriatrics.* Vol. 42, No. 6, 33-42.

Tragere, J. (1988). Castelli unabashedly pro-oatmeal. *Medical Tribune.* 11/88, 15.

Verschuren, W.M.M., et. al (1995). Serum total cholesterol and long-term coronary heart disease mortality in different cultures. *JAMA.* Vol. 274, No. 2, 131-135.

Wallis, C. (1984). Hold the eggs and butter. *Time.* 3/26/84, 56-63.

Weinberg, R.B. (1987). Lipoprotein metabolism: Hormonal regulation. *Hospital Practice.* 6/87, 223-243.

Work, J.A. (1987). Treating patients who have high cholesterol levels: The role of screening tests, drugs and exercise. *The Physician and Sports Medicine.* Vol. 15, No. 8, 113-122.

Writing Group for the DISC Collaborative Research Group. (1995). Efficacy and safety of lowering dietary intake of fat and cholesterol in children with elevated low-density lipoprotein cholesterol. *JAMA.* Vol. 273, No. 18, 1429-1435.

Weight and Body Composition Management:

Bierman, E.L. (1991). Why treat obesity? Contemporary management of the overweight patient, *Symposium Proceedings.* Tempe, Arizona.

Brownell, K.D. (1991) Behavior modification initiatives. Contemporary management of the obese patient, *Symposium Proceedings.* Tempe, Arizona.

Brownell, K.D. and Steen, S.N. (1987). Modern methods for weight control: The physiology and psychology of dieting. *The Physician and Sports Medicine.* Vol.15, No. 12, 122-137.

Dwyer, J.T. (1991). Nutrient needs in weight loss and maintenance. Contemporary management of the obese patient, *Symposium Proceedings.* Tempe, Arizona.

Eastman, P. (1994). Obesity: The search for a "satiety factor." *Cardiology World News.* 12/94, 7.

Griffin, K. (1989). Body fat: How much is too much? *Hippocrates.* 7/89, 92-94.

Horton, E.S. (1991). The exercise prescription. Contemporary management of the obese patient, *Symposium Proceedings.* Tempe, Arizona.

Jackson, A.S. (1985). Practical assessment of body composition. *The Physician and Sports Medicine.* Vol. 13, No. 5, 76-89.

Laino, C. (1994). Experts advocate individual weight loss programs. *Medical Tribune.* 4/94, 2-3.

Lavie, C.J., Milani, R.V., Squires, R.W., et. al. (1992). Exercise and the heart: Good, benign, or evil? *Postgraduate Medicine.* 9, 130-134.

Nicolosi, R., et. al. (1994). American Heart Association guidelines for weight management programs for healthy adults. *Heart Disease and Stroke.* 7/94, 221-232.

Parker, D.F. and Bar-Or, O. (1991). Juvenile obesity: The importance of exercise--and getting children to do it. *The Physician and Sports Medicine.* Vol. 19, No. 6, 113-125.

Pi-Sunyer, F.X. (1991). Etiologic factors in obesity. Contemporary management of the obese patient, *Symposium Proceedings.* Tempe, Arizona.

Roach, M. (1993). Advice from the world's biggest weight experts: Their gain can be your loss. *Hippocrates.* 3/93, 50-60.

Schelkun, P.H. (1991). The risks of riding the weight loss roller coaster. *The Physician and Sports Medicine*. Vol. 19, No. 6, 148-156.

Shenk, L. (1990). Fats and figures. *Women's Sports and Fitness*. 7/90, 14.

Skelton, N.K. (1993). 8 questions on obesity management. *Hudson Monitor*. 2/93, 71-76.

Stamford, B. (1987). What's the importance of percent body fat? *The Physician and Sports Medicine*. Vol. 15, No. 3, 216.

Wing, R.R. (1992). Behavioral treatment of severe obesity. *American Journal of Clinical Nutrition*. 55, 545-548.

Yanovski, S.Z. (1993). A practical approach to treatment of the obese patient. *Archives of Family Medicine*. 2, 309-316.

Zoler, M.L. (1989). A billion dollar bulge: Obesity. *Medical World News*. 11/98, 32-38.

Supplements:

Aronson, V. (1986). Vitamins and minerals as ergogenic aids. *The Physician and Sports Medicine*. Vol. 12, No. 3, 209-212.

Cowart, V. (1992). Dietary supplements, alternatives to anabolic steroids? *The Physician and Sports Medicine*. Vol. 20, No. 3, 189-198.

Frankle, M.A. (1989). Anabolic-androgenic steroids: A guide for the physician. *The Journal of Musculoskeletal Medicine*. 11/89, 69-87.

Greenberg, E.R. (1994). Antioxidant vitamins and cancer: An open question. *The Columbia University School of Public Health Newsletter*. 11/94, 1-2.

Johnson, L.E. (1994). The emerging role of vitamins as antioxidants. *Archives of Family Medicine*. 3, 809-816.

Kleiner, S. (1994). Antioxidants, vitamins that do battle. *The Physician and Sports Medicine*. Vol. 22, No. 2, 23-24.

Long, P. (1993). The vitamin wars. *Hippocrates*. 5/93, 32-41.

Long, P. (1994). Vitamin E: Should you believe in it? Here's all you need to know. *Hippocrates*. 121/94, 46-53.

Morgan, B.L.G. (1986). Minerals, myths and facts. *Rx Being Well*. 3/86, 27-32.

Offermann, M.K. and Medford, R.M. (1994). Antioxidants and atherosclerosis: A molecular perspective. *Heart Disease and Stroke*. 1/94, 52-57.

Zuckerman, S. (1985). Vitamins, who needs them and when? *American Health*. 11/85, 49-55.

Index

A

Academic credit for health, 315
Acceptance, 22
Accidents, 25
Acknowledgement, 22
Activity, 41
Adaptation, 29
Adversaries to change, 23
    Homeostasis, 23
    Inertia, 23
    Generational compulsion to repeat, 23
Aerobic exercise, 103
    Achieving the training effect, 107
    Aerobic fitness, 107
    Aerobic fitness test, 315
    Aerobic training zone, 108
    Efficiency, 104
    FIT principle, 109, 129
    Mitochondrion, 104
    Other sites of adaptation, 104
    Primary fuel, fat, 105
    Primary site of adaptation, 103
    Rate of gain and decline, 110
    Writing your prescription, 129
Aggressive behavior, 28
Aggressive communication, 151
Allen, Robert G., 35
Allow, 37
Alternative solutions, 11
Altitude and exercise, 115
Amino acids, 52
    Essential, 52
Anatomy of digestive tract, 48
Anger, deal with it as the Japanese do, 165
Anger-In Personality Screening Test, 339
Antioxidant vitamins, 275
    Atherogenesis and, 276
    Carcinogenesis and, 277
    Eye disease and, 278

Free radicals, 275
Specific vitamins, 279
    Selenium, 280
    Vitamin A, 279
    Vitamin C, 279
    Vitamin E, 280
Appel, Charles Albert, 209
"Apple" shape, 252
Aristotle, 304
Arizona Heart Institute, 210
Articulate change, 38
Ask, 34
Assertive behavior, 27, 28
Assertive communication, 151
Atherosclerosis (hardening of arteries), 214
ATP (energy currency), 99, 104
"Atta-boys", 329
Attitudes and expectations, 31, 38
Automaticity of behavior, 20
Awareness, 10, 21, 34, 257

B

Behavior change, 17
    (see behavior modification)
    Choosing to change, 33
Behavior development, 19
Behavior modification, 17, 21
    Acceptance and acknowledgement, 22
    Awareness, 21, 34
    Capacity to change, 21, 33
    Certificate of Title, 22, 37
    Execution, 22
    External motivation, 21, 36
    Internal motivation, 22
Bell, Annie, MS, RD, 46
Benefits of exercising, 95
Benefits of good nutrition, 47
Bernard, Claude, 145
Black Dog, the, 187
Body Mass Index (BMI), 251
Borg scale of perceived exertion, 107
Buring, Julie, 282
Burnout Inventory, 334

367

C

Calorie requirement, computing, 72, 240
Calories, 232
    Alcohol, 235
    Carbohydrate, 235
    Fat, 235
    Protein, 235
Canon, Walter, 145
Capacity (to change), 21, 33
Carbohydrates, 49
    Complex, 49, 50, 72
    Disaccharide, 49
    Glycogen, 49
    Monosaccharide, 49
    Polysaccharide, 49
    Sources, 51
    Starches, 49
Castelli, William, MD, 45, 230
Catalysts, social, 321
Catalytic behaviors, 41, 199
Celente, Gerald, 320
CEO, be your own, 161
Certificate of Title (to behavior), 22, 37
Charitable groups, financial sources, 331
Charity, 313
Cholesterol, 213
Cholesterol Lowering Athero Study, 219
Cholesterol (a poem), 209
Choosing behaviors, 33
"Circle the Wagons," 162, 185
Communication, assertive, 313
Conditioned responses, 19
    Operant conditioning, 19
    Stimulus-response conditioning, 19
Confidence, social, 308
Connolly, Cyril Vernon, 231
Contact, physical and verbal, 304
Contract, sign one, 38
"Cool", being healthy must be, 311
Coronary Primary Prevention Trial, 218
Corporations, source for finances, 330
"Crisis team", 162
Cronkite, Kathy, 187

D

Daisies (a poem), 207
Denial, 41
Depression, 41, 187
    Classification, 192
        Atypical, 192
        Bipolar disorder, 193
        Catatonic, 192
        Depressive disorder not otherwise specified (DDNOS), 193
        Melancholic, 192
        Post-partum, 193
        Psychotic, 192
        Seasonal affective disorder (SAD),192
    Depression Questionnaire, 195
    Preventing and combating, 198
        Beauty, seek it, 205
        Choice, 202
        Daisies, pick them, 206
        Delegate, 205
        Depressants, avoid, 204
        "Eat the elephant", 205
        Exercise, 201
        Face forward, 206
        Help, ask for it, 204
        Isolation, avoid, 203
        Laugh, 208
        Leonardo da Vinci, 206
        Listen, 200
        Love, 206
        Middle man use, 205
        Newness, 205
        Newsbreaks, 204
        Nutrition, 201
        Preventive philosophy, 202
        Six months to live game, 205
        Socialize, 203
        Talk, 199
        Therapist, 207
        Write, 202
    Recognition, 194
    Social costs, 190
    Symptoms, 191
Determining your Nutritional Health, 336
Diets, 253
    Diet Center, 254
    High protein, 253

Jenny Craig, 254
Nutri Systems, 254
Starvation, 253
Very low calorie (VLCD), 254
Weight Watchers, 254
Digestive tract, anatomy of, 48
Disraeli, Benjamin, 299
Dissonance, 24, 26, 36
Dryden, John, 91
Duke University, 10
Dunne, Finley Peter, 135
Duodenum, 48

E

Eating at home, 68
How to establish good habits, 71
Kitchen tips, 70
Presentation, tricks, 74
Recipe modification, 73
Stocking your kitchen, 68, 69
Storage of food, 69
Tools, 69
Eating outside the home, 75
Economy, 76
Healthy choice selections, 76
Restaurant dining dilemma, 77
Appetizer and soup as meal, 79
Assertive ordering, 79
Brown bag it, 78
Eat at home, 78
Ethnic dining, 80
Exclusively healthful, 80
Mindless pig, eat like one, 80
Modify and substitute, 79
Nutrition sense, 79
User friendly restaurants, 78
Education, 10
Ego defense mechanisms, 33
Einstein's Bagel Shop, 15
Eliot, Robert S., MD, 10, 163
Ellison, Curtis, 46
Emotional Inventory, 335
Empty calories, 50
Energy availability from food sources, 235
Energy balance equation, 235
Energy sources, chart, 106

Energy storage, 235
Engel, George, 1
Esophagus, 48
Execution (of change), 22, 38
Exercise, 91
Aerobic (see aerobic ex), 103
Anaerobic (see strength training), 101
Benefits, 95
Children, 115
Depression and, 201
Energy sources, 106
Energy replenishment, 106, 112
Environmental considerations, 113
How to implement your program, 117
Attitude, 118
Be in touch with your body, 120
Choose your activity, 118
Commit to two months, 119
Contract, sign it, 119
Contract, sign a new one, 121
Develop an active lifestyle, 122
Exercise where you happen to be, 120
Expectations, 118
Motivate yourself, 117
Nutrition, 119
Picture, 119
Plateaus, expect them, 122
Record workouts, 119
Review, modify, communicate, 121
Rewards, 120
Schedule, 119
Social conscience, 122
Socialization, 120
Success, expect it, 121
Trick yourself, 122
Integrating activities, 133
Lipids and, 215
Metabolism, 99
(see Metabolism)
Muscle structure and physiology, 98
(see Muscle structure and function)
Nutrition specifics, 111
Risks, 96
Sample form for recording, 131
Seniors, 116
Strength training, 101
(see Strength training)
Stress, 160
Teaching, 305
Whom to trust, 135

Why we don't, 94
Women, 116
Expectations (see attitudes), 31, 38
Expressive emotions, 41

F

Fast twitch fiber, 98
Fat burning fallacy, 260
Fats, 54
    Energy (caloric) from, 54
    Essential fatty acids, 55
    Free fatty acids, 54
    Monosaturated, 54
    Polyunsaturated, 54
    Saturated fats. 54
    Triglyceride, 54
Fat soluble vitamins, 55, 270
Fiber, 55
    Sources, 56
    Water soluble, 56
    Water insoluble, 56
"First team", 39, 162
FIT principle (aerobic training), 109, 129
Flight 1601, 6
"Flavors" of behavior, 27
Flower oils, 55
Food diary, 71, 255
Food, fundamentals of, 49
French paradox, 46
Freud, Sigmund, 145
Frustration, 41

G

Gall bladder, 48
General adaptation syndrome (GAS), 138
Generational compulsion to repeat, 20, 23
"Get a Life, America!", public health, 299
    Health education across America, 304
        Pregnant mothers, 304
        Grades 1-3, 306
        Grades 4-8, 310
        High school, 312
        College years, 316
        Work environment, 316

        Adult education, 317
        Nursing homes, 318
        Corporate programs, 319
        Central facility, 320
    Changing society's attitudes, 321
        "Go Hollywood", 324
        Healthy role model program, 322
        Who else?, 325
    Nationwide marketing campaign, 327
        Societal rewards, 329
        Money? Sutton's Law, 329
    Why this program will work, 303
Glossary, 344
Guided visual imagery, 161

H

Happiness, 41
Harvard alumni study, 93
Health and wellness programs (work-site),
    316, 319, 327
Health, fitness, and wellness, 93
Health management, 7
Healthy People 2000, 8, 92, 302
Hear, 36
Heart rate, 107
    Determination, 107
Hecht, Harvey, MD, 210
Helsinki Heart Study, 214
Hermit crab concept of business, 331
Homeostasis, 23, 29
"Hot reactor", 163
How do you eat an elephant?, 158
Humidity and exercise, 114
Hydration and exercise, 112
Hydrogenation, 55

I

Identify behaviors to change, 38
Illness, physical, 25
Imus, Don, 325
Inertia, 23
Insurance companies, source for finances,
    330

Intestine (large and small), 48
Investment House Illnesses, 12

J

Jordan, Michael, 188
Judge, don't, 37

K

Kabat-Zinn, Jon, Ph.D., 165
  (see mindfulness meditation)
Koop, C. Everett, MD, 10, 213
Kubler-Ross, Elisabeth, MD, 10,17,44, 156

L

Labor force, 331
Laugh, 208
Legacy for exercise, none, 95
Let go, 37
Letter to colleagues, 9
Lifestyles, 7
Lipids (fats), 210
  Cholesterol profiles, 216
  Desirable, 212
  Elderly, 225
  Epidemiologic studies, 218
  Estrogen, 226
  Exercise, 215
  Genetic predisposition, 221
  HDL, 213
  How to control cholesterol, 227
    Drink only moderately, 229
    Eat smart, 228
    Get lean, 228
    Monitor you own cholesterol, 229
    Responsibility, take it, 228
    Smoke, don't, 229
  Hyperlipidemia, 212
  LDL, 213
  Low cholesterol diet dangers, 220
  Transport, 213

Valerio Dagnoli, story of, 223
  Women and Children, 224
Listen, 35, 37
Listen (a poem), 200
Liver, 48
Look, 37
Lucci, Susan, 91

M

Major League Players of Health, 16
Margerines, 55
MCI approach, 24
Meditate, 35, 176
Metabolism, 99
  Aerobic, 99
  Anaerobic, 99
  Anaerobic threshold, 99
Metropolitan Insurance actuarial data, 233
Mindfulness, 26
Mindfulness meditation, 26,155, 161, 165
  Be aware, 169
  Breathing, 168
  Complete, you are, 168
  Depression and anxiety, be alert for, 170
  Ebb and flow, allow it, 170
  Emotions, connect with, 169
  Intuitive knowing, 169
  Judgmental feelings, 168
  Nature, be in concert with, 171
  Past and future, don't be there, 169
  Peaceful mind, maintain it, 170
  Present, where you are, 170
Minerals, 272
  Calcium, 272
Iodine, 274
  Iron, 274
  Magnesium, 273
  Phosphorous, 273
  Selenium, 274
  Sodium (potassium and chloride), 273
  Zinc, 274
Mitochondrion, 99, 103
"Monkey see, monkey do", 325
Motivation, 15
  External, 21, 36
  Internal, 22, 37

Mount St. Helens, 40
Mouth, 48
Movement, joy of, 308
Muscle structure and function, 98
    Energy replenishment, 106, 112
    Fiber types (fast, slow), 98
    Motor unit, 98

N

"Naked-in-the-mirror" test, 40, 251, 258
National Cholesterol Ed. Prog., 219
National debt theory of living, 284
National Health and Nutrition Survey, 232
National Heart Lung and Blood Inst., 218
Nature, forces of, 40
Nature abhors a vacuum, 40
Newman, Paul, 325
Nicklaus, Jack, 326
Non-assertive behavior, 28
Non-assertive communication, 151
Nutrition, 45
    Benefits of, 47
    Depression and, 201
    Exercise and, 111
    Good nutrition, 47
    Healthy Nutrition Score, 337
    Teaching, 305
    Tips for quick and healthy eating, 80
        Brush your teeth, 82
        High fiber cereal, 81
        Muffins, steer clear, 81
        Pizza, make your own, 82
        Prepared pasta dishes, avoid, 81
        Skim milk, 81
        Vegetables, microwave, 82
    Recipes, 83
        Curried Turkey Salad, 84
        Oriental Pasta and Snow Peas, 85
        Spinach Lasagna, 86
        Chicken Baked in Parchment, 88
        Mandarin Orange Chicken, 89
        Zesty Lentil Stew, 90
    Weight management and, 238

O

Oasis, personal, 162
Obesity, 232, 243
    Deleterious effects, 246
        Cardiovascular diseases, 247
        Diabetes, 247
        Gallbladder disease, 248
        Mortality, 246
        Structural problems, 248
        Surgical risk, 248
    Theories of origin, 243
        Fat cell theory, 243
        Genetics, 243
        Impaired thermogenesis, 245
        Metabolic theories, 245
        Neural theories, 245
        Set point theory, 244
        Thyroid abnormalities, 244
Ornish, Dean, MD, 10, 12
Oslo Study Group, 214
Ownership (of behavior), 37

P

Paffenbarger, Ralph, 92, 94
Palmer, Arnold, 326
Pancreas, 48
Paradigm, new, 7
Parental involvement in teaching, 312
Paris, 46
Peace, 41
Peak performance, 152
    Burnout, 152
    Burnout Inventory, 334
    Flameout, 152
    Flameout Screening Test, 153
"Pear" shape, 252
Peer pressure, 20, 311
Percentage body fat (PBF), 250
Perception of control, 30, 241
Personal empowerment, 10
Personal oasis, 162
Physical illness, 25
Plato, 307
Player, Gary, 326

Pollution and exercise, 115
Popular diets, 253
Practice, 39
Principles and philosophy, 10
Prospective awareness, 24
Proteins, 51
    Complete, 52
    Complimentary vegetable sources, 52
    Incomplete, 52
    Requirements, 53
    Sources in common foods, 53
Proximal muscles, 125
Public health (see Get a Life ...), 299
Putting it all together, 283
    Attitudes and expectations, 289
    Behavior modification process, 289
    Body composition and weight, 293
    Choices, 288
    Exercise, 291
    Family history, 286
    Full Monty, the, 296
    Journal entries, 295
    Lessons to pass along, 284
    Lipids, 293
    Nutrition, 290
    Periodic review, 296
    Psychologic well-being, 292
    Recidivism, 296
    Self, 295
    Stress, 291
    Vitamins and supplements, 294
Pylorus, 48

R

Recidivism, 30
Recipe modification, 73
    Elimination, 73
    Reduction, 73
    Substitution, 73
Recommended dietary allowances, 267
References, 347
Remind yourself that change is good, 40
Resting metabolic rate, 236
Retrospective awareness, 24
Rewards, 39, 327, 329
Roadblocks to change, 34

Rochester, University of, 1
Role models, 38, 92, 305, 307, 309, 312, 315
Role models, students as, 313
"Running for public office," 15

S

Salmonella, 66
Satcher, David, MD, 299, 322
Screening test, take one, 35
Secrets, 8, 10
Sedentary lifestyle, 41
Selye, Hans, MD, 137, 138, 171
Shalala, Donna, 322
Sharkey, Brian J., Ph.D., 265
Skin fold measurements, 251
Slow twitch fiber, 98
"Small stuff, it's all small stuff", 164
Snacks, 72
Social conscience, 122
Socialize, 203
Societal changes, 8
Spokesperson for health, 321
Stanford University, 92
Stewardship, two-year, for change, 29
Stomach, 48
Stop, 36
Strength training, 101
    Drop sets, 125
    Duration, 102
    Example sequence of exercises, 126
    Formula, 102
    Optimal tension, 102
    Recovery, 103
    Strength training stimulus, 102
    Technique, 125
    Writing your prescription, 125
Stress, 137
    Abnormal thought patterns, 146
        All or nothing thinking, 147
        Arbitrary interference, 148
            Mind reading, 148
            Negative prediction, 148
        Being right, 149
        Control fallacies, 149
        Disqualification of the positive, 147

Emotional reasoning, 148
Fallacy of change, 149
Fallacy of fairness, 149
Heaven's reward fallacy, 149
Labeling and mislabeling, 149
Magnification or minimization, 148
Overgeneralization, 147
Personalization, 149
Selective negative focus, 147
Should statements, 148
Accumulation of stressors, 142
Attitude and social support, 143
Be your own CEO, 161
Caffeine, 143
"Circle the Wagons," 185
Communication styles, 150
Aggressive, 151
Assertive, 151
Passive, 151
Definition – yeah, right!, 140
Eliot, Robert S.' thoughts, 163
Exercise and, 160
Five T's of stress management, 164
Guided visual imagery, 161
Hermit crab concept, 185
Holmes-Rahe Scale, 142
"Hot reactor", 163
How to live with stress, 155
Maladaptations to stress, 146
Meditation (see mindful med.), 161, 165
Modulation, 139
Peak performance (see peak perf.), 152
Physiologic response, 139
Physiology of stress, 145
Preventive efforts, 156
Assertive communication, 159
Be your own CEO, 161
Choices, 156
Downtime, shorten it, 157
Eat the elephant, 158
Exercise and nutrition are key, 160
Guided visual imagery, 161
Isolation, don't, 160
Learn to live with stress, 160
Perception, that's stress, 160
Thinking distortions, eliminate, 159
Principles of stress management, 156
Ripple effect, 143
Selye, Hans, MD prescription, 171
Frustration, release, 171

Hierarchy, recognize, 171
Natural code of conduct, adopt, 172
Altruistic egotism, 172
Earn thy neighbor's love, 172
Find your own stress level, 172
Simplicity, embrace, 171
Pleasantries of life, enjoy, 172
Prioritize, 171
Procrastinate, don't, 172
Successes, take stock, 172
Socialization, 160
Social toll, 141
Stress busters, a great list, 174
Accept your own authority, 179
Acknowledge the negative, 185
Ask for help, 181
Be where you are, 178
Biofeedback, 183
Caffeine and alcohol, reduce, 182
Change your environment, 174
"Circle the Wagons", 185
Colors, choose them well, 176
Consider negative outcomes, 182
Credit for past accomplishments, 182
Diet, improve it, 176
Distract yourself, 174
Don't expect future failures, 182
Don't magnify your failures, 182
Don't worry, be happy, 177
End of day stress busters, 179
Float your blues away, 175
Flowers, buy, 184
Get to the root of the problem, 175
Happy face, put one on, 177
Hermit crab concept, 185
Hike, take one, 177
Humor and fun, 182
I love stress, 186
If your not mad now, why later, 185
Intermediary, use one, 184
Journal, 183
Let go of your fantasies, 178
Lists, get rid of, 184
Look positively at yourself, 183
Massage, have one, 184
Meditate, 176
Minimize expectations, 183
Newsbreaks, 184
"No", learn to say it, 180
Organizational skills, use, 181

Overload, be aware, 179
Play, 179
Procrastinate, do it well, 175
Realize an event has passed, 184
Relax and observe, 176
Seize the moment, 179
Self tolerance, develop, 182
Simplify, 184
Six months to live game, 185
Stressors, identify and eliminate, 185
Sunshine, try some, 177
Take 15 min., shut out the world, 181
Time, take control, 179
Touch, reach out and, 175
Tuition concept of learning, 185
Tune in, 176
Two solutions for each complaint, 181
Stress is perception, 139
Teaching, 310
Test your job stress, a survey, 341
Thinking distortions, 159
Tuition concept of learning, 185
Stress Index Test, 144
Stretching, 100
Writing your prescription, 123
Student involvement in teaching, 313
Supermarket shopping survival, 58
Abused terms, 62
Dairy products, 67
Food labeling, 60
Fish and shellfish, 66
Guided tour, 63
Breads, 64
Cereals, 64
Dairy products, 67
Fish and shellfish, 66
Fruits and vegetables, 63
Legumes, 64
Meats, 65
Pasta, 65
Rice, 65
Soups, 65
Tofu, 64
Vegetable oils, 65
Guiding principles, 59
Carbohydrate hunt, 60
Educate, 59
Five aisles worth visiting, 59
Hungry, never go, 60
Labels, read, 60
List, prepared, 59
Storage items, 59
Sell-by date, 66
Supplements, 274, 280, 282
Support systems, 38, 72
Sutton's Law, 256, 330
Synergism, 43, 199

T

Talk, 34, 199
Temperature, and exercise, 113
Thermic effect of food, 236
Thermic effect of physical activity, 236
Think, 35
Thirst, 57
Tigris Eatalotofus, 138
Trends 2000, 320
Trickle down theory of behavior, 323
Tropical oils, 55
"Two-Year Stewardship" of change, 29

U

US Military, 329
US Public Health Service, 92, 251

V

Vitamins, 265
Fat soluble, 270
A (retinol), 270
D, 271
E (tocopherol), 271
K, 271
Recommendations, 282
Top ten foods for vitamins, 272
Toxicity, 278
Water soluble, 268
B-1 (thiamine,), 268
B-2 (riboflavin), 268
B-3 (niacin), 268
B-6 (pyridoxine), 269

B-12 (cobalamin), 269
Biotin, 269
C (ascorbic acid), 269
Folic acid, 269
Pantothenic acid, 269

W

Waist hip ratio (WHR), 251
Wake-up calls, 24
Water, 41, 56
    Adequate intake, 57
    Exercise and, 57
    Hydration, 57
Water soluble vitamins, 268
Weight and body composition, 231
    Benefits of weight loss, 248
    Body fat and risk status, 251
    Caloric requirements, 240
    Energy balance equation, 235
    Exercise and, 241
    How to manage, 255
        Attitudes and expectations, 255
        Awareness, practice, 257
        Body composition indices, 256
        Calculate energy balance deficit, 256
        Calories, cut, 256
        Changes, one at a time, 256
        Eating, confine to meals, 257
        Energy use diary, 255
        Exercise, 257
        Extremes, avoid, 259
        File card system, 257
        Food diary, 255
        Lapse, accept an occasional, 257
        Naked in the mirror test, 258
        Plan ahead, 257
        Read, 259
        Recidivism, 259
        Relationships, 259
        Simplify, 257
        Snack wisely, 257
        Sublimate, 258
        Weigh, not often, 258
    Nutritional considerations, 238
    Optimal rate of weight loss, 239

Percentage body fat, 250
Resting metabolic rate, 236
Thermic effect of food, 236
Thermic effect of physical activity, 236
Weight-energy relationship, 234
    Energy available from foods, 235
Wonder Chow From a Cow, 61
Write, 35
Written records, 39

Y

"Yes", say it, 38
Yo-Yo dieting, 242

Z

ZZ Top, 283

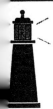

Sabec Publishing Co.
P.O. Box 82545
Portland, OR 97282-0545
www.Getalifeamerica.com

PURCHASE ORDER

PO #:
Date:
Customer ID:

To:

In case we need to contact you about your order:

Daytime phone:

E-mail address:

Req By

Qty	Description	Dsc %	Tax	Unit Pr	Total
	Get a Life, America!			$24.99	

Subtotal	
Tax	
Freight	
Bal Due	

Payment by cash, check, or money order

Quantity discounts available

Download order form at www.Getalifeamerica.com